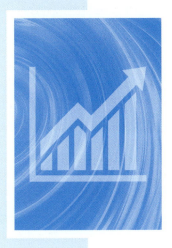

The Business of
Physical Therapy

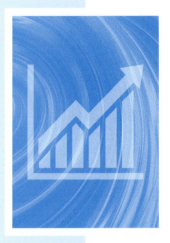

The Business of Physical Therapy

Mark Drnach, PT, DPT, MBA

Professor of Physical Therapy
University of Findlay
Findlay, Ohio

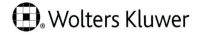

Philadelphia • Baltimore • New York • London
Buenos Aires • Hong Kong • Sydney • Tokyo

Acquisitions Editor: Lindsey Porambo
Senior Development Editor: Amy Millholen
Editorial Coordinator: Anju Radhakrishnan
Editorial Assistant: Lauren Bala
Marketing Manager: Danielle Klahr
Senior Production Project Manager: Catherine Ott
Manager, Graphic Arts & Design: Stephen Druding
Art Director, Illustration: Jennifer Clements
Manufacturing Coordinator: Margie Orzech
Prepress Vendor: S4Carlisle Publishing Services

Copyright © 2025 Wolters Kluwer.

All rights reserved. This book is protected by copyright. No part of this book may be reproduced or transmitted in any form or by any means, including as photocopies or scanned-in or other electronic copies, or utilized by any information storage and retrieval system without written permission from the copyright owner, except for brief quotations embodied in critical articles and reviews. Materials appearing in this book prepared by individuals as part of their official duties as U.S. government employees are not covered by the above-mentioned copyright. To request permission, please contact Wolters Kluwer at Two Commerce Square, 2001 Market Street, Philadelphia, PA 19103, via email at permissions@lww.com, or via our website at shop.lww.com (products and services).

9 8 7 6 5 4 3 2 1

Printed in Mexico

Library of Congress Cataloging-in-Publication Data

ISBN-13: 978-1-975195-84-7

Cataloging in Publication data available on request from publisher.

This work is provided "as is," and the publisher disclaims any and all warranties, express or implied, including any warranties as to accuracy, comprehensiveness, or currency of the content of this work.

This work is no substitute for individual patient assessment based upon healthcare professionals' examination of each patient and consideration of, among other things, age, weight, gender, current or prior medical conditions, medication history, laboratory data, and other factors unique to the patient. The publisher does not provide medical advice or guidance and this work is merely a reference tool. Healthcare professionals, and not the publisher, are solely responsible for the use of this work including all medical judgments and for any resulting diagnosis and treatments.

Given continuous, rapid advances in medical science and health information, independent professional verification of medical diagnoses, indications, appropriate pharmaceutical selections and dosages, and treatment options should be made and healthcare professionals should consult a variety of sources. When prescribing medication, healthcare professionals are advised to consult the product information sheet (the manufacturer's package insert) accompanying each drug to verify, among other things, conditions of use, warnings and side effects and identify any changes in dosage schedule or contraindications, particularly if the medication to be administered is new, infrequently used or has a narrow therapeutic range. To the maximum extent permitted under applicable law, no responsibility is assumed by the publisher for any injury and/or damage to persons or property, as a matter of products liability, negligence law or otherwise, or from any reference to or use by any person of this work.

shop.lww.com

Dedication

To my children, Alek, Grace, Luke, and Rachel. You four have made me the richest man in the world. All my love, always. **Dad**

Contributors

Mark Drnach, PT, DPT, MBA
Professor of Physical Therapy
University of Findlay
Findlay, Ohio

Grace Drnach-Bonaventura, EdD, MPH
Chief of Staff
School of Public Health
University of Pittsburgh
Pittsburgh, Pennsylvania

David Edwards, PT, EdD
Assistant Professor
Wheeling University
Wheeling, West Virginia
Owner, Edwards Absolute Kinetics
St. Clairsville, Ohio

Ken Erb, PT, MPT, BS
President
Erb Physical Therapy PC
Pittsburgh, Pennsylvania

Preface

Every student who endeavors to study the art and science of a health care profession is aware of the time, effort, and responsibility that go into acquiring that knowledge in order to practice effectively in the US health care system. The volume of information to absorb and then master is daunting. On the periphery, and often thought of as secondary, are the external factors that significantly influence the practice, delivery, and reimbursement for the services rendered. Many times, it is only when one has worked in the health care system for a period of time that the influences of these external factors are understood, and the provider's behavior is shaped accordingly.

This textbook is organized to provide the reader with a working knowledge of the business aspect of health care, using the perspective of the profession of physical therapy, the author's profession. It is intended to give the reader a jumpstart in the practice of physical therapy, either as an employee or as a proprietor of a small business. The textbook begins with the setup or foundational elements of business: basic economics (Chapter 1), accounting practices, and the common financial documents used by all small businesses (Chapter 2). Understanding the language of business allows the health care practitioner to engage in conversations on cost-effectiveness, productivity, value-based outcomes, budgeting, and the allocation of financial resources, bringing into the discussion both the needed professional knowledge of the health care provider and the business knowledge of cost. In addition to understanding the language of business, it is helpful for the practitioner to understand some of the history of health care in the United States (Chapter 3) and the major influencer of health care today, the third-party payer (Chapter 4). This information can put into perspective the discussions and decisions that are made to provide optimal care to the patients served today.

The second section of the textbook addresses the many decisions a practitioner has to make when starting to practice or setting up a business. Employment options are presented in Chapter 5 to provide a basic understanding of the opportunities that are available. Chapter 6 focuses on entrepreneurship and starting a private practice or small business. The elements of the structure of a private practice as well as how to market the practice are addressed in Chapters 6 and 7. An important skill, probably the most important, is the skill of communication. Chapter 8 presents information on communication in health care including interprofessional communication, oral and written communication (including electronic delivery), and the basics of coding for services, which is a means of communication with a third-party payer.

The third section of this textbook addresses the necessary components of a plan to be successful and sustainable in business. Obtaining the professional knowledge of physical therapy, and understanding and applying basic business principles are important, but monitoring and measuring outcomes, costs (Chapter 9), and risks (Chapter 10) are vital to achieve sustained success. This success is built upon honest engagement with employees, patients, payers, and the community. Civic engagement (Chapter 11) highlights the role of the physical therapist in public health and provides the reader with a basic understanding of global health metrics, the social determinants of health, and the basic process of grant funding. Chapter 12 veers somewhat from the practice or business and focuses on personal financial literacy and the management of personal finances, including debt. An important motivator to the owner of any small business is personal financial wealth.

I hope the reader finds the information contained in this textbook, along with the ancillary items (ie, assignments, internet resources, review questions, tutorials), valuable and helps the reader to become a better participant in the health care system. We need business-educated health care practitioners to improve the outcomes of our current health care system. Thank you for your interest in becoming one of those leaders.

Mark Drnach

Acknowledgments

There are many people who inspire and support the creative process of writing. These people are invaluable in producing a piece of work that presents a perspective and understanding on the framework and thought process of entrepreneurial endeavors. I am inspired by my brothers Robert Drnach and Joe Drnach and sister-in-law Sharon Drnach, who are successful entrepreneurs. They took the initiative and risk to venture into self-employment to provide services to their respective communities where they could apply their values and work ethic. They are an inspiration to me. I encourage the readers of this book to seek out the entrepreneurs in their lives and obtain inspiration from their work.

The contributors to this textbook, David Edwards, Ken Erb, and Grace Drnach-Bonaventura, are entrepreneurs who have a desire and vision to provide a service to their communities in an efficient, professional, and value-based manner. Their enthusiasm provides the fuel to their seemingly endless supply of energy and effort in creating, providing, and sustaining a business. They are remarkable. Their contributions, insights, edits, and recommendations to the content of this textbook provide a real-life application of the business aspect of health care. If the readers of this textbook are fortunate to have such business-minded people in their lives, I would encourage them to learn from these hard-working individuals.

Creating a piece of written work is not a solo endeavor. I am fortunate to work with Juliana Kepple, who is completing her degree in English Writing. She assisted me by reading and editing the final drafts of the chapters and providing feedback on the content and presentation of the information. Her perspective and insights were helpful in organizing the information in the chapters so that the reader would have a better understanding of the chapters' content and topic.

The people at Wolters Kluwer have been very supportive and patient. I appreciate their willingness to allow me to write this textbook, which addresses an important aspect of health care. Their guidance in the production of this textbook, and willingness to discuss the various steps involved in publishing, is appreciated. I could not have done this without their help and kindness.

I would like to thank all these people, and you the reader, for taking the time to better understand the business aspect of physical therapy.

Mark Drnach

Contents

Contributors vi
Preface vii
Acknowledgments ix

SECTION 1   The Setup   1

1. The Language of Business: Economics   1

Economics of Health Care   2
The Role of Government 3
Capitalism 4

Basic Economic Principles   5
Wants and Needs 5
Scarcity 6
Value and Utility 7
Supply and Demand 8
Elasticity of Demand 9

Competition in the Market   11
Understanding the Market 12

Cost   13
Pricing 17
Break-Even Analysis 18
Cost-Effectiveness Analysis 19

Summary   20

2. Accounting and Finance   23

Accounting   24
Chart of Accounts 26
Double Entry 28
Debits and Credits 28
Asset, Liability, and Equity 28
Accrual and Cash 30
Revenues and Expenses 30

Fundamental Financial Statements   31
Balance Sheet 33
Income Statement 33
Cash Flow Statement 33
Retained Earnings Statement 35

Budgeting   36

Financial Analysis   39
Financial Ratios 39
Performance Indicators 42
Productivity 43

xii Contents

Revenue and Expense Management   45
Revenue Management   45
Expense Management   48
Summary   48

3. The History of Health Care in the United States: From Service to Business   50

Early Development of the Hospital, Physician, and Physical Therapist   51
Early Developments in Physical Therapy Treatment   53
Federal and State Laws   56
A Call to Change   58
From Paternalism to Partnership   60
Value-Based Care   60
Summary   62

4. The Influencer in Health Care: Health Insurance   65

Components of Health Insurance   66
Types of Health Insurance   68
Productivity   73
Clinical Decision-Making   73
Frameworks   74
The Steps in Clinical Decision-Making   76
Frequency and Duration of Services   78
Documentation   80
Utilization of Daily Documentation   80
Outcomes   82
Communicating With the Payer   83
Summary   84

SECTION 2   The Decision   87

5. Employment Options   87

Independent Contractor   88
The Contract   88
Business Structure   90
The Employee   90
Setting Options   93
Acute Care Hospital   93
Inpatient Rehabilitation   95
Outpatient Rehabilitation/Outpatient Clinic   98
Home Health Agency/Home Care   99
Hospice   101
Schools and the Individuals With Disabilities Education Act   103
Skilled Nursing Facilities   107
Higher Education/Faculty   108
Summary   109
Appendix 5A: An Evaluation: Early Intervention Physical Therapy Evaluation   112
Appendix 5B: School-Based Evaluation, Documentation, and Outcome Forms   120

Contents **xiii**

6. Entrepreneurship 130

Basic Entrepreneurial Skills and Attributes 130
Action Minded 130
Leadership Skills 131
Resilience/Tenacity 131
Willingness to Work Hard 132
Comfortable Being Uncomfortable 132
Basic Finance Skills 132
Communication Skills 134
Branding/Marketing 134

Small Business Administration 135

Practice in the Digital Age 136
Web Page Basics 136
Electronic Communication 137
Social Media Marketing 138
Basics of Virtual Visits 139

How to Begin 140
Components of a Business Plan 140
Staff Selection 141
Profit Centers 145
Vendor Relationships 145
Creating and Keeping a Great Team 146
Subcontracting 147

A Few Tips From the Author 148
Grit Matters 148
Getting the Right Help 148
Honesty With Staff and Customers 149
Private Pay or Insurance-Based Reimbursement? 149
Monitor Spending 149
Direct Access and Practitioner of Choice 150
First Impressions Matter 150

Summary 151

7. Marketing 153

Marketing 153
SWOT Analysis 154
Basics of Marketing 155
Marketing Mix 160
Product 160
Price 160
Place 160
Promotion 161
Packaging 161
Physical Evidence of Effectiveness 161
Processes 162
Personnel 163

Digital Marketing 163
Marketing Yourself 165
A Personal SWOT Analysis 168
Personal Marketing Mix 168

xiv

Passion 169
Practice 169
Place 170
Payment 170
Summary 171

8. Communication in Health Care 173

Basic Elements of Communication 174
Verbal Communication 174
Nonverbal Communication 177
Written Communication 177
Interprofessional Communication 179
Patient Communication 180
Payer Communication: Coding 182
Coding the Procedure 182
Coding Other Services 183
Coding the Disease 184
Billing 184
Independent Contractor 186
Participating With the Third Party 187
Summary 188

SECTION 3   The Plan to Succeed 191

9. Monitoring and Measuring 191

Key Performance Indicators 192
Metric Timing 192
Metric Scope 192
Leading and Trailing Indicators 193
The Physical Therapy Revenue Equation 193
Benchmarking 194
Monitoring and Reporting 194
General Practice Metrics 195
*New Patients (NP): The Heart Rate of a Practice 195
*Visits per Week (V/wk): The Respiration Rate of a Practice 197
*Average Visits/Plan of Care: The Rate of Metabolism of a Practice 198
*Arrival Rate (AR) %: The Hematocrit Level of a Practice 199
General Financial Metrics 200
*Payment per Visit (PPV): The Blood Pressure of a Practice 200
*Profit and Loss Statement: The Oxygen Saturation Level of a Practice 200
*Cost/Visit and Profit/Visit: The Caloric Intake of a Practice 202
Payer Mix: The Diet of a Practice 202
Expense Reporting: Salary—The Calories of a Practice 203
Billing and Collection Metrics 204
Account Aging: The Body Weight of the Practice 204
Days That a Sale Is Outstanding (DSO): The Body Mass Index of a Practice 205
Individual Physical Therapist Metrics: Managing by the Numbers 208
Average Weighted Timed Units per Visits (TU/V) × RVU: A Measure of Efficiency 208
Revenue/Visit per Therapist (Compare to TU/V-W): A Great Teaching Tool 209

Contents

Relative Value Units Billed per Visit (RVU/V): What Do Your Payers Think Is Most Beneficial? 209
Visits/POC per Individual Therapist 209
Patient Register, Plan of Care Completion, and Patient Drop-Off % 210
Reactivation Rate 211

Marketing Metrics 211
Referral Source Reporting 211
Return on Investment (ROI) 212
Cost of Acquisition (CoA) 213
Rate of Customer Return (RCR; Unique Episode) 213
Lifetime Value of a Patient (LVP) 214

Customer Satisfaction Metrics 214
Net Promoter Score (NPS®) 214
Google Reviews 215

Developing Multisite Physical Therapy Practices 215
Profit and Loss by Location (or Profit and Loss by Class) 216
Place of Service Summary 217

Monitoring the Market 218
Summary: Putting It All Together—How Often to Review Your Metrics. . . and What to Do About Them 218

10. Risk Management 220

Identifying Risk 221
Regulations 222
Revenues 224
Reputation 224

Risk Options 225
Avoid Risk 225
Accept Risk 226
Mitigating Risk 226
Transfer Risk 226

Risk Management 228
Protection 228
Improvement 235

Summary 235

11. Civic Engagement 237

History of Physical Therapy in Public Health 237
Health Metrics and Global Agenda 239
Global Targets 241
Challenges and Considerations With Achieving Sustainable Development Goals 245
Grant Funding 246
Social Determinants of Health 246
Health Equity, Health Equality, and Health Disparities 254
Providing Services to Vulnerable Populations 256
Domestic and International Outreach 256
Service-Learning and the Role of Physical Therapy 256
Documentation 259
Ethical Considerations 259
Summary 260

xvi

12. Financial Literacy   263

Financial Literacy   263
Needs and Wants   265
The Paycheck   266
Budgeting   268
   Debt Management   271
   Personal Financial Advisors   274
   Monitoring   276
Summary   277

Index   279

SECTION 1
The Setup

CHAPTER 1

The Language of Business
Economics

MARK DRNACH

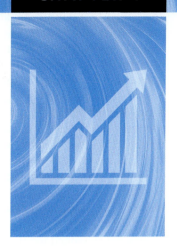

Learning Objectives

The reader will

1. Understand the basic economics of health care in the United States.
2. Describe basic economic principles commonly encountered in health care.
3. Understand the role of competition in the market and the common economic indicators that reflect key aspects of the market.
4. Identify the various costs and their behavior associated with the delivery of health care in the clinical setting.

Health care has evolved into a multibillion-dollar business that now includes not only the providers of care but a myriad of people who support the delivery of that care, pay for that care, and monitor the compliance with established standards and outcomes of care. The need of a business to remain financially profitable requires that providers have a working knowledge of those additional factors associated with the delivery and sustainability of care, such as financial profitability, productivity, efficiency, the cost of services, a unit of production, and outcome expectations. Health care providers must broaden their understanding of the clinical treatment of patients and have a working knowledge of the efficient utilization of resources, the various types of costs, and other economic factors associated with the delivery of services and the maintenance of a business's operations. To engage in the conversation and decision-making process, health care providers must have a basic understanding of the terminology of business and of basic economic principles.

Economics is the study of economies. The term *economy* refers to the amount of services and goods that are produced and available, how services and goods are distributed, and how many and what types of services and goods are consumed. This chapter is intended to provide the reader with a fundamental understanding of commonly used economic terms and the principles that drive the US economic system, especially as they apply to the service of health care.

1

Economics of Health Care

The systematic interactions between producing, distributing, and consuming wealth can be applied to a country or any segment of business. Economists investigate how people use their limited resources to fulfill their wants and needs under conditions of scarcity (ie, limited supply), together with the interaction of the consumers, producers, and the government. How the economic system (the economy) is functioning is one of life's important domains. The national economy influences the quality of life through macroeconomic policies (eg, monetary policies influencing the supply of money and the interest rate and fiscal policies influencing taxes and government spending), which are concerned with the economy as a whole. Microeconomic principles help predict how specific markets will respond to certain policies such as how an individual or business will respond to a policy that limits access to specific resources, prices, or incentives. Additional examples include the supply and demand of a specific service or good in a given market, inflation and unemployment status, and, in turn, the standard of living.[1] Economics is often presented in terms of the production of a good or service and is commonly understood in relationship to the buying and selling of consumer goods, like food or other tangible objects, in which money is exchanged for the service or product. The application of basic economic principles to the behavior of the health care industry is not as straightforward given the complex nature of health care as a product or service.[2] Folland et al[3] suggest that what makes health care a distinctive economic system is the following:

1. The presence of uncertainty inherent in a person's health, making demand irregular for the individual. Consumers of health care are uncertain of their needs for any specific period in the future, which makes demand for health care irregular from the individual's or individual practice's perspective.
2. The presence of health insurance, which guards against uncertainty but also reduces the costs of health care at any one point in time. The demand for a costly health service (eg, orthopedic surgery) may rise in the presence of health insurance, since that insurance costs less than surgical intervention. This affects demand for health care by those consumers who may be candidates for the intervention and, depending on the insurance coverage, may affect the incentives of the health care provider through payment systems such as diagnosis-related groups, prospective payment systems, and resource utilization groups.
3. The lack of information on what constitutes good or needed health care is also problematic. Consumers may have limited knowledge of what they need to regain health without the advice of health care professionals like physicians or physical therapists. The professional also does not know with absolute certainty the outcome of any specific intervention or episode of care and may perform several diagnostic tests or evaluations to guide the diagnostic process and subsequent provision of care.
4. The restriction on competition through states' legislation, licensure laws, Certificate of Need programs, professional education requirements and educational costs, as well as

economics – systematic study of the production, conservation, and allocation of resources in conditions of scarcity and the interaction of the consumers, producers, and government

macroeconomic policies – monetary policies that influence the supply of money and interest rate, and fiscal policy that influences taxes and government spending

microeconomic principles – principles that predict how markets and consumers will react to policies such as the price of goods or services

Chapter 1 / The Language of Business

other imposed regulations can impact the supply of health care by restricting the number of people who can become health care providers.

5. The lack of health care in another individual often evokes feelings of sadness or concern, leading people to believe that something should be done to provide health care, although exactly how that should be accomplished is debatable.

6. Government subsidies and programs in most major countries provide a structured means of service delivery at a certain level and are funded primarily by mandatory taxes on the citizens. With government-sponsored programs comes the basic economic problem of what type and level of health care to provide (eg, vaccinations, preventative services, comprehensive or limited rehabilitation), how to provide it (eg, through government or private clinics or facilities), and who is eligible for the government program (eg, economically poor, people with limited or no access to services, people with disabilities requiring a variety of services).

7. The fact is that health cannot be bought with money; health care can be bought and the factors or influences that produce health, or a return to a healthy state, are sought by the consumer. Health is desired because it makes people feel better, promotes their functional independence, and allows them to participate in gainful employment, thereby increasing their income and providing tax revenue for the government.

Similarly to providing for financial health (eg, Social Security), providing for a citizen's physical health may also be viewed as the responsibility of the government. Given the distinctive features of health care, and the rising demand and costs, some governmental intervention is warranted, but how that intervention is structured is debatable.

The Role of Government

What is the role of the government, and why do people organize themselves with a central governing body? This is a fundamental question that is crucial to understanding why people form governments and what is expected of them. Intervention by a government in regard to the citizens' health and safety comes mainly through three activities: provision, distribution, and regulation.[3] First, a government has the duty to protect the people from violence, both within its borders and from external attacks. This is done in part by the establishment of a national defense system, a legal system, and a police force that are responsible for protection and the maintenance of order. Secondly, a government has the duty to establish certain social practices that protect the people from oppression or injustice, which, in turn, promote internal order and general satisfaction among the people. This is addressed in part by the establishment of rules and regulations and a system of justice, including a system of incarceration and rehabilitation of individuals who break the established laws. Thirdly, a government has the duty to establish and maintain a system of public goods. Public goods are services and products for the benefit of the people. No one is excluded from accessing them regardless of who paid for them. Public goods include such things as the building and maintenance of public highways, harbors, airports, and railways for public use. These systems support and promote trade among people and factor into the economic growth of a society.[4]

Prior to the 1900s, the role of the government in the United States, as well as other developing countries, was minor, with relatively low taxation and few regulations.[4] And then governments started to change, instituting more social programs such as public education,

public goods – services or goods that benefit all the people in a country and that are available to all regardless of the ability to pay

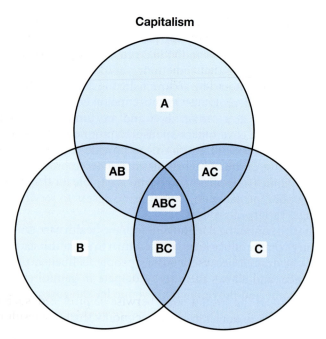

Figure 1.1 **Capitalism.** The controlling powers in a society: (A) individuals with private control; (B) governments with state control; (C) natural resource constraints or property control. (If A > B then AB = democracy. If B > A then AB = dictatorship.) The four pillars of capitalism: (AB) democracy; (AC) free markets; (BC) governmental regulations; (ABC) private property rights.[1] (Adapted from Hajiran H. Interdisciplinary teaching tools for economics 101: gateway concepts of quality of life & capitalism. Papers.ssrn.com. Published December 13, 2004. https://ssrn.com/abstract=643384. Reprinted with permission from Homayoun Hajiran.)

workers' compensation for work-related injuries, old-age pension, and the funding of health care. This broadening of the role of government has brought about profound changes, not only in the programs that the government has to offer but also in the amount of funds needed to financially support and maintain the various social programs that have been developed. The availability of funds is influenced by many factors, including the economic system that is adopted by a government or country, the system and level of service provision, and the utilization of the services by the people.

Capitalism

Capitalism can be defined as an economic system based on private ownership of capital, in which the production and distribution of goods are done in a relatively free (limited government influence) market for profit (Figure 1.1). It is the main economic system in North America. It is based on four main pillars: a democratic or freely elected government; free markets for economic competition and the pursuit of an improved quality of life; private property rights that empower profit motives by owners/entrepreneurs; and governmental regulations regarding enforcement of commerce-related contracts both nationally and internationally.[1]

The US government, which is part of the world's largest and most successful capitalistic society, is faced with the problem that most industrialized nations have: how to provide basic health care to all of its citizens. Through a system of taxation and governmental

> **capitalism** – an economic system based on private ownership of capital in which the production and distribution of the goods are done in a relatively free market for profit

Chapter 1 / The Language of Business

programs (ie, Medicare, Medicaid, and the Affordable Care Act) the US government has tried to provide health care for its citizens, but the debate continues on the questions of who should receive health care; who should pay for it; and what level of care should be provided while maintaining a balance between government regulations, free markets, and private rights in a capitalist society. When a central authority such as a government answers these questions based on a master plan, it is a command economy. A modification of the command economy is one in which the consumer has some limited choices. Through the price systems in a market economy, consumers and producers interact to determine what, how, and for whom goods will be produced. In the case of public goods (eg, law enforcement, military, and transportation services), they may be better provided by a government rather than by individual (private) producers. The forum for consumer and producer interactions/transactions is referred to as a market (see Figure 1.1, AC). The right to own property, and the consumer's and producer's freedom of choice characterize a market economy (see Figure 1.1, ABC and AC). Consumers have the freedom to spend their resources as they see fit. Producers (providers) are free to allocate their resources to produce the type and amount of services and/or products they desire. The role of government (see Figure 1.1, B) in a market economy is to:

1. Provide goods or services that would not otherwise be produced, such as public safety.
2. Accommodate for weaknesses in the market economy that may result in misallocation of resources, such as health care.
3. Establish restrictions to the free market that are in the interest of the public good or health.

In support of a market economy, there is a core set of economic principles and related concepts. The following sections discuss these principles and concepts.

Basic Economic Principles

Wants and Needs

A basic discussion on economics can begin with an understanding of a human being's wants and needs. Maslow[5] presented a human-centered theory on motivation that categorized a human's basic needs in a hierarchical fashion, where the appearance of one need rests on the prior satisfaction of another. Every drive or motivation is related to the state of satisfaction or dissatisfaction of other needs or desires. These basic needs are categorized as: (1) physiologic needs such as food, clothing, and shelter; (2) safety needs such as safety from harm, tyranny, or extreme temperatures; (3) love needs, both giving and receiving such things as affection, belonging, or the need for a life partner; (4) esteem needs such as personal achievement, independence, or prestige; and (5) self-actualization needs such as the feeling of self-fulfillment, living a life that one was meant to live, or the actualization of one's full potential. The emergence of these needs rests on the satisfaction of the preceding or more fundamental need.

command economy – an economic system where the goods and resources are owned by the government and their distribution is determined by a centralized authority

market economy – an economic system where the consumers and producers interact to determine what, how, and for whom the goods will be produced and delivered

market – a forum for the consumers and producers to interact

needs – the basic requirements of a person in a society such as shelter, safety, love, esteem, and self-actualization

A **want** can be defined as things that a person desires or would like to have. These wants can also be motivating to a person, especially if the person has the financial means to obtain them. Understanding the difference between what a person needs and what a person wants is important in the delivery of health care services, in marketing a business, and in personal financial decisions.

Scarcity

Scarcity is an economic condition when human wants and needs exceed the available supply. A society cannot fulfill all of the wants or needs of the people simultaneously; there has to be a point where the supply of one item is sufficient given the total amount of all the various wants and needs that can be identified. Whenever resources are limited in the presence of unlimited wants, it can be said that there is a scarcity of the resource. Goods and services are scarce because of limited availability (due to production or natural constraints) along with the limits of technology and trained people to provide the goods or service relative to the total amount of the item desired.

The concept of **opportunity cost** is related to scarcity of resources. Consumers have finite resources. When expending limited resources, consumers strive to gain the maximum value (best outcome for the lowest cost). They cannot afford all of the goods and services they might desire. As a result, they must choose between all of the possible goods and services available to them. The goal is to make the choice that results in the greatest added value to them. To do this, the consumer must compare the relative value of alternative purchases under consideration. The opportunity cost of a decision or acquisition is the lost value of the alternative decision or acquisition that was not chosen.[6]

In the United States, most people may not believe that health care resources are scarce. A general hypothesis is that everyone is entitled to live as long as possible and as healthily as possible and that this is attainable given enough health care resources. When combined with the opinion that health care resources and the money to buy them are readily available, it may become clearer why some individuals resist restrictions on health care, even though they might agree that health care resources are not being used efficiently. Few people will tolerate limits on health care when the limit is viewed not as a result of scarcity but as someone else's refusal to spend money on available care.[7]

But is health care really scarce, or do the shortages of health care personnel and technology result from limited government funding or other market barriers to accessing health care services, such as the price of the professional education or practice costs? A problem with the current health care system may not be associated with scarcity but rather resource allocation: how to allocate limited resources to people who have unlimited wants. This is based on opportunity cost more than financial cost, the main concerns being the efficiency, choice, and distribution of health care.[2] If the allocation is efficient, then the quantity and type of health care that the consumer wants would be available and produced at the lowest possible cost. The value that is placed on a service or good will be reflected in the allocation of funds to produce an adequate supply of those services or goods. How money is allocated toward resources is a reflection of the importance placed

---

want – a thing that a person desires or wants to have in excess of need

scarcity – an economic condition where people's wants and needs exceed the available supply

opportunity cost – the lost cost, tangible or intangible, associated with the relative value of an alternative choice

Chapter 1 / The Language of Business

on those resources. In the United States, only a portion of the available government funds are allocated to health care. How we allocate resources reflects how we value, and then prioritize, funding of different resources such as national defense, Social Security programs, and public education.

Value and Utility

Value is the importance that an individual good or service attains for a person because he is dependent on it for the satisfaction of a want or need.[8] Value may be tangible (quantifiable), intangible (not quantifiable), or both. Consider the process of deciding on a vacation. Assume that the alternatives have been narrowed down to a ski trip or a tropical cruise. If the ski trip and cruise are the same price, then both trips will result in the same decline in the vacationer's resources. Their final choice will be based on their assessment of intangible value. Intangible value might be a measure of expected enjoyment or prestige. If the cruise were twice as expensive as the ski trip, then the vacationer would have both tangible and intangible value to consider. Intangible value may weight a decision in favor of the costlier alternative. The concept of intangible and tangible value applies to organizational decisions as well. When an organization has the opportunity to invest in one of two alternative business ventures, management will use financial information to identify the resource requirements (cost) and projected value to the organization. Often, they want to determine which venture will yield the greatest projected financial return. However, under some circumstances, the venture with the lower financial return may be selected based on intangible value. For example, a community hospital may select a venture that does the most to further its mission of community service or that has a lower short-term return but positions it for greater return to the community in the long run.

In these types of decisions, the monitoring and analysis of the costs associated with the decision and the benefits received from enacting those decisions are important in obtaining the greatest financial return.

Marginal analysis is used to solve microeconomic problems by looking at the cost and benefit associated with the next, or marginal, unit that is either bought or sold. In order to maximize profits, producers must produce at a level at which the marginal cost is equal to the marginal revenue. If the marginal revenue is greater than the marginal cost, then there is potential to make more profit, so the producer will produce more. If the marginal cost is greater than the marginal revenue, then the producer is overproducing and losing profit on each unit. The marginal value of a good or service is the value, tangible or intangible, of the last increment of the good or service sold or purchased.

Utility is a measure of satisfaction or benefit one receives from a product or service. People will attempt to maximize their utility (satisfaction) given their unique constraints (eg, available funds). This helps to determine how much a person would be willing to pay for a good or service. *Marginal utility* is defined as the extra utility or satisfaction achieved by consuming one more unit of a good. Utility will increase for bottled water, as an example, up to a certain point; it then increases at a decreasing rate as the addition of one more bottle of water decreases the satisfaction or benefit of having bottled water. This concept

value – the importance of an individual good or service to a consumer who desires the good or service to fulfill a need or want

marginal analysis – used in microeconomics to identify the cost and benefit associated with the next unit that is either bought or sold

utility – a measurement of satisfaction a consumer receives from a product or service

is formally known as the law of diminishing marginal utility. As a person increases their consumption of a service or product, there is a diminishment of satisfaction or benefit with each additional unit consumed. This may be seen in a physical therapy plan of care that shows decreased patient satisfaction or perceived benefit with the plan/interventions/exercises as time progresses, the patient recovers, and the additional satisfaction received from the next visit diminishes. How consumers go about choosing the mix of services and goods that maximize their utility is based on their needs, wants, and preferences; the amount of money they have to spend; and the price of the goods or services available to them in the market. By collecting relevant data on the individual consumer's choices based on various determinants of demand such as price, income, and price of alternatives, a market demand can be estimated.

Supply and Demand

According to the Department of Labor, the demand for physical therapists is expected to grow by 21% until 2030, much faster than the average for all occupations (8% expected growth).[9] This increase is facilitated by the growing older adult population, the aging of people with chronic illnesses, and the advancements in technology that saves the lives of people who experienced a traumatic accident or infants born too soon or with life-threatening disabilities. The supply of physical therapists in the United States is increasing, with a surplus expected by 2030.[10] A basic concept in economics is the relationship between the quantity supplied of an item, such as a physical therapy service, and its relationship to the quantity demanded of such an item in a market. This is commonly represented in a supply and demand curve (Figure 1.2).

In economics, this is one of the simplest ways to explain the price behavior resulting from the willingness of consumers to buy and the willingness of producers to produce. Basically, at a given level of demand, as the supply of an item or service increases, the price that a consumer is willing to pay for that item decreases. This explanation of a consumer's

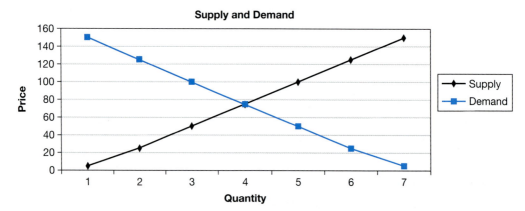

Figure 1.2 **Supply and demand diagram.** A basic economic representation of the relationship between the quantity supplied of a good or service and the quantity demanded and its relationship to price. As demand increases, the price decreases. As the price increases, the supply increases.

---

law of diminishing marginal utility – a decrease in the level of satisfaction with the addition of one more unit of a good or service

supply and demand curve – a curve created by the supply and demand relationship that shows that the variables are inversely related

Chapter 1 / The Language of Business

9

behavior assumes that all other factors in the market are held constant, such as an individual's income, perceptions, and the price of other items in the market at that time.

An example of a supply and demand relationship could be applied to the demand for physical therapy services in a local community or market. If the services are available and provided for free, the quantity demanded would be expected to be at its maximum, with other factors held constant. If the price for a physical therapy service were increased to $100, the quantity demanded would be expected to drop as the consumer makes a decision that the service is not valued at $100, or, living on a finite amount of dollars, chooses to spend their $100 on something else that is of value to them in the market. If the price of a physical therapy service increases to $150, the demand will continue to drop. That is why the demand curve slopes downward. The **law of demand** states that the quantity demanded will decrease as the price increases.

Supply can be looked at similarly. As the price (payment) that is paid to the physical therapy provider increases, the supply (the number of physical therapists providing services) will also increase. For example, if physical therapists were not paid to perform a service, the supply of physical therapists would be expected to be very limited given that other factors remain constant. If the price paid to a physical therapist were increased to $100 per service, the supply of physical therapists would be expected to increase. If the price paid for a service increased to $150, the supply would continue to rise. That is why the supply curve slopes upward. The **law of supply** states that the quantity supplied will increase as the price increases.

Under ideal conditions, the point at which the supply and demand curves meet is the point of equilibrium in the market. This is the point where the supply of physical therapists meets the demand for physical therapy services. If the quantity of physical therapy services supplied exceeds the quantity demanded, theoretically, the price for a physical therapy service is forced to decline, leading to a decrease in the quantity supplied. Conversely, if the quantity of physical therapy services falls short of the quantity demanded, the price of physical therapy services will rise, leading to an increase in the quantity of physical therapists willing to supply their services to the market. Theoretically, in a free market without government control, supply and demand vacillate until an equilibrium point is reached.

Elasticity of Demand

A basic economic question is, as the price of a health care service rises, how will the quantity demanded be affected? This question reflects the economic concept called elasticity. **Elasticity** is a term used to describe the responsiveness of any variable to a change in another variable. Relating this to health care services is to observe how the demand for a health care service is affected by a change in some other variable like price. The sensitivity of demand to changing price is called price elasticity. Price elasticity of demand (PED) is calculated by dividing the percentage of change in the quantity demanded by the percentage change in the price.

$$\text{PED} = \frac{\text{Percentage change in quantity demanded}}{\text{Percentage change in price of the product}}$$

law of demand – a behavior seen in consumers where the demand for a good or service decreases as the price of the good or service increases

law of supply – a behavior seen in producers where the supply of a good or service increases as the price of the good or service increases

elasticity – the responsiveness of any variable to a change in another variable

The absolute value of the price elasticity reflects the relationship between price and the quantity demanded and is not expressed in any particular units. Demand is price inelastic when the percentage of change in price results in a smaller percentage of change in quantity demanded, resulting in a PED less than 1 in absolute value (ie, ignore the negative sign). Demand is price elastic when the percentage of change in price results in a larger percentage change in demand, resulting in a PED greater than 1. As an example, suppose that a physical therapy business offers evaluations for fall risks to the older adult population in the community. The business charges $50 for the evaluation and currently provides 10 evaluations per month. What if they increase their charge to $55 (+10%) and only get requests for seven evaluations per month (−30%)?

Then:

PED = −30%/+10%

PED = −3

The PED indicates that the price of the evaluation is very sensitive to the change in price.

The price elasticity of a service or product will dictate the shape of the demand curve for any specific service or product. Demand may be inelastic or insensitive to price changes when the service or product is essential to the consumer, such as gasoline or home heating fuel. Compared to luxury products, basic necessities are price inelastic. Demand may also be inelastic because the consumers have sufficient resources (income) to buy the needed items when there is a substantial price change. This is seen when the cost of luxury products such as personal use technology increases but the demand stays high. When the quantity demanded changes significantly in response to a price increase, demand is said to be highly elastic. Under conditions of high elasticity, price increases may result in an overall decrease in the quantity demanded or, in a competitive market, the consumer may switch to a competitor's service or product or an alternative service or product. When consumers turn to an alternative source or product, it is called a **substitution**. The closer the alternative service or product to the original, the more likely it is that the consumer will turn to a substitution when prices increase. For some consumers, chiropractic physicians, athletic trainers, occupational therapists, and massage therapists are substitutes for physical therapists.

Income will also have an impact on demand by causing a shift in the demand curve to the right. This might happen if income growth provides consumers with more disposable personal income (income available after taxes are paid) to spend on desirable services or products. For example, as income rises, the overall demand for high-end day spa services might increase. Conversely, if disposable income declines, the demand for high-end day spa services may decline while the demand for less expensive personal care services may increase.

The impact of price on profit is of great interest to producers. Producers desire to maximize their profit. Their goal is to charge a price that gives that greatest net income (after expenses are paid) or profit.

Total revenue = Price per unit × Quantity of units sold

Total expense = Cost per unit × Quantity of units produced

Net income (profit) = Total revenue − Total expense

substitution – when consumers choose an alternative good or service from the one being observed or studied in the market

Chapter 1 / The Language of Business

Producers attempt to maximize their net income (profit) by:

1. Identifying and charging the highest price that consumers are willing to pay.
2. Producing goods or services at the lowest per unit cost of production.

As price rises, producers are motivated to increase the amount of service or product they provide to consumers. However, price elasticity may result in diminishing demand as prices rise. As price increases, demand will decrease. At some point, total revenue (units of service or product provided multiplied by the price per unit) will reach a maximum and then begin to decline. Producers must determine how much of which products to produce based on their available resources and price.

At market equilibrium, the demand for a product equals its supply. The interaction between price, supply, and demand works in concert to maintain a demand-supply balance. For example, holding supply constant, when demand increases, some consumers are willing to pay more, and this drives the price upward. A new equilibrium between quantity supplied and quantity demanded will be achieved. The increase in price will also act as an incentive for producers to increase the quantity supplied. As long as there is a positive impact on total revenue and net income, producers will be motivated to increase the quantity supplied.

In health care, the supply and demand relationship is influenced by unique factors. The consumer doesn't necessarily know what makes a good physical therapist or what constitutes appropriate physical therapy services. A physical therapist provides both the information and the service, which affects the concept of supply by influencing the consumer's perception of the value and expected benefits of the service. In addition, the demand from the consumer is influenced by the consumer's expectation of the benefit and need for health care at a certain period of time.

Other factors that influence supply and demand are the availability of physical therapy services in a local market, the cost associated with becoming and practicing as a physical therapist, the consumer's health care insurance structure, the consumer's personal income, and other prices in the market. The supply and demand model, as it applies to the business of health care, does provide a basic understanding of the forces of supply and demand in a free market and allows the physical therapist to better understand the behavior of the consumer and the factors that influence their decisions.

Competition in the Market

A competitive market is characterized by multiple producers each having a minority share of the market. In a competitive market, consumers have a choice of services/providers and products/producers from which to choose. If one provider or producer raises their price or decreases production, the consumer has the ability to substitute another or similar providers or producer. The result is that price increases are constrained. When one provider or producer dominates a market, it is called a monopoly. In a monopoly market, the consumer is unable to substitute. As a result, demand is price inelastic.

At times, a free market economy may find a monopoly (ie, natural monopoly) desirable because of the lower cost per unit of producing essential services or products resulting from the economy of scale. Economy of scale is the decrease in the cost of producing a unit

competitive market – a market where there are a variety of providers for a certain good or service

monopoly – a market where there is only one provider for a certain good or service

economy of scale – the decrease in the cost of producing one more UOS or goods due to an efficient use of fixed costs (eg, equipment, machines)

of service (UOS) with an increase in the volume of production, resulting from the efficient use of fixed costs (eg, equipment, physical assets) that produce more output. For example, a community may have only one source for utilities, internet, or hospital care because the cost of supporting multiple service providers of the same service or product is prohibitive. When a monopoly for an essential service is present in a market, the government may impose regulations on the monopoly to control production, the price, and to ensure equitable distribution of the services.

Understanding the Market

The practice of physical therapy in the health care market requires the physical therapist to demonstrate skills in business management, leadership, professionalism, and administration, including skills with economic relevance.[11] Focusing on specific aspects of the market, the physical therapists can make business decisions based on what is happening in the market, both nationally and locally. Environmental scanning is the behavior of collecting information about the current status or changes in the market and prices in order to make decisions about the direction of a particular business or service. It includes both searching for information and viewing information and can range from information gained from casual conversations to formal marketing research.[12] Environmental scanning can cover several environmental sectors, such as attributes or needs of the customer, advances in technology, pending or possible regulatory issues, sociocultural-political demographics or trends, competitors' statistics, and economic indicators. It is a behavior (environmental assessment) that new physical therapists should have as they begin clinical practice.[11,13]

To gain information on the local market, information from patients, durable medical equipment suppliers, referral sources, or other physical therapists is valuable and should be captured and recorded. This information can be obtained during one-on-one conversations where the physical therapist can note common themes or concerns of patients, such as the price of health care in the community, the access to services on the weekend, or the outcomes of certain health care providers. Information on the local market can also be obtained through the local government or business organizations such as the Chamber of Commerce[14] or through the U.S. Census Bureau.[15] Local information about the number and type of health care facilities in an area, the local unemployment rate, the average household income, and the population demographics and trends can aid in strategic planning and decision-making regarding the type of services to develop or expand. Some basic ways to gain information about the national health care market are to read the American Hospital Association's Annual Environmental Scan[16] and follow aggregate data provided by the government, such as the U.S. Census Bureau or the U.S. Bureau of Labor Statistics.[9] At the national level, there are many economic indicators that are monitored and periodically reported. Some of the more common indicators are the following:

- *Consumer Price Index (CPI)*: An economic indicator that measures the change in the cost of a fixed collection of goods or services. Typically includes housing, electricity, food, and transportation. It is a widely used measure of inflation (ie, an increase in price is a decrease in purchasing power, or as inflation increases, purchasing power decreases).
- *Gross Domestic Product (GDP)*: The total dollar value of all goods and services produced in a country in a given year. It is one indicator of a country's economic size and health.

environmental scanning – a behavior of monitoring, collecting, and analyzing information about the current status and trends in a market in order to make strategic decisions

Chapter 1 / The Language of Business

Typically, the US economy grows at around 2.5% to 3% per year. If growth varies from this expected range, the federal government typically steps in to try to influence the economy (eg, by changing interest rates, imposing taxes, restricting government spending). The GDP should grow at least as fast as the population if the standard of living is to be maintained.

- *Unemployment rate*: Defined as the level of unemployment as a percentage of the labor force. Monitoring the monthly unemployment rate is a good guide to economic development. For every 1% rise in the unemployment rate, over 1 million beneficiaries are added to the Medicaid program.[17] The cost of this program is shared by the federal and state governments, and the additional cost can have an effect on the federal and state budgets for health care and other social programs.
- *Population demographics/trends*: The aging population with its higher utilization rates and increasing rates of chronic diseases point to increasing demand for health care services.[18] The changing ethnic and cultural diversity of people requires services and efficient deliveries that are responsive to the needs of this population.

Cost

Cost is defined as a measure of economic sacrifice.[19] It is what is given up in order to obtain something else. The issue of the cost of health care has been in the forefront of the public debate on universal health care coverage and the cost of the employee benefit for businesses as the cost continues to rise. Since the late 1960s, health care spending has increased significantly as a percentage of the GDP, from 5% to 19%.[20] Workers with employer-sponsored health insurance often experience a reduction in wages in response to increasing health care costs. Increased cost is also offset by direct wage reductions, increased employee cost sharing, or, in cases where wages are fixed (ie, contractual obligations), by increasing the number of hours worked.[21] Increasing cost means a shifting of resources toward health care and away from other goods and services, which impact the economy at a local, national, and international level. This is expected to continue in the United States as health care costs continue to rise at a rate faster than the GDP.[22]

Cost as a factor in the price of a service is an important component in the decision-making process of both the consumer and the producer. An understanding of the cost associated with the service or goods must be identified and understood by the provider in order to set a price that is acceptable to the consumer and that is conducive to the financial viability of the business.

Identification of the most commonly treated conditions in a physical therapy practice is the first step in the cost identification process. Once the common conditions are identified, the cost associated with the interventions and treatment of the people with these conditions can follow, and a general picture of how much it costs to provide services to a person with a specific condition can become clearer.

Cost can be divided into various categories. *Implicit costs* are those costs that are more intangible and related to things like time and effort put into the maintenance of a company by the owner or the use of assets for which no payment is made or value reduced. The most common implicit cost is opportunity cost, the cost of the next best alternative. Although not recorded in financial statements, opportunity cost should be considered when discussing or evaluating alternative courses of action in a business. For example, if a practice owner is considering what to do with the additional space in their clinic, they may consider expanding their current outpatient services, which will allow them to provide

cost – a measure of economic sacrifice

services to an additional three patients per hour. Another alternative would be to make the space a pediatric treatment gym, which would allow the practice to expand its current services into the area of pediatrics and to provide additional programs to the community. One factor in the decision on what to do would be to estimate the opportunity cost associated with each decision.

The other category of cost is *explicit costs*. These are tangible costs that can easily be accounted for, such as wages and supply costs. There are two types of explicit costs: direct and indirect costs. *Direct costs* are those costs directly associated with the production of goods or services. In a physical therapy clinic, these would include such things as the salary and benefits given to the physical therapist; the supplies and equipment that are used in the delivery of physical therapy services; and the tools that are used in the examination, evaluation, and treatment process. These are clearly directly related to the production of the physical therapy service. *Indirect costs* are those costs that are indirectly associated with the production of goods or services, often referred to as overhead costs. Indirect costs may not be so readily identified. These costs include such things as administrative salaries, utility bills, building and grounds maintenance, or laundry services. In larger organizations, indirect costs are generally allocated to departments within the organization based on the size of the department, the number of employees in the department, the revenues the department generates, or some other formula derived by the organization's management. Indirect cost allocations can vary depending on the type and size of the organization.

In order to determine the total cost associated with some cost group or cost center, a worksheet can be completed to help determine the total cost. Figure 1.3 contains an example of a cost worksheet.[22] This is one method of calculating current costs or expenses of an employee in the delivery of a service. The direct costs associated with an employee would be the salary of the employee plus the additional costs of employer-paid taxes, contributions to a retirement fund, professional liability insurance, and the associated employer costs for health care, short- and long-term disability insurance, and life insurance, as a few examples. In addition, there are costs associated with mileage reimbursement, if that is a requirement of the job, and additional expenses that may be part of an employee package (eg, continuing education funds). Indirect costs include those expenses associated with the support of the delivery of the service (eg, utilities, administration salaries, maintenance costs). An indirect cost rate (ICR) is the ratio between the total indirect expenses associated with a set of direct expenses.[23] The ICR can range significantly, depending on the size of the organization, the organizational structure, the overhead costs, and the physical location of the business. Once the total direct and indirect costs are identified, the cost of providing services based on 2,080 hours for full-time employment (40 hours per week $\times$ 52 weeks = 2,080 hours) can be determined. This information can be used to determine the cost per hour associated with this employee. This will factor into the price for the service and productivity expectations.

Identifying costs provides a baseline to work from when calculating how much revenue is needed to reach a target profit level. Generating a profit is important to maintaining the practice, updating equipment, increasing salaries, or expanding a current practice into a new market. It is important to include all expenses when making expense projections. Often, independent practitioners may forget the obvious expenses such as home-office space, office supplies, traveling expenses, and continuing education expenses. It is important, however, to be able to provide an explanation or support, in the form of receipts, or purchase orders, to justify the expense to an outside agency.

Once expenses have been identified, they can be classified as fixed, variable, or semivariable. This will help identify how the expenses behave and how much control the physical therapist has over certain expenses.

Explicit costs can also be classified as fixed, variable, or semivariable. *Fixed costs*, such as salary and wages, rent, interest expenses on loans, and depreciation of equipment, are set

Chapter 1 / The Language of Business

Cost Worksheet

DIRECT COST:

1. Salary

a.	Base		$95,620[1]
b.	Overtime		0
c.	**Total salary** =		$95,620

2. Fringes (approx. 30% of 1c.)

a.	FICA (7.65% of 1c.)		$ 7,315
b.	Workman's comp. (4% of 1c.)[2]		$ 3,825
c.	State unemployment (av. $250/yr)[2]		$ 250
d.	Fed. unemployment ($56/yr)[2]		$ 56
e.	Pension plan (av. 2% of 1c.)[3]		$ 1,912
f.	Professional liability (1% of 1c.)		$ 956
g.	Insurance (health, life, disability) (12% of 1c.)		$11,474
h.	**Total fringes** =		$25,788

3. Other

a.	Mileage[4]		$ 300
b.	Continuing education		$ 500
c.	Tuition reimbursement		$ 0
d.	Licence/dues/subscriptions		$ 500
e.	**Total other** =		$ 1,300

4. **Direct total** (1c + 2h + 3e) = $122,708

5. INDIRECT COST RATE (allocation)[5]:
   Private clinic or Home health agency
   (add 65% of direct total)
   Hospital based (add 30% of direct total) $ 36,812

TOTAL COST (4 + 5) = $159,520

TOTAL COST of 159,520/2,080 **HOURS PAID TO WORK PER YEAR** =
COST PER HOUR of $76.69
Typically 2,080 hours per year for a 40-hour workweek. 1,950 for a 37.5-hour workweek
For a 10-month school year, 7 hours per day: 1,400 hours.

---

[1] Median annual earnings for a physical therapist. Bureau of Labor Statistics; U.S. Department of Labor. *Occupational Outlook Handbook.* 2022
[2] May vary depending on the state, profession, and paid to date amount.
[3] Varies depending on organization benefit package. Will vary depending on employer matching programs.
[4] Depends on federal reimbursement for mileage and the job description, if driving in required once the employee is at work.
[5] Includes nonrevenue-generating staff and overhead costs. The ICR can range significantly depending on the size of the organization, the organizational structure, the overhead costs, and the physical location of the business. 30% was used in this example.

Figure 1.3 **Cost worksheet.** (Reprinted with permission from Drnach M. The basics of billing. In: Drnach M, ed. *The Clinical Practice of Pediatric Physical Therapy: From the NICU to Independent Living.* Wolters Kluwer Health/Lippincott Williams and Wilkins; 2008:339-349.)

and do not change over an extended period of time or with service volume. Fixed costs are more easily budgeted and managed because they are not affected by service volume. *Variable costs* are the costs that do vary, depending on volume. These are the costs over which a physical therapist exerts the most control. Variable cost items could include supplies such as home exercise program forms, office supplies, printing costs for brochures and pamphlets, and the costs of small equipment or any item that is "used up" in the process of service provision. Because variable costs are the easiest to control, they are generally the first to be affected in order to meet short-term financial goals. A business owner's request to turn off lights when not in use and copying on both sides of a piece of paper may sound insignificant to an employee, but it is one way to control variable costs. Decreasing salaries or limiting benefits would be a more drastic measure. *Semivariable costs*, sometimes referred to as mixed costs, fall between fixed and variable costs. Semivariable cost items have a fixed cost component and a variable cost component, which is affected by volume. Examples of these items include the cost of fuel and public water, which has a fixed monthly rate for a specific amount but can increase when more fuel (for either heating or transportation) or water is used. If the user exceeds the basic amount, an additional cost is incurred. The *total cost* can be determined with the following formula:

Total costs = Total fixed costs + Total variable costs

Identifying the total costs associated with the provision of services provides necessary information in the calculation of needed revenue to sustain a business. Generating revenue in excess of total costs (a profit) is important in maintaining the business, updating equipment, increasing salaries, or expanding into new markets.

In health care, cost is usually associated with a *unit of service*, which can mean different things to different organizations (Table 1.1). A UOS may be defined as a patient encounter, a 15-minute increment of physical therapy service, a specific treatment intervention, or the length of the episode of care. Understanding how an organization defines a UOS is an important aspect of understanding and calculating costs.

Marginal cost (or incremental cost) is the additional cost required to provide one more UOS. This is an important piece of information when deciding to see one more patient or providing services for one more day (or UOS). How much money will be spent? How much additional revenue will be realized? The difference in total cost before a change is made and after the change has been made represents the marginal cost of that change. In addition, many managers or owners of a practice may want information on the cost per diagnostic group or cost per intervention or treatment modality. This represents average cost and is calculated using the total volume of the UOS provided for the target segment. *Average total cost* can be determined with the following formula:

Average total cost = Total cost/Total volume of UOS

For example, if the total cost associated with providing physical therapy services for 1 year was $95,000 and the total UOS delivered in that year was 1,560, then the average total cost for the provision of services would be $60.90 per UOS. Similarly, marginal cost is:

Marginal cost = Change in total cost/Change in UOS output

Table 1.1 Examples of UOS	
Service	*1 Unit Equals*
Inpatient	15 min
Outpatient	Intervention CPT code
Skilled nursing facility	8 min
School-based therapy	30 min
Home care	One patient visit

CPT, Current Procedural Terminology; UOS, unit of service.

Chapter 1 / The Language of Business **17**

Table 1.2 Costs					
Volume	**Fixed Cost**	**Variable Cost**	**Total Cost**	**Average Cost**	**Marginal Cost**
1	200	100	300	300	
10	200	1,000	1,200	120	100
15	200	1,500	1,700	113	100
20	200	2,000	2,200	110	100

Note that as volume increases, the average cost decreases (economy of scale).
Marginal cost = Change in total cost/Change in UOS
When the volume goes from 1 to 10, MC = 900/9 = 100

If it costs $50 to provide one more UOS (Table 1.2), then the marginal cost would be:

MC = 50/1

MC = 50

The marginal cost to produce one more UOS is less than the average cost in this example.

Pricing

Before a business can estimate the expected revenues from services rendered, a fee schedule needs to be created. The fee schedule is a listing of the services provided and the charge for each of those services. The fee can be based on a per hour or minute of service, on the type of service or treatment, or per session for a set number of sessions. A flat fee is a fee that is charged to the patient no matter how long or complicated the intervention. Flat fees can be useful in contracts to provide services in a school or hospice setting, whereby a physical therapist agrees to provide services for a specific number of hours per week for a flat fee, regardless of the number of students/patients seen. A per hour or minute fee is the more common type of fee used by most professionals, especially in hospital outpatient settings or private practice. Fees are charged to patients in time increments, usually minutes. Fees can also be based on the number of sessions or the number of patient consults. For example, in the case of a patient who needs 10 treatment sessions, the first evaluation session is charged at $150, but each subsequent treatment session is only $100. This is common in practices where multiple sessions over a short period of time are expected, such as with physical therapy.

The actual dollar amount of the fees can be calculated using several different methods: market or going rate, breakeven, or markup. The market or going rate, also referred to in health care as the usual, customary, and reasonable rate (UCR), is what others in the marketplace are charging for the same or similar service. This method is easily established but runs the risk of not covering all of the cost of the individual practice, since those may be significantly different from others in the marketplace. The break-even, or cost method,

fee schedule – a listing of the services or goods provided and the charge for each of those items

flat fee – a fee that is charged no matter how long or complicated the delivery of the good or service

market or going rate – a fee determined by what other competitors are charging in the market

break-even cost method – a fee determined by the revenue needed to cover the cost, without consideration of a profit

requires the physical therapist to identify all of the expenses of their practice so the appropriate fee can be calculated to cover all of the costs. This method will cover costs but may not provide the money to be able to update or expand the practice. The most common method is a markup method. The markup method is similar in most industries, whereby a fee or price is estimated based on several factors such as cost, time, location, and type of service provided, and then a markup or additional percentage is added onto the fee to cover any unanticipated costs or to allow for additional revenue to fund updates or practice expansion.

Fee for service is the term used to describe the amounts charged by a physical therapist, or any health care provider, per the fee schedule. The revenues are service specific and generally reflect the market value of the service provided. Fee for service revenue can vary by the type of service (eg, private or hospital based) or the location of a service (eg, rural or urban area). Typically, health care providers create a fee schedule, which is a listing of all their services and the corresponding fees for those services. The practice then sets fees for certain services based on what the market will bear. Thus, for example, a physical therapist who practices in a city where the demand for physical therapy is high might set a fee of $145 for 15 minutes of services, whereas another physical therapist practicing in a rural setting might set the same service at a fee of only $85 per 15 minutes of services. Every practice can have only one fee schedule, and thus one fee for each type of service. It is illegal to charge different fees for the same services unless a true cost difference can be proven with the delivery of that service.

Identifying the revenue and expenses and establishing a fee schedule are the starting points of an independent practice. The sale price for a UOS, the costs associated with the delivery of that service, and the volume needed to break even then to make a profit are other important aspects of a business.

Break-Even Analysis

Identifying and categorizing the costs of doing business can lead to a better understanding of the behavior of a UOS in making money, losing money, or breaking even. This is not simply looking at the average cost and the revenue generated but also looking at the volume of patients or UOS that are provided with the fixed costs for the program or service. Fixed costs are not influenced by volume, but as the volume increases, the fixed costs per UOS as a percentage of total cost decrease because of the sharing of the fixed cost with an increasing number of patients. This is referred to as economy of scale: the reduction in the cost of providing services with increased volume because fixed cost is used more, thereby decreasing the average cost per UOS (see Table 1.2).

The break-even analysis is a technique to find the specific volume at which a business neither makes nor loses money.[24] It is based on the following formula:

Break-even quantity = Fixed costs/Price per UOS − Variable cost per UOS

markup method – a fee determined by the revenue needed to cover the cost, plus the addition of a profit margin

break-even analysis – a calculation of a specific volume at which a business covers costs but does not make a profit. A point in production where a business neither makes nor loses money

Using the information in Table 1.2, a manager would want to know how many UOS it would take to break even given a program that has a fixed cost of $200 and a variable cost of $100 (eg, supplies used, hourly labor costs). The price for one UOS is $150. Using the formula:

Break-even quantity = $200/150 − 100

= $200/50

= 4 units

Therefore, until four UOS are provided, the business will be operating at a loss; once four UOS are provided, the business will be making neither a profit nor a loss but will break even; after four UOS, the business will be operating at a profit. Note that Figure 1.4 can be used to estimate the break-even point.

When trying to achieve the break-even point, a manager has several options. One is to lower the fixed cost associated with the UOS. As stated previously, this may be difficult to do given the nature of fixed costs and those items associated with them, such as salary and benefits. The appropriate utilization of a less costly employee, such as a physical therapist assistant instead of a physical therapist, is one way of lowering fixed costs. Lowering variable cost or the price for the service is another option, although lowering the price in an insurance-driven industry is not always prudent. The easiest way to achieve the break-even point and beyond is to increase volume, recruiting more patients.

Operating at breakeven may sustain a business for a short period. Unfortunately, a business must have some level of profit to maintain its current financial position over time. Additional resources will be required for nonroutine expenses such as equipment replacement or routine building maintenance. Over time, reserves will be depleted, and the break-even business will be unable to sustain operations. The bottom line is that in order to exist into the future, a business must bring in more money than it spends.

Cost-Effectiveness Analysis

All players in the health care system, such as employers, insurers, providers, and consumers, as well as federal and state policymakers, need objective, scientifically based information to help them make decisions about the allocation of the scarce health care resource. Physical therapists have to make decisions every day regarding the allocation of resources and the effectiveness of the services they provide. The Agency for Healthcare Research and

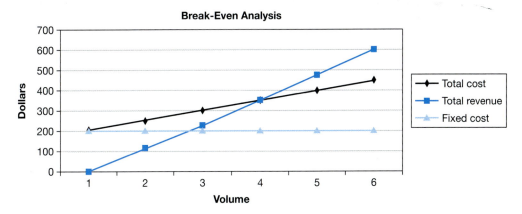

Figure 1.4 Graphic representation of a break-even analysis.

Quality, Department of Health and Human Services Public Health Service,[25] is the federal government's agency charged with supporting research designed to improve the quality of health care, reduce its cost, address patient safety and medical errors, and broaden access to essential services.

Once a physical therapist understands costs, costs can be factored into clinical decision-making regarding the most cost-effective method to produce an outcome in a given patient population or program. Articles are now appearing in the literature that address or include the concept of cost-effectiveness in the study of the effectiveness of certain physical therapy interventions.[26-29]

A cost-effectiveness analysis (CEA) is done to promote an efficient use of finite resources. It is the measurement of the relative costs and outcomes associated with a particular activity or program in comparison with another similar program that produces the same outcome. It is important that the outcome measurement tool is consistent between the two programs under consideration to ensure that patients achieve the same result. When performing a CEA, the costs (both direct and indirect) for each program are identified, categorized, and monitored along with other quantitative and qualitative data. After the provision of services for the duration of the program is complete, patient outcomes are obtained and decisions made regarding the efficient use of resources to produce the optimal outcome for the patients. A problem that may arise in the clinic is the inclusion of less costly services or the exclusion of more costly services in an attempt to control cost, without looking at the effects such substitutions have on the outcomes of the services provided. If a new approach produces the exact same outcome for less money, then it can be concluded that the new approach is cost-effective. Being less costly is not the sole goal of physical therapy intervention. Being cost-effective and producing the same outcome for the patient over alternative interventions is the ultimate goal.

Summary

Economics studies how people use their limited resources to fulfill their wants and needs. In a free market economy, consumers interact with producers to determine what, how, and for whom services and goods will be produced. Some goods and services (ie, public goods) are produced by governments. Historically, it has only been recently that governments have expanded their role into more social programs such as health care, in addition to public education and national defense. This expansion has created opportunities as well as challenges as capitalistic economies balance the influence of government with individual and private control.

The need for providers (such as physical therapists) to have a basic understanding of economic principles such as scarcity, resource allocation, value, utility, and demand has become more important in clinical decision-making as health care cost continues to rise and cost containment measures are discussed and implemented in the health care industry. Such measures often introduce the concept of opportunity cost and the value associated with the foregone alternative action. Consumers have finite resources. When expending limited resources, consumers strive to gain maximum value. Value is often associated with price, which has an interesting elastic component and is important in determining the effect a change in price would have on the quantity demanded by the consumer. Supply of a resource affects quantity demanded as well as the price. Assuming all other factors

cost-effectiveness analysis – a calculation of the relative costs and outcomes associated with a particular service typically compared to other similar services that produce an equivalent outcome

Chapter 1 / The Language of Business

are constant, as the price of a product or service increases, the quantity demanded by the consumer is likely to decrease, and vice versa. Less expensive substitutes become more attractive to buyers.

When there are alternative providers of services and products, there is competition in the market. A competitive market is characterized by multiple producers, each having a minority share of the market. In a competitive market, consumers have a choice of products/producers from which to choose. Having a basic understanding of how to scan the market or environment provides information about the current status or changes in the market and aids in strategic planning for a business.

The cost associated with the provision of health care is an important component in the decision-making process of both the consumer and the producer. An understanding of the various costs associated with the service or goods (ie, fixed costs, variable costs, and mixed costs) must be identified and understood by the provider in order to set a price that is acceptable to the consumer and that is conducive to the financial viability of the business. Activities such as a break-even analysis and CEA can aid the physical therapist in maximizing their economic potential while maintaining quality care made evident through clinical outcomes.

REFERENCES

1. Hajiran H. Interdisciplinary teaching tools for economics 101: gateway concepts of quality of life & capitalism. Published December 13, 2004. https://ssrn.com/abstract=643384
2. Scott RD 2nd, Solomon SL, McGowan JE Jr. Applying economic principles to health care. *Emerg Infect Dis.* 2001;7(2):282-285. doi:10.3201/eid0702.010227
3. Folland S, Goodman AC, Stano M. *The Economics of Health and Health Care.* Routledge; 2016.
4. Lipford JW, Slice J. Adam Smith's roles for government and contemporary U.S. government roles: is the welfare state crowding out government's basic functions? *Indep Rev.* 2007;11(4):485-501. http://www.jstor.org/stable/24562411
5. Maslow AH. A theory of human motivation. *Psychol Rev.* 1943;50(4):370-396. doi:10.1037/h0054346
6. Finkler SA, Ward DM. *Essentials of Cost Accounting for Health Care Organizations.* 2nd ed. Aspen; 1999.
7. Mariner WK. Rationing health care and the need for credible scarcity: why Americans can't say no. *Am J Public Health.* 1995;85(10):1439-1445. doi:10.2105/ajph.85.10.1439
8. Menger C. *Principles of Economics.* Ludwig von Mises Institute; 2007.
9. U.S. Bureau of Labor Statistics. *Physical Therapists: Occupational Outlook Handbook.* Published February 22, 2019. Updated April 18, 2022. Accessed July 8, 2022. https://www.bls.gov/ooh/healthcare/physical-therapists.htm
10. American Physical Therapy Association. APTA physical therapy workforce analysis. Published December 2020. Accessed July 8, 2022. https://www.apta.org/contentassets/5997bfa5c8504df789fe4f1c01a717eb/apta-ptworkforcereport2021.pdf
11. Schafer DS, Lopopolo RB, Luedtke-Hoffmann KA. Administration and management skills needed by physical therapist graduates in 2010: a national survey. *Phys Ther.* 2007;87(3):261-281. doi:10.2522/ptj.20060003
12. Choo CW. Environmental scanning as information seeking and organizational learning. *Inf Res.* 2001;7(1). Accessed July 8, 2022. http://informationr.net/ir/7-1/paper112.html
13. Schafer DS. Environmental-scanning behavior among private practice physical therapy firms. *Phys Ther.* 1991;71(6):482-490. doi:10.1093/ptj/71.6.482
14. Chamber of Commerce. The most trusted online business community. Updated 2022. Accessed July 8, 2022. https://www.chamberofcommerce.com
15. U.S. Census Bureau. Updated July 2022. Accessed July 8, 2022. https://www.census.gov
16. American Hospital Association. 2022 Environmental Scan. Published 2022. Accessed July 8, 2022. https://www.aha.org/environmentalscan
17. Holahan J, Garret B. Rising unemployment and Medicaid. *Health Policy Online.* 2001;(1):1-9. Accessed July 8, 2022. https://www.urban.org/sites/default/files/publication/61631/410306-Rising-Unemployment-and-Medicaid.PDF
18. U.S. Bureau of Labor Statistics. *Healthcare Occupations: Occupational Outlook Handbook.* Published February 22, 2019. Updated April 18, 2022. Accessed July 8, 2022. https://www.bls.gov/ooh/healthcare/home.htm
19. Morse W, Roth H. *Cost Accounting: Processing, Evaluating, and Using Cost Data.* Addison-Wesley Publishing Co; 1986.

20. Centers for Medicare & Medicaid Services. Historical. Published December 2020. Accessed July 8, 2022. https://www.cms.gov/data-research/statistics-trends-and-reports/national-health-expenditure-data/historical
21. Office of the Assistant Secretary for Planning and Evaluation. Effects of health care spending on the U.S. economy: executive summary. Published 2005. Accessed July 8, 2022. http://aspe.hhs.gov/health/costgrowth/index.htm
22. Centers for Medicare & Medicaid Services. NHE fact sheet. Updated 2021. Accessed July 8, 2022. https://www.cms.gov/data-research/statistics-trends-and-reports/national-health-expenditure-data/nhe-fact-sheet
23. U.S. Department of Labor; Cost and Price Determination Division; Office of Strategy and Administration. A guide for indirect cost rate determination. Published October 2021. Accessed July 9, 2022. https://www.dol.gov/sites/dolgov/files/OASAM/legacy/files/DCD-2-CFR-Guide.pdf
24. Finkler S, Kovner C, Jones C. *Financial Management for Nurse Managers and Executives.* Saunders Elsevier; 2007.
25. Agency for Healthcare Research and Quality. Healthcare costs. Accessed July 9, 2022. https://www.ahrq.gov/topics/healthcare-costs.html
26. Hon S, Ritter R, Allen D. Cost-effectiveness and outcomes of direct access to physical therapy for musculoskeletal disorders compared to physician-first access in the United States: systematic review and meta-analysis. *Phys Ther.* 2021;101(1):pzaa201. doi:10.1093/ptj/pzaa201
27. Bove A, Smith K, Bise C, et al. Exercise, manual therapy, and booster sessions in knee osteoarthritis: cost-effectiveness analysis from a multicenter randomized controlled trial. *Phys Ther.* 2018;98(1):16-27. doi:10.1093/ptj/pzx104
28. Rhon DI, Kim M, Asche CV, Allison SC, Allen CS, Deyle GD. Cost-effectiveness of physical therapy vs intra-articular glucocorticoid injection for knee osteoarthritis: a secondary analysis from a randomized clinical trial. *JAMA Netw Open.* 2022;5(1):e2142709. doi:10.1001/jamanetworkopen.2021.42709
29. Khodakarami N. Treatment of patients with low back pain: a comparison of physical therapy and chiropractic manipulation. *Healthcare (Basel).* 2020;8(1):44. doi:10.3390/healthcare8010044

CHAPTER 2

Accounting and Finance

MARK DRNACH

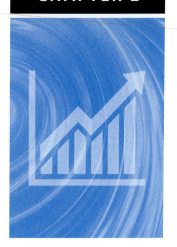

Learning Objectives

The reader will

1. Define the basic terms, aspects, and processes of accounting.
2. Demonstrate an understanding of the application of standard accounting practices.
3. Compare the contents of the four fundamental financial statements.
4. Understand the process of budgeting.
5. Apply the basic aspects of accounting in the financial analysis of financial information.
6. Understand management's role in revenue and expense management.

The constant need to achieve and maintain a positive bottom line (making a profit) in the health care industry has expanded the role and responsibilities of the providers of health care, including the physical therapist, in the delivery of services. Whether it is a sole proprietor practice or part of a larger group or organization, such as a hospital, the need to organize, manage, and understand financial information is now an important aspect of health care. Understanding the established rules and regulations for identifying, recording, and reporting financial information allows the health care provider to participate in the business of health care, program evaluation, cost-effectiveness analysis, value outcome measurements, and in the development of plans that contribute to long-term organizational sustainability. Having a basic understanding of the terms and processes used in accounting is one of the first steps in this process, and it is necessary in order to participate in the conversations about health care finances. Basic accounting practices are used to develop four fundamental financial statements:

1. Balance sheet
2. Income statement
3. Cash flow statement
4. Retained earnings statement

An understanding of the information in these statements will allow the reader to better understand the relationship between the delivery of patient care services and the revenues and expenses of operating a health care business. Decisions about new or expanded programs, staffing, and purchases that would otherwise be based on a "best guess" will become clearer and more objective. Application of objective information about the performance of an organization as compared to what was planned (the budgeting process) and/or what competitors are doing will help the organization stay on target with performance objectives.

In addition, every health care provider should have a basic understanding of how to maximize revenues. It is necessary to understand the payment options available for services rendered, either by the first party (the patient/client), the second party (the provider), or the third party (an insurance company), and how to balance work expectations, providing quality care, producing valuable outcomes, and maximizing revenues. Once the principles of health care accounting and financial planning are understood, financial management skills can be applied to health care operations to maximize an organization's productivity and financial performance.

This chapter will cover the basic accounting and financial issues that can help a health care provider understand these fundamental aspects of an organization. In doing so, he or she will be better equipped to effectively participate in this important aspect of health care. The accounting concepts have direct application to personal financial management as well.

Accounting

Accounting is a system of record keeping that allows an organization to keep an account of its financial activity. It is a process of identifying, recording, summarizing, and reporting in monetary terms information about an organization during a specific period of time. Accounting is not a science but rather a set of rules and conventions that apply to the way an organization identifies, records, summarizes and reports financial information. These rules and reporting requirements are established by the Financial Accounting Standards Board (FASB) and are called the Generally Accepted Accounting Principles (GAAP).[1] The GAAP provide some consistency to the accounting process, allowing an individual or investor to analyze or compare companies' financial statements. Examples of some of the more common accounting principles include the following:

1. The *identification of the entity*, which is the business unit, the person, or business that is the focus of attention and for which the financial statements are being prepared
2. The *expectation of going concern*, which is the belief that the business is going to continue into the future. If the entity is planning on going out of business, then disclosing that information is required.
3. The *matching principle*, which states that a business must record the expenses that are associated with the revenues generated for a given period. Matching is the only way an organization can determine if a specific product and/or service is contributing to the organization's financial performance.
4. The *identification of the cost* of any quantifiable resource, which is typically the amount the organization paid for that resource (historical or acquisition cost). This may significantly understate the current value of a resource (compared to its replacement cost or market value). It is the easiest and most objective way to capture a resource's value.
5. The *availability of objective evidence*, which means that the information in the financial statement is based on objective and verifiable evidence (eg, receipts)
6. The *acceptance of materiality* or tolerance of the inherent errors or omissions (eg, the small stuff; the useful life of a paper clip or pen.) in the financial statement. Some error cannot be avoided, and, therefore, financial statements are not expected to be error free, but the error or intentional omission should not be sufficient (or material) to cause the user of the financial statement to change his or her decision based on the information provided.

accounting – a system of record keeping that allows a business or entity to keep a record of its financial activity

Chapter 2 / Accounting and Finance

7. The *application of consistency* in the accounting methods used in the business from year to year
8. The *trust in full disclosure* of the financial position and results of operations of a business, in accordance with GAAP[2]

Because these common principles are expected to be followed by all organizations, reporting transactions and the results of such activity will allow a potential investor, peer reviewers, or other external entities to better understand the financial aspects of an organization.

Many organizations hire a certified public accountant (CPA) once a year to examine their financial statements because of their importance to the organization as well as to ensure compliance with various US taxation requirements. The credential of CPA is a designation given by the American Institute of Certified Public Accountants to those individuals who successfully pass the Uniform Certified Public Accountant Examination and meet the state's requirements for licensure, indicating a level of expertise in accounting, financial planning, and auditing (a process of examining the accuracy and completeness of a financial statement). CPAs are required to report whether the financial statements have been prepared in accordance with GAAP.

In certain circumstances, the GAAP are modified by specific accounting conventions. The accounting conventions common to health care are allowances for contractual deductions and fund accounting. The convention of *allowances for contractual deductions* addresses the difference between the price charged for a service and the price paid by third-party payers. This approach reflects the utilization of a variety of contractual third-party payers by an organization, which leads to differences in the payment for such services. The amount of payment may vary significantly between payers and is seldom under the control of the health care provider. To capture and account for the difference between the amount charged and the amount paid, an account called allowances for contractual deductions is used. This account will show the organization how much money it could have received if the third-party agreement was not in effect and the patient paid directly for the services rendered. This information helps the organization to evaluate the benefit of having a contractual agreement with the insurance company. Contractual allowances are accepted by an organization often based on volume of people with that type of insurance in the target market. For example, an organization may accept Medicare insurance even though the payment for services is less than the organization's fee, in order to increase patient volume by providing services to the people in the area. In this agreement, the business agrees to accept the payment of the insurance company as payment in full, for the services rendered. *Fund accounting* is often found in not-for-profit hospitals and health care organizations (HCO). An HCO may need to separate financial information of one or more of its sections or programs into a specified category or fund to be examined separately from that of the total entity, especially when funds are provided for a specific purpose. For example, if an HCO received a philanthropic gift to be used only for the support of a pediatric program or building project, a separate fund would be set up to account for this donor-restricted gift. This separation prevents the comingling of restricted funds with general funds. Types of accounting funds that may be seen in health care are endowment funds, plant replacement and expansion funds, and specific-purpose funds.[3] Each fund is considered an independent entity with its own set of accounts but is part of the larger financial entity; therefore, the performance and condition of the fund accounts are included in the financial reports of the total entity.

Accounting involves the creation of an internal system of record keeping and reporting, which ultimately results in the creation of financial statements for the business. These systems include such aspects as the creation of a chart of accounts, adherence to a double entry system of accounting, and the classification of financial activities such as debits, credits, assets, and liabilities.

Chart of Accounts

The process of accounting begins with the identification of the entity for which the financial information will be gathered and then the identification of the entity's accounts. An account is a category of assets, liabilities, owner's equity, revenues, and expenses. A chart of accounts is the foundation for accounting information systems within an organization and serves as the nucleus for the development of standard financial statements.[4] It is simply a listing of all of an organization's accounts by title and corresponding numerical code. The chart of accounts is often arranged in the order that the accounts appear on the balance sheet (assets, liabilities, then owner's equity) and income statement (revenues then expenses).[4] A numerical code is used to classify and to differentiate accounts. The number and types of accounts will depend on the size, type, and complexity of the business. The information needs of the management will influence the number and degree of specificity of the chart of accounts. For example, management may wish to have one general account to record revenue from equipment sold. If it is important to know the sales revenue for each type of equipment sold, management may choose to have one account for each type or category of equipment. The total of these equipment revenue accounts would then be combined to determine total revenue from equipment sold. Table 2.1 provides an example

Table 2.1 Outline of a Chart of Accounts at the Primary Classification Level as of September 30, 20XX			
Code	Type	Subcode	Fund
100–199	Assets	110	Operating
		120	Capital equipment
		130	Other
200–299	Liabilities	210	Operating
		220	Capital equipment
		230	Other
300–399	Capital	310	Operating
		320	Capital equipment
		330	Other
400–499	Revenue	410	Patient services
		420	Deductions from revenue
		430	Other
500–599	Expense	510	Patient services
		520	Support services
		530	Management services
		540	Purchased services

Adapted with permission from Drnach M. Accounting and finance. In: Nosse LJ, Friberg DG, eds. *Management and Supervisory Principles for Physical Therapists*. 3rd ed. Wolters Kluwer Health/Lippincott Williams and Wilkins; 2010:405-428.

account – a category of assets, liabilities, owner's equity, revenues, and expenses of a business or entity

chart of accounts – a listing of all of a business' accounts in the order that the accounts appear on the Fundamental Financial Documents

Chapter 2 / Accounting and Finance

of a chart of accounts at the primary classification level. Each of the major account types from the balance sheet and income statement are assigned a series of numbers that define the characteristics of the account (eg, revenue or expense). Within each numerical series, the major accounts are further defined by subgroupings of funds or subgroupings of accounts (eg, revenue from patient services; expenses for support services).

Table 2.2 contains a more detailed example of numeric coding for the expense category of salaries and benefits. The logic that has been used to assign a numeric code to each of the subclasses, such as employee type, is provided. Once the logic of the numeric coding is provided, it should be easily understood and used as reference for the accounts included in budgets and other financial statements. The chart of accounts is specific to an organization and can vary depending on the information needed to make financial decisions. Having an understanding of an organization's chart of accounts provides information on how the organization categorizes, allocates, and monitors its revenue and expenses.

Table 2.2 Example of a Chart of Accounts for Expenses, Expanded

Chart of Accounts Logic

500–599	Expense
	Salaries
531.10	Management
511.10	Therapist
511.12	Technical
521.10	Billing
521.12	Clerical
	Benefits
532.10	Management
512.10	Therapist
512.12	Technical
522.10	Billing
522.12	Clerical
	FICA
533.10	Management
513.10	Therapist
513.12	Technical
523.10	Billing
523.12	Clerical

Summary-Coding Logic

Digit	Meaning	Code	Technical Salaries
First	Type of account	5	Expense
Second	Subgroup/fund	1	Patient services
Third	Account class	1	Salaries
Fourth and Fifth	Subclass/department	.10/.12	Technical/billing

FICA, Federal Insurance Contribution Act.
Reprinted with permission from Drnach M. Accounting and finance. In: Nosse LJ, Friberg DG, eds. *Management and Supervisory Principles for Physical Therapists*. 3rd ed. Wolters Kluwer Health/Lippincott Williams and Wilkins; 2010:405-428.

The development and utilization of the chart of accounts is a significant aspect in the generation of uniform financial statements, which in turn are vital in the analysis of outcomes, cost effectiveness, and comparative studies.[4]

Double Entry

When a financial event occurs, it is recorded (posted) in a spreadsheet of accounts, also referred to as a ledger. This event, considered a transaction, has two aspects, the change in the entity's assets and the change in the entity's liabilities. For example, if a patient owes a practice $75 and is billed for the service that would be recorded in the account for *accounts receivable* (what is owed). When payment is made, the account for cash on hand will go up, while the account for accounts receivable will go down. Both aspects of a transaction should be recorded. The accountant debits the transaction to one account and credits it to another.

Debits and Credits

Debits and credits – from the Latin words *debere*, which means to owe, and *credere*, to entrust – preceded the concept of positive and negative numbers. Historically, the posting of debits is done on the left-hand side of the ledger, and the posting of credits is done on the right-hand side. Debits and credits are not assigned negative values, nor is the sum of the debits or credits assigned a negative value. They are terms used to describe the basic accounts in a *double entry accounting system*, in which one account is debited, whereas another is credited. Whether or not this has a positive or negative effect on the organization's financial statements depends on what type of account is involved (eg, revenue accounts increase with credit postings, and expense accounts increase with debit postings).

Asset, Liability, and Equity

Assets are economic resources that are owned by a business and are expected to benefit future operations.[5] Assets include such things as:

- Prepaid expenses
- Inventories
- Account receivables
- Capital assets
- Intangibles
- Cash
- Investments

Prepaid expenses include such things as salary advanced or insurance payments made for a future period. *Inventories* represent the value of supplies or products that will be used or sold during future periods. Accounts receivable are a type of asset in which the patient or client has an obligation to pay the organization for a product or service rendered on credit. (Some transactions are done "on account." This means that payment was not made when the service or product was delivered; instead, an account was opened and is tracked until payment is made in full.) Capital assets include land, buildings, and equipment. Sometimes, assets are called *intangible*, meaning the asset has no physical substance. Patents, trademarks, copyrights, and goodwill (eg, reputation for excellence, good relationships with community partners) are examples of intangible assets.[5]

Assets – economic resources that are owned by a business

Chapter 2 / Accounting and Finance 29

Assets are important in determining the financial health of the organization. For the purposes of reporting, the value of an asset represents its current value to the organization and its ability to continue the operation of the business. Potential creditors view assets as resources available to cover the organization's debt, including the creditor's investment. For the creditor, more assets mean a better chance of repayment if the operation of the organization does not produce enough income to cover expenses. Creditors value assets based on the value and the speed with which the asset can be converted to cash. Cash and assets that can be readily converted to cash are referred to as liquid assets (eg, checks, cash in savings accounts, easily converted securities). Assets that require a long conversion period are referred to as fixed assets (eg, real estate, equipment, furniture).

Liabilities are debts of the organization. Total liabilities are the amount of the organization's assets that are owned by its creditors. Liabilities that are repayable within 1 year are considered to be short term. Liabilities not due or payable for greater than 1 year are considered to be long-term liabilities. Liabilities include things such as:

- Accounts payable
- Accrued expenses
- Notes payable

Accounts payable are debts payable to individuals who have provided products or services to the organization on credit. Outstanding bills for supplies and professional and cleaning services are examples of debts that would fall under accounts payable.

Accrued expenses represent the value of debts that are held for payment in the future.[6] The time or need for payment may not be known. Vacation time or Paid Time Off (PTO) is an example of an accrued expense. The organization owes its employees the value of their accrued time off. Often, employees are able to bank or use accrued time off at their discretion. Should they terminate their employment, they may or may not be able to claim the value of their banked time. If accrued PTO is paid at prevailing wages instead of the wage at the time of accrual, the value to the employee and size of this accrued debt can grow over time. As long as the employer has the potential to pay for this accrued debt, it is listed as a liability.

Notes payable are promises (notes) to pay a certain amount of money at a certain time in the future. Generally, these are loans evidenced by loan agreements, indicating the loan amount, repayment schedule, and the interest due at future dates. Amounts owed for lines of credit, start-up capital, and mortgages are examples of debts that would fall under the category of notes payable.

Equity, or ownership, is often associated with a publicly traded stock but is also the value of an organization beyond its liabilities or what it owes (net worth = what is left after debts were paid). The owner's equity is the difference between the organization's total assets and its total liabilities. It is the portion of the assets that the owner owns as opposed to what he or she borrowed. The net worth of the owner can increase in two ways. First, the owner can invest additional resources into the organization, or the net worth can increase as a result of profitable operations (an increase in income greater than an increase in expenses).

liquid assets – assets that can be quickly converted to cash

fixed assets – assets that cannot be quickly converted to cash

liability – debts

notes payable – a promise or note to pay a certain amount of money at a certain time in the future

equity – the amount of money an owner would receive after selling an asset and paying any liabilities associated with the asset

Accrual and Cash

The concept of accrual refers to the practice of recording financial transactions within an appropriate period of time. The accrual basis of accounting requires that revenue be recorded within the period it is earned. Likewise, expenses must be recorded in the period when the resources are consumed for the production of related revenue. For example, an organization using the accrual method would record the cost of PTO earned by and employee as a liability in the period it is earned. This liability is then carried until the employee takes the PTO benefit. When the PTO is used, the liability is reduced. In this way, the expense of the PTO is recorded in the time period it was earned, not when it is paid out. If it was not recorded (accrued) in this manner, the expense for the period when the PTO was earned would be understated, and the expense for the period when the PTO was actually paid to the employee would be overstated, and the organization's real liabilities would be understated by the total amount of PTO owed to the employee.

For an employee who is paid $25 per hour, a bank of 20 PTO days (160 hours) would represent a liability of $4,000 to the organization. Capturing this liability and planning for it in the future ensures adequate cash on hand to cover expenses. Consistent recording procedures allow for accurate financial management during any specific period of time. The basic rules for transaction recording are: (1) revenue and expenses should be recorded when services and/or products are sold, or costs are incurred, and (2) expenses should be recorded during the time period in which the item purchased is used in the production of the entity's goods or services.

The cash basis of accounting is used as an alternative to the accrual method. Under the cash basis for accounting, revenue is recorded when cash is received, and expenses are recorded when bills are paid. This approach fails to match revenue and expenses. It will not support management efforts to determine the costs of individual products and services and is used on a limited basis in health care, most commonly in small private practices and partnerships.[5]

Revenues and Expenses

Revenue is gross income (gross = before anything is taken out or paid). An HCO has several potential sources of revenue:

- Income from the sale or delivery of a service or product
- Seminars or continuing educational programs provided
- Income from grants or philanthropic gifts
- Income from investments

Under the accrual basis of accounting, revenue is recorded in the period the revenue is earned. Under a cash basis, revenue is recorded when the money is received. Revenue from the sale of a service or product is calculated by multiplying the price of the service or product times the number sold. The revenue recorded for items sold at discounted or a third-party payer's established and agreed upon price should be adjusted by recording a deduction to revenue. For example, a $150 evaluation provided under a contract with a third-party payer requiring a 10% discount would be record with two entries. The first

---

accrual basis – the practice in accounting that records revenues and expenses in the period in which they are earned

cash basis – the practice in accounting that records revenues when they are received and expenses when they are paid

Chapter 2 / Accounting and Finance

entry would record revenue of $150. The second entry would record a $15 deduction from revenue. The revenue net deductions would equal the $135 discounted price. This allows the HCO to capture the amount of revenue (or cash) lost due to the contractual arrangement. Revenue is also classified by its origin. Revenue for the sale of a service or product provided by the company is referred to as revenue from operations or, simply, operating revenue. Revenue from all other sources is referred to as nonoperating revenue.

An *expense* is money spent to produce or purchase a service or product that is sold. Under the accrual basis of accounting, expense is recorded in the time period the service or item is produced. Under a cash basis, expense is recorded when the bill is paid.

An HCO has several potential expenses related to the provision of services:

- Salary
- Benefits
- Equipment
- Supplies
- Utilities

When an organization's revenues exceed expenses for a scheduled period of time, the excess is classified as a *profit*. When expenses exceed revenue, the difference is classified as a *loss*. Making a profit allows the organization to increase salaries to keep up with inflation, purchase new or updated equipment, or to expand the practice if so desired. Having excess cash or a profit is beneficial to the livelihood of any organization. Understanding the financial aspect of health care is necessary in order to generate sufficient revenue to sustain a business. Understanding the basic financial statements that capture the financial aspect of an organization is vital to this process.

Fundamental Financial Statements

The fundamental financial statements are a set of financial reports that generally include a balance sheet, an income statement, a cash flow statement, and a retained earnings statement. Each statement is interrelated and is collectively used to view the financial health, stability, and growth potential of an organization. Financial statements can also be used to compare past to current performance, revealing trends that can be used to evaluate current performance or to predict future performance. These statements can be as simple or complex as the business and should be prepared with the aid of a professional, such as a CPA.

Projected financial performance is reflected in financial plans or budgets that are referred to as "pro forma" (for the sake of form) statements. Pro forma statements present financial information in advance or in the future. An annual financial business plan or budget represents management's best estimate of what will happen in the future. It is the internal benchmark against which day-to-day performance can be assessed.

The FASB sets the standards for accounting and financial reporting.[7] The FASB defines the objectives of financial reporting, which include the provision of information:

1. That is useful to present and potential investors, creditors, and other users in making a rational investment, extending credit, and similar decisions
2. That lists the economic resources of an organization; the claims to those resources; and the effects of transactions, events, and circumstances that change resources
3. That describes an organization's financial performance during a stated period

fundamental financial statements – the financial statements that reflect the financial health, stability, and growth potential of a business

4. That identifies ways in which an organization obtains and expends cash, about its borrowing and repaying of borrowed funds, about its capital transactions, and about other factors that may affect its liquidity or solvency
5. That states how management has discharged its stewardship responsibility for the use of the organization's resources
6. That is useful to managers and directors in making decisions in the interest of owners

Financial statements are typically prepared to represent the financial activity for a specific period of time. The specific date of the statement is the last date for which information was included. The time frame may vary based on the needs of the organization. Common time frames are yearly, quarterly, monthly or every 2 weeks. Detailed activity tracking reports may be produced weekly or even daily. Financial reporting does not always follow the chronological year, depending on the nature of the business, but follows a *fiscal year (FY)*. A FY follows any established 12-month cycle, ending historically when the organization experiences a decrease in the volume of activity (ie, the lowest time in a 12-month cycle). This allows additional time to be spent on closing the books and preparing the financial statements. Once an organization has established its FY, it will continue to operate and report performance on that FY cycle. The FYs of related organizations are often the same, which allows for the comparison and cumulative reporting of financial results among related businesses.

Some additional basic accounting practices that are used in creating financial statements include the justification or alignment of all numerical information. All of the decimal places for the numbers in the statement must be vertically aligned. In addition, if the statement includes specific information on the cents for one account, it is assumed that all of the accounts are correct to the cent. This is typically done with personal checking account balances. However, by contrast, financial statements round off to the nearest dollar amount. The dollar sign ($) is generally used only with the top and bottom figures in a financial statement; at the bottom indicating the total figure for a group of accounts. Double lines underneath a number indicate the final figure in the statement (Table 2.3). Financial statements also use parentheses to indicate a negative number as opposed to the dashed line. Understanding these basic accounting practices can lead to a better understanding of the fundamental financial statements, which include the balance sheet, the income statement, the cash flow statement, and the retained earnings statement.

Table 2.3 Balance Sheet for Fiscal Year Ending September 30, 20XX

Balance Sheet for September 30, 20XX

Assets		Liabilities and Owner's Equity	
Cash	$45,000	Liabilities:	
Investments	60,000		
Prepaid expenses	2,000	Accounts payable	$50,000
Inventories	10,000	Accrued expenses	5,000
Accounts receivable	60,000	Notes payable	225,000
		Total liabilities	$280,000
Land	$40,000		
Buildings	90,000		
Equipment	200,000	Owner's equity	$227,000
Total	$507,000	Total liabilities and owner's equity	$507,000

Reprinted with permission from Drnach M. Accounting and finance. In: Nosse LJ, Friberg DG, eds. *Management and Supervisory Principles for Physical Therapists*. 3rd ed. Wolters Kluwer Health/Lippincott Williams and Wilkins; 2010:405-428.

Chapter 2 / Accounting and Finance

Balance Sheet

The first statement in the set of financial statements is the balance sheet, a statement of an organization's financial *condition*. A balance sheet is a listing of assets, liabilities, and owner's equity. At all times, the total assets will equal the total liabilities plus the owner's equity, which is called the balance sheet equation:

Total assets = Total liabilities + owner's equity

The balance sheet is for a past period of time, prepared to reflect the organization at a certain point in time, giving a picture of an organization's pluses (assets and owner's equity) and minuses (liabilities) at a glance. Table 2.3 depicts a balance sheet for a physical therapy practice ending September 30, 20XX. The clinic runs from October 1 to September 30. This balance sheet represents an end of the year status but includes all activity of the organization prior to that date.

Income Statement

The income statement is a report on the *financial performance* of an organization over a specific period of time. It provides a comparison of monies earned (revenues) to monies spent (expenses). The difference between revenues and expenses is the *net income* or *loss* from operations during the reporting period. In an income statement, revenues are listed first, followed by allowance for contractual deductions to revenue, then expenses.

Revenues in physical therapy practices are typically volume driven, so an increase in the number of patients treated increases the revenue the business generates.[8] Revenues can also be contractually based, meaning that for a stated service, a negotiated amount of revenue will be paid to the organization.

Expenses follow revenue on the income statement. Some expenses are volume driven, whereas others are fixed. The income statement is a summary of revenues generated minus the expenses incurred resulting in net income. Income statements are also known as *Profit and Loss Statements* or a *Statement of Operations* because net income (revenues − expenses) shows how much of a profit or how a big loss has been generated for a specific period of time, typically in the past not the future. The income statement is represented by the equation:

Revenue − Expenses = Net income

Table 2.4 is an example of the income statement for a physical therapy practice for the FY ending September 30, 20XX. This is an annual income statement. Income statements can be prepared to cover any increment of time but should be prepared at a minimum of once per year. Net income (profit or loss) from the income statement will affect the owner's equity on the balance sheet. Accrued expenses on the income statement will affect accounts payable on the balance sheet.

Cash Flow Statement

The cash flow statement is a mandatory part of an organization's financial statements. It reports on the cash that flows through the business from core operations, financing, or investing. It reports on the actual cash and not any future incoming or outgoing cash on

balance sheet – a financial statement of a business' financial condition

income statement – a financial statement of a business' operations and performance

cash flow statement – a financial statement of the cash that flows through a business at any period in time

Table 2.4 Income Statement for Fiscal Year Ending September 30, 20XX		
Income Statement Year Ending September 30, 20XX		
Revenue:		
Gross revenue		
Services	$832,818	
Equipment	60,000	
Total operating revenue		$892,818
Less:		
Allowance for deductions		203,563
Gross revenue net deductions		689,255
Nonoperating revenue		23,000
Total revenue		$712,255
Expenses:		
Salaries	$361,421	
Benefits	65,056	
FICA	28,191	
Education	6,300	
Recruitment	5,000	
Professional services	11,000	
Purchased services	600	
Supplies	51,095	
Travel	4,000	
Dues	2,000	
Equipment	1,200	
Rent/lease	20,000	
Utilities	9,000	
Communication	3,375	
Environmental services	5,300	
Accrued expenses	40,083	
Insurance	6,100	
Total expenses		$619,721
Net income (loss)		92,534
Taxes		30,536
Net income after taxes		$61,998

FICA, Federal Insurance Contribution Act.
Reprinted with permission from Drnach M. Accounting and finance. In: Nosse LJ, Friberg DG, eds. *Management and Supervisory Principles for Physical Therapists.* 3rd ed. Wolters Kluwer Health/Lippincott Williams and Wilkins; 2010:405-428.

account. The availability of cash to cover short-term liabilities, such as payroll, is of critical importance especially for a small business that cannot borrow against future profit like a large business. This financial statement will show how an organization's cash position changes over time and provides a basic report on the financial health of an organization. Table 2.5 is the cash flow statement for a physical therapy practice for the period October 1,

Chapter 2 / Accounting and Finance

35

Table 2.5 Cash Flow Statement for Fiscal Year Ending September 30, 20XX			
Cash Flow Statement Year Ending September 30, 20XX			
Cash balance, October 1, 20XX			
Cash in bank		$39,517	
Petty cash		500	
Cash balance			$40,017
Sources of cash			
Cash from operations	$51,613		
Accounts receivable	751,910		
Owner investment			
Total sources of cash		$803,523	
Uses of cash			
Accounts payable	$213,110		
Payroll	495,568		
Owner withdrawal	25,000		
Capital purchase	4,862		
Cash Flow Statement			
Land and building	60,000		
Total uses of cash		$798,540	
Increase (decrease) in cash			$4,983
Cash balance, September 30, 20XX			$45,000

Reprinted with permission from Drnach M. Accounting and finance. In: Nosse LJ, Friberg DG, eds. *Management and Supervisory Principles for Physical Therapists*. 3rd ed. Wolters Kluwer Health/Lippincott Williams and Wilkins; 2010:405-428.

20XX, through September 30, 20XX, of the following year. Cash flow statements can be prepared for past, present, and future time periods. Cash flow statements that look to the future (called a pro forma statement) can help management identify potential problems in available cash before they happen. The cash flow statement is represented by the equation:

$$\text{Current cash balance} = \text{Beginning cash balance} + \text{Cash received} - \text{Cash spent}$$

The cash flow statement is useful in financial planning and is usually required when seeking financial support from a bank or other financial institutions. It is prepared from the information on the balance sheet and income statement and captures the changes in cash over a period of time. For example, if the cash balance on the balance sheet has increased over the year, the cash flow statement indicates the reason. It may show that the accounts receivable balance was reduced or that payments are being stretched out over a longer period of time, reflected as a growth in the accounts payable.

Note that the cash balance on the cash flow statement always equals the cash asset on the balance sheet.

Retained Earnings Statement

A retained earnings statement is also referred to as an owner's equity statement. Retained earnings are commonly influenced by the organization's net income and the payment of

retained earnings statement – a financial statement of the owner's equity in the business

Table 2.6 Retained Earnings Statement for Fiscal Year Ending September 30, 20XX

Beginning balance	$190,002
Net income	61,998
Dividends paid	(25,000)
Current balance	$227,000

Reprinted with permission from Drnach M. Accounting and finance. In: Nosse LJ, Friberg DG, eds. *Management and Supervisory Principles for Physical Therapists*. 3rd ed. Wolters Kluwer Health/Lippincott Williams and Wilkins; 2010:405-428.

dividends to stockholders or owners of the company. The retained earnings statement explains the differences in an owner's equity on the balance sheet and provides information on how profits are used in a business, either distributed to the owners or reinvested into the business. Table 2.6 is the retained earnings statement for a physical therapy practice for the period October 1, 20XX, through September 30, 20XX, of the following year.

In the early years of a business, the owners may reinvest more of the profits into the business for growth and development. As the business matures, the owners may take out a larger portion of the profits for their personal income. Net income on the income statement will affect the retained earnings on the statement of retained earnings.

The retained earnings statement is represented by the equation:

Current retained earnings = Beginning retained earnings balance + (Revenues − Expenses) − Dividends paid

The balance sheet of an organization presents the financial position of the organization at a particular date with the other three statements contributing to that financial picture. The four documents are related, and any discrepancies between them should be further evaluated (Table 2.7).

Budgeting

Financial planning often includes the creation of a budget. A budget is a financial statement of the estimated income and expenditures for an organization or an aspect of the organization, covering a specified future period of time. The format of a budget

Table 2.7 Relationships Between the Financial Documents

Statement	Relationship
Income	Net income affects owner's equity on the **Balance Sheet** Net income affects retained earnings on the **Retained Earnings Statement**
Cash Flow	Reports the movement of money recorded on the **Balance Sheet**
	Current cash balance equals cash assets on the **Balance Sheet**
	Net income equals the net income on the **Income Statement**
Retained Earnings	The retained earnings on the beginning **Balance Sheet** is the beginning retained earnings on the **Retained Earnings Statement**

budget – a financial statement of the estimated or allocated revenues and the anticipated expenses of a business or aspect of a business, such as a department

follows the income statement format but reflects the anticipated performance of the organization, a discrete department or program, or a major capital undertaking. There can be several types of budgets, such as an operating budget, a strategic budget, a capital budget (eg, for buildings or equipment), a cash budget, or a special purpose budget (eg, pediatric services only), to name a few.[2] The focus of this section is the operating budget that plans for the operating revenues and expenses of an organization within a period of 1 year. (Strategic budgeting is done for a long-range plan, typically 3-5 years.) All of the budgets of an organization make up the budget for the whole organization or practice.

Budgeting requires the manager to plan ahead, forecast, and anticipate what will happen in the next year from a financial point of view. It is a dynamic process that requires monitoring and making revisions as the revenues and expenses fluctuate for any given month. Budgeting is an important process that establishes an organization's financial or activity goals along with benchmarks to measure progress throughout the year.

There are a variety of ways to prepare a budget for the upcoming year, depending on the size of the organization and the program for which the budget is being prepared. Typically, the budgeting process would include the following:

- **Environmental scanning**. In preparing a budget, the manager should be aware of what is happening in the local and national markets of health care in order to anticipate any significant changes that may occur within the next year, to identify opportunities for growth, or to make adjustments for anticipated changes in reimbursement or revenue levels. This would also include the identification of any anticipated changes such as the need to acquire new equipment, the need for additional personnel, the need to increase salaries, or to cover the expected increase in the cost of a provided benefit, such as health care insurance.
- **Identification of goals and objectives**. Clear financial goals and objectives should be determined and understood by all parties in the budget-making process so that all participating parties are working toward the same goals and have a clear understanding of what those entail. If the organization wishes to increase its profits in the upcoming year so it can expand its services by opening up a new clinic, or create a library for staff and patients, or to cover the rising cost of benefits, the amount of funds needed and the rationale for the objective should be clear and appropriate.
- **Identify the relationship between the established goals and objectives with the organizations' mission, structure, strategic plan, and current policies and procedures**. The goals and objectives identified in the previous steps should clearly relate to the mission of the organization. The relevant policies and procedures and the positions in the organization (organizational chart) responsible for the functions that will be affected by the goals and objectives related to the proposed budget (both revenues and expenses) should make sense to the organization as a whole and to the employees individually (eg, spending money to update equipment, which is in line with the mission to provide current and up-to-date interventions). The financial information contained in a budget should reflect the mission and strategic growth of the organization.
- **Gather data on estimated costs and revenues**. A manager or team should develop specific measurable operating objectives. How much revenue would be needed to support the expenses of the department or program? What profit margin would be necessary in order to make the budgeted program viable and add to the overall financial success of the organization? What would be the break-even point? How much time will it take to reach the break-even point? Is there enough cash to start up a new program? What is the expected fee for the program or service? What are other organizations currently charging for this service? These are just a few questions that would facilitate the investigation and acquisition of information in the development of a budget.

- **Develop a proposed budget.** The next step is to develop a budget that will then be used in the overall decision-making process for the development of the program or service. The accounts in the budget should be from the established chart of accounts of the organization. The expenses should be accounts (or subaccounts) that are also listed on the income statement. The source of the proposed revenues should be identified. How will the anticipated revenues be generated? Are they coming from an established source, or will the organization need to take out a loan? Note that revenues provided to an aspect of an organization may not reflect the total revenues generated from that aspect or department. Physical therapy departments or programs often bring in more revenues than their expenses, contributing a significant profit for the overall organization. They are referred to as *profit centers or loss centers* depending on their net income. Therefore, the program or department may only get a portion of the total revenue that is generated from the programs or services provided, with the additional revenue going to offset the costs of another aspect of the organization. This is not necessarily negative. There are many aspects of a business that do not generate revenue but that are necessary for the delivery of services, such as building maintenance, administrative personnel, or housekeeping. The amount of operating revenues provided to such a department or program is considered the allocated operating revenue for a specific period of time (Table 2.8).

Table 2.8 Annual Operating Budget for the Fiscal Year Ending September 30, 20XX

Annual Operating Budget Year Ending September 30, 20XX			
REVENUE		YTD	Variance
Operating revenue	$619,721		
EXPENSES			
Salaries	$361,421	$361,421	0
Benefits	65,056	65,056	0
FICA	28,191	28,191	0
Education	6,300	7,000	(700)
Recruitment	5,000	5,000	0
Professional services	11,000	11,000	0
Purchased services	10,600	10,600	0
Supplies	51,095	50,000	1,095
Travel	4,000	5,250	(1,250)
Dues	2,000	2,000	0
Equipment	21,283	21,083	200
Rent/lease	30,000	30,000	0
Utilities	9,000	9,300	(300)
Communication	3,375	4,125	(150)
Environmental services	5,300	5,300	0
Insurance	6,100	6,100	0
Total expenses	$619,721	$621,426	$(1,705)

Note: Variance is the difference between what was budgeted and what was spent. This practice is over budget by $1,705. Why do you think this happened?
FICA, Federal Insurance Contribution Act; YTD, year to date.
Reprinted with permission from Drnach M. Accounting and finance. In: Nosse LJ, Friberg DG, eds. *Management and Supervisory Principles for Physical Therapists*. 3rd ed. Wolters Kluwer Health/Lippincott Williams and Wilkins; 2010:405-428.

Chapter 2 / Accounting and Finance

Once a budget has been developed and approved, it has to be implemented and monitored. Basic accounting practices are applied to the budget as with other financial statements. Capturing the variances in what was budgeted versus what is actually happening is an important aspect in financial management.

Financial Analysis

A key to effective financial management is the ability to analyze projected to actual performance. This is referred to as *variance analysis* (see Table 2.8). Variance analysis compares the actual entry to the projected or budgeted amount. The difference between the two is considered a variance, which is listed as a positive number if the variance is less than expected or a negative (noted by parenthesis instead of a negative sign) when the variance is over what is expected (see Table 2.8). Variance analysis identifies the difference between the actual and the projected for a specific period of time. More detailed information is often necessary to determine causal factors.

Information in financial statements can also be subjected to a variety of analytic techniques to assess a company's performance, financial position, and relative financial viability. These techniques include *common-sizing, comparative, and ratio analysis.*[6] More often than not, financial statements are used for comparative analysis. Comparison can be made between the elements of one financial statement for one period of time, between two or more time periods, or between planned (budgeted) and actual performance. To aid in the comparison of financial statement entries, numbers are expressed as a percentage of a total category. For example, in Table 2.9, salary expense for FY 20XX could be expressed as an amount, namely, $361,421, or 58.3% of the total expenses. When comparative percentages are used to define elements of a financial statement, it is referred to as a *common-size statement.*[9] Information on a financial statement can also be expressed for more than one date or period of time and are called *comparative statements.* Table 2.9 is an example of both a common-size and a comparative financial statement.

Comparative analysis allows for the identification of trends and financial patterns. It is up to management to determine the value of the information relative to the performance of the business. In the example in Table 2.9, the statement shows an improved financial performance between FY 20XX and FY 20XX, 1 year later. Note that although gross revenues from services increased $166,564 (a 25% increase), it still continued to make up 93% of the total operating revenue owing to the increase in gross revenues from equipment (which also increased 25%). Using common-size percentages also allows a comparison *between* organizations based not on absolute numbers in dollar amounts, but on percentages of totals, which eliminates the size of the organizations being compared. This allows an investor to compare such attributes of an organization such as the percentage of gross revenues from services as a percentage of total operating revenue or the percentage of total expenses paid to salaries.

Financial Ratios

Another technique that can be used to compare financial performance over time between elements or between similar organizations is the use of *financial ratios*. The purpose of ratio analysis is to find two ratios that when compared, provide some beneficial insight into the financial health of the organization. Financial ratio analysis refers to the use of the relationships between two mathematical quantities that have management significance. The idea behind the use of financial ratios is to summarize key financial data in a format that is easy to understand and evaluate.[6] Common-size, liquidity, efficiency, and profitability ratios are examples of ratios used to evaluate an organization's performance.

Table 2.9 Comparative Common-Size Income Statement for FY Ending September 30, 20XX, and September 30, 20XX (ie, 1 Year Prior)

Comparative Common-Size Income Statement, Year Ending September 30, 20XX and September 30, 20XX

	FY 20XX	FY 20XX	Common-Size Percentages	
			FY 20XX (%)	FY 20XX (%)
REVENUE:				
Gross revenue				
Services	$832,818	$666,254	93	93.3
Equipment	60,000	48,000	6.7	6.7
Total operating revenue	892,818	714,254	100.0	100.0
LESS:				
Allowance for deductions	203,563	162,850	22.8	22.8
Gross revenue net deductions	689,255	551,404	96.8	96.8
Nonoperating revenue	23,000	18,400	3.2	3.2
Total revenue	$712,255	$569,804	100.0	100.0
EXPENSES:				
Salaries	361,421	335,124	58.3	55.6
Benefits	65,056	60,322	10.5	10.0
FICA	28,191	25,805	4.5	4.3
Education	6,300	4,500	1.0	0.7
Recruitment	5,000	5,000	0.8	0.8
Professional services	11,000	15,000	1.8	2.5
Purchased services	10,600	8,480	1.7	1.4
Supplies	51,095	40,876	8.2	6.8
Travel	4,000	2,500	0.6	0.4
Dues	2,000	1,500	0.3	0.2
Equipment	21,283	15,500	3.4	2.6
Rent/lease	30,000	63,300	4.8	10.5
Utilities	9,000	9,000	1.5	1.5
Communication	3,375	3,375	0.5	0.6
Environmental services	5,300	5,300	0.9	0.9
Insurance	6,100	7,100	1.0	1.2
Total expenses	$619,721	$602,682	100.0	100.0
Net income (loss)	92,534	(32,878)	10.4	−4.6
Taxes	$30,536	0	33.0	0.0
Net income after taxes	$61,998	($32,878)	6.9	−4.6

FICA, Federal Insurance Contribution Act; FY, fiscal year.

Reprinted with permission from Drnach M. Accounting and finance. In: Nosse LJ, Friberg DG, eds. *Management and Supervisory Principles for Physical Therapists*. 3rd ed. Wolters Kluwer Health/Lippincott Williams and Wilkins; 2010:405-428.

Chapter 2 / Accounting and Finance

41

Common-size ratios allow comparison of one account to the total account (eg, accounts receivable to total assets). They also allow the comparison of an organization to other organizations of different sizes, as discussed previously (eg, common-sized financial statements). Common-size ratios answer the question: what percentage of account x is made up of the subaccount y? Several financial accounts can be common sized, including:

- Cash to total assets = Cash/Total assets
- Current liabilities to total equity = Current liabilities/Total equity
- Operating income to total revenues = Operating income/Total revenues

Common-size ratios put absolute dollar amounts into perspective by eliminating the factor of the quantity or size and are also helpful in the analysis of historical information or trends.

Liquidity ratios are used to assess an organization's ability to meet its short-term financial obligations (liabilities). Does the organization have available cash to pay off current liabilities when they come due? Two of the more common liquidity ratios are:

Current ratio is the ratio of current assets to current liabilities. It is a common index of liquidity. The higher the ratio, the better a business is positioned to meet its current obligations.[6] Generally, this ratio is considered healthy at approximately 2:1.[10]

Current Ratio = Current assets/Current liabilities

The *acid test ratio* is the most rigorous test of liquidity. It takes into consideration only cash or those assets that can be immediately liquidated for cash. The higher the ratio, the better the organization's potential to meet its current obligations.[6]

Generally, this ratio is considered healthy at approximately 1:1.[10]

Acid test ratio = (Cash + Marketable securities)/Current liabilities

Efficiency ratios can provide some information on how efficiently the organization is run. A common efficiency ratio is the *days receivable,* that is, a measurement of the average time taken to collect the cash from the accounts receivable. Days receivable is calculated by first finding the net patient revenue per day (net patient revenue for the year/365 days per year), then dividing that number into net accounts receivable.

Days receivable = Accounts receivable/Patient revenue per day

Days receivable will have a direct effect on the cash flow statement and the amount of available cash to meet expenses, such as payroll.

Another common efficiency ratio is *revenue to assets*, which provides information on how many dollars of revenues have been generated by each dollar invested in assets.[2] It is calculated by the following formula:

Revenue to assets = Total revenues/Total assets

If Business A generates $1 of revenue for each dollar invested in assets, compared to Business B which generates $2 of revenue for each dollar invested in assets, Business B would appear to be more efficient in its use of assets than Business A.

Profitability ratios are other ratios used in both for-profit and not-for-profit organizations. The need to make a profit is vital in both types of organizations in order to keep up with inflation, the cost-of-living expenses, and to sustain growth. The operating margin

operating margin – the ratio of net income (total revenue minus expenses, including taxes) to total revenue

is the ratio of net income to total revenue. Operating margin can be calculated for all or discrete parts of an organization. Good financial performance results in a high operating margin. This ratio provides a basis for comparison of the economic performance of one organization to industry standards, previous performance, and other investment opportunities. Operating margin can also help an organization assess the relative contribution of one operating unit to another.

$$\text{Operating margin} = (\text{Total revenues} - \text{Total expenses})/\text{Total revenues}$$

Return on assets is the relationship of total income to the total investment (assets) of the organization. Return on assets can be calculated for all or discrete parts of an organization. A higher return on assets indicates good performance. This ratio also provides a basis for comparison of the economic performance of one organization to industry standards, previous performance, and other investment opportunities. Return on assets may be used as a criterion for selecting between alternative business strategies.

$$\text{Return on assets} = (\text{Income} + \text{Interest expense})/\text{Total assets}$$

It should be noted that a variety of ratios can be developed or used other than those described earlier.

Performance Indicators

Financial ratios offer a set of standardized assessment tools that allow for the comparison of current financial performance to past performance, current expectations, as well as the performance of similar organizations on an individual or industry-wide basis. Some additional financial performance indicators that may be of particular value for assessing the performance of a physical therapy practice are the following:[11]

Volume
  number of referrals
  number of scheduled treatments or unit of service (UOS)
  number of completed (billed) treatments or UOS
  number of visits
  case mix
Revenues
  net revenue per referral
  net revenue per visit
  net revenue as a percentage of charge
Costs
  labor cost per volume measure
  nonlabor cost per volume measure
  employee benefits as a percentage of salary
Efficiency
  productive hours paid per billed UOS
  nonproductive hours paid per billed UOS
  number of visits per referral
  number of visits per referral by diagnosis, age, or another defining factor
  number of billed UOS per patient visit

Performance indicators can be used to create a report card for organizational performance. Management should use performance indicators that are meaningful to its success. Through careful selection, clear performance expectations, sometimes called performance

Chapter 2 / Accounting and Finance **43**

benchmarks, can be established and communicated to members of the organization. Organizational performance indicators should be tracked and trended, and the outcome should be shared with everyone who has a role in meeting performance targets (Chapter 9).[12]

There is an increasing trend in health care toward the use of industry performance standards to evaluate the performance of individual HCO. Medicare law includes value-based payments as an aspect of an HCO's quality improvement program in clinical practice. It is a move away from payment based on quantity to payment based on quality. Improving communication and care coordination between providers, targeting specific health care practices (eg, management of specific patient diagnoses, reduction of hospital-acquired conditions, and incentive payments based on quality of care) are aimed at rewarding HCOs and providers who demonstrate a level of quality in the care they provide to people with Medicare insurance (Chapter 3).[13]

Industry performance standards can help management assess performance in a rapidly changing environment when historical performance has less relevance, set reasonable improvement targets, and for competitive positioning. However, the use of external performance standards should be done only with a complete understanding of the source and applicability of the standard. Care should be taken to be sure that selected industry standards are clearly applicable, represent comparable data, and that regional and organizational differences have been identified. A common performance indicator is the measurement of an employee's productivity. Additional performance indicators that address the value of the services provided could include the following:

1. Number of hospital readmissions for the management of congestive heart failure or total joint arthroplasty
2. Incidence of pressure ulcer development in residents of a long-term care facility
3. Frequency of self-medication errors in the home care setting
4. Percentage of patients discharged from outpatient services who met a cutoff score on a standardized functional test or measurement

Productivity

Productivity refers to the amount of a resource consumed in the production of an increment of output, historically viewed in health care as the volume or number of billable units for a specific period of time.

$$\text{Productivity} = \frac{\text{Output (eg, number of billable services provided)}}{\text{Input (eg, cost of providing those services)}}$$

When viewing productivity as a measurement of quantity, increasing the number of billable units provided would increase productivity, given a fixed cost of the input.

Maximizing productivity would maximize profits and, ultimately, wages of the employees. This is one view of productivity that focuses on volume for profit, which is seen as the value of the outcome.

As health care payers shift from a quantity-based payment model to a quality-based payment model, it is vital that health care providers are included in the discussion and give input to the structure of the organization's system of productivity measurement. Productivity is

productivity – amount of resources consumed in the production of an increment of output

more than the number of billable units produced. It encapsulates the use of evidence-based practice, adherence to ethical principles,[14] respecting clinical judgment, and the unique aspects of the model of care delivery in the specific setting that optimizes patient outcomes.[15]

Value is added when the health care provider's expertise is efficiently utilized; when the time to effectively educate the patient, family, and caregivers is viewed as important; and when consulting with other experts and collaborating with the health care team[16] are recognized as a necessary and valuable use of time.

As with any other aspect of organizational performance, an objective performance target will help direct management and staff efforts in the right direction. *Productivity standards* are performance targets. To be of maximum benefit, productivity standards should be:

- Based on a measurable unit of output
- Objectively measured
- Readily available
- Understandable
- Achievable

Management, in consultation with key members of the health care delivery, are responsible for setting productivity standards (performance expectations) for resources consumed. Where productivity standards do not exist or are out of date, new standards should be set using internal data and external benchmarks or standards. Internal data will demonstrate how well the organization is performing in comparison to historical performance. Comparison of *external benchmarks* to internal performance measurements will show how the organization is performing in comparison to other similar organizations. External benchmarks may be available through professional organizations, business associations, consultants, proprietary databases, or directly from similar business (see Chapter 9).

Productivity standards are historically based on financial activity or billable time (Table 2.10). A physical therapist could be productive in the historical sense of the word but not financially productive. For example, researching the latest evidence of the effectiveness of an intervention commonly used in the practice, learning to use a new database system, learning to use new technology to supervise support personnel, or a piece of assistive technology may be productive in that these activities promote the knowledge and skills of a physical therapist or the efficient delivery of services but may not be billable to a third-party payer. Financial productivity will become clearer and more understandable if the physical therapist understands the importance of providing cost-effective services in a productive manner. If the activity is associated with increasing referrals (by providing a more cost-effective and efficient intervention, thereby improving outcomes), decreasing nonlabor cost (by decreasing the need for support staff for certain activities), or maximizing the amount of billable time available (by the use of technology to complete a supervisory visit of a support personnel), for example, the relationship of these activities to financial productivity will become clearer and more understandable to all persons involved.

Productivity, or the number of billable hours available, is also influenced by several additional factors, which can include the following:

- Patient cancellation rate
- Utilization of appropriate personnel and resources
- Physical plant design and layout
- Documentation requirements and access procedures
- Supervisory requirements of paraprofessionals
- Use of technology

To become more productive does not automatically mean to "see more patients" and should begin with an examination of current practices and making them more efficient.

Chapter 2 / Accounting and Finance

45

Table 2.10 Calculating Financial Productivity		
Time	*PT*	*PTA*
Hours paid/year[a]	2,080	2,080
Nonproductive hours:		
PTO: 15 d	120	120
Continuing education: 3 d	24	24
Required meetings: hours/year	40	40
Total nonproductive/year[b]	184	184
Available productive hours/year	1,896	1,896
Billable hours		
6 h billable/8 h worked[c]		
75% productivity expectation	1,422	1,422
UOS (=15 min)/year[d]	5,688	5,688
UOS/day	24	24
Cost[e]		
Salary	47,008	37,918
Benefits	8,461	6,825
FICA	3,596	2,901
Education	500	300
Human resources	200	100
Total cost	59,765	48,044
Total cost/hours paid	28.73	23.1
Total cost/productive hour	42.03	33.79
Total cost/UOS	10.51	8.45

FICA, Federal Insurance Contribution Act.
[a]A full-time employee gets paid for 40 hours per week for 52 weeks per year or 2,080 hours. This is considered a full-time equivalent (FTE).
[b]In-home care time should be allocated for travel, which is nonbillable and would significantly affect the available productive hours per year.
[c]Six hours per day takes into consideration 1 hour for a paid lunch and 30 minutes at the beginning and end of the day for documentation and other patient management activities. 6/8 = 0.75 75% of the available productive hours 1,896 = 1,422.
[d]1 UOS = 15 minutes. Four 15 minutes units = 1 hour. 1,422 hours × 4 units per hour = 5,688 UOS.
[e]Cost accounts may vary. See Figure 1.3, Cost Worksheet.
Reprinted with permission from Drnach M. Accounting and finance. In: Nosse LJ, Friberg DG, eds. *Management and Supervisory Principles for Physical Therapists*. 3rd ed. Wolters Kluwer Health/Lippincott Williams and Wilkins; 2010:405-428.

Revenue and Expense Management

Revenue Management

For most HCOs, revenue management is the management of accounts receivable. It is the actions taken to increase total revenue and improve the collection of accounts receivable. Revenue management is a lengthy process that involves several activities. including:

1. Measuring services and products for sale
2. Setting prices (fees)
3. Identifying the payer(s) for each service or product
4. Establishing policies and procedures that address the provision of the service, recording the delivery of the service, and collecting reimbursement

5. Estimating expected payment
6. Following procedures for payment receipt, account reconciliation, and cash management
7. Financial reporting

The goal of revenue management is to maximize income from operations and investments. This can be done by increasing the volume of patients seen or maximizing the payer mix to optimize reimbursement (ie, have more patients with better paying insurance; requires marketing), decreasing the cost of services provided, raising the fees charged for services rendered, or improving the collection of accounts receivable.

Fees

Under the current US health care reimbursement system, most of the health care payments come from private health insurance and governmental health payment plans. A minor but growing percentage of payment is self-payment (patients paying out of pocket). Commercial (private) health care insurance plans typically use standardized payment schedules that determine the amount that they will pay for a specific health care service. This is called the *usual, customary, and reasonable rate (UCR),* which is consistent with the average rate or fee for similar services in a particular geographic area. Often, commercial health care insurance will pay the provider charges up to the UCR. The patient is sometimes required to pay the difference. Governmental payers, such as Medicare, use a variety of payment methods that range from paying some percentage of the provider cost (expenses) to paying a fixed amount per service regardless of the health care provider's cost. Who is paying and how the service is provided will influence the organization's fee schedule (see Chapter 1).

The *fee schedule* is a listing of the services provided and the charge for each of those services. The established fee can be based on an amount of time, on the type of service, on a per session or per visit basis, a per day basis (per diem), or a set number of sessions.

Typically, each listing on a fee schedule is defined by:

1. Numeric charge code
2. Description
3. Unit of measure for the product or service
4. Price

An organization's fee schedule will vary based on the size and complexity of its business. It will also vary based on management and customer information needs. The more specific the information needs of management, the more specific the charges on the fee schedule.

Decisions about fee setting need to balance the desire to maximize net income against market sensitivity to the price for the service. All organizations must also be mindful of laws that govern pricing. The Robinson-Patman Act of 1936 prohibits organizations from charging similar customers different prices unless the differences are based on differences in production cost, transportation, or sale, or quantities in which commodities are sold.[17] Differential pricing must be based on real cost differences. As a result, the organization must set charges to maximize the potential payment from all sources while using one level charge for all patients. All of these factors can be accommodated if the fee is set somewhere above the highest payment rate.

Billing and Collections

Although patients have the option of paying cash to the provider on the day that service is rendered, a high percentage of health care services are provided on credit, an aspect of accrual accounting. Credit purchasing occurs when the customer is billed through the use of an invoice for money owed after the service or product is provided. This is considered an accounts receivable, an asset for the organization. The faster a business collects its accounts receivable (eg, days receivable; an efficiency ratio), the more financial resources will be available to pay its bills, for investment, or to meet other business needs.

Organizations that provide services on account should have clear policies and procedures regarding the extension of credit that are discussed with the person at the time of admission/registration.[6] This would include the expectation to be paid for services provided, authorization to bill a patient's health insurance, and the production of the necessary documents if a patient would like to be considered for a reduced fee based on a *sliding scale fee schedule*. This type of adjusted fee schedule takes into account a person's income and the number of dependents in the home. It is created based on the organization's costs and the federal government established poverty levels, published by the Department of Health and Human Services.[18] Sliding scale fee schedules are done to promote fairness in the ability of people within a target market to access services. It should be remembered that a physical therapist is ethically obligated to seek remuneration for services rendered to provide *pro bono publico* (Lat. "for the public good") care when appropriate.[19] Services provided pro bono do not release the PT from their legal obligations under the State's Practice Act, applicable government laws, documentation requirements, or ethical responsibilities.[20] Physical therapists are encouraged to provide pro bono services when appropriate by:

- Providing professional service at no fee or at a reduced fee to persons of limited financial means when allowable by law.
- Donating professional expertise and service to charitable groups or organizations.
- Engaging in activities to improve access to physical therapist services.
- Offering financial support for organizations that deliver physical therapist or other health services to persons of limited financial means.[21]

The benefits of engaging in these types of activities can include an enhanced public image and an increase in both personal and collective work satisfaction, both intangible assets of an organization.[22]

When a third-party payer is involved, services should not be provided until the payer authorizes them. This is called *preauthorization*. Preauthorization does not guarantee payment, but it may limit loss of payment resulting from technical or contractual issues. Usually, it is the responsibility of the *enrollee or beneficiary* (patient or person who bought the insurance plan) to understand and comply with the terms of his or her health care insurance. In practice, it is in the provider's best interest to assist the patient with benefit verification and preauthorization compliance. Not only is it good customer service (another intangible asset), but preauthorization of service coverage also has the potential to increase the speed and rate of payment (Chapter 4).

Key factors that can improve the collection of payments for services rendered include the following:

- A clear understanding by both the patient and the provider on how payment will be made prior to the delivery of services
- An appropriate understanding of the benefits and limits of an individual's health care insurance prior to the delivery of services
- Clear and appropriate documentation of services rendered and the patient's response to the intervention
- Timely submission of invoices
- Timely provision of documentation needs of the third-party payer or medical claims reviewer
- Adherence to an established plan of care
- Clear communication with both the patient and the third-party payer on the benefits and limitations of physical therapy interventions

Expense Management

Expense management is controlling operating and capital expenses. Operating expenses are associated with the cost of resources used in the production of goods and services in a limited (typically 1 year) period of time (ie, expenses in the income statement). Capital expenses are associated with the purchase of equipment, facilities, and other high-priced items that contribute to the delivery of the service or product over an extended period of time (typically more than 1 year). An organization will often use a dollar threshold, such as $500, to differentiate between operating and capital expenses. Equipment with an extended life and a value greater than the threshold will be classified as a capital expense. Controlling operating or capital expenses requires close attention to the variances that may occur in budgets for operations (operation budget) or capital ventures (capital budget). Management may also attempt to control operating expenses by influencing the utilization of mixed or variable cost items such as utilities, supplies, or recruitment.

The goal of expense management is to maximize net income. To reach that goal, the spread between gross revenue and total expenses must become wider. Armed with a working knowledge of cost characteristics, managers should be able to predict the impacts of their decisions regarding the purchase and use of resources on net income. The importance of efficiently managing resources has increased as payment cuts reduce the net income of most HCOs. As health care costs continue to rise, the need and payment for services will continue to be scrutinized. HCOs will need to continuously improve revenue and/or decrease cost. To manage expenses effectively requires knowledge of the types of expenses, what expenses can be controlled, how expenses are controlled, and how expenses behave in relation to volume of service and/or goods provided. Some basic activities associated with expense management include the following:

- Monitoring budgets and investigating variances
- Implementing policies and procedures and monitoring the utilization of mixed or variable cost items (including overtime pay to nonexempt employees)
- Monitoring the market (environmental scanning) in anticipation of increases in benefits, salaries, or other expense items
- Engaging in cost-effectiveness analysis of services provided[23]

Summary

This chapter provided a financial and accounting background for PTs to enhance their ability to participate in business financial discussions and decision-making. The discussion stressed the importance of accounting and financial information to support organizational decisions. The application of standard accounting practices ensures that financial reports have a consistent meaning between time periods and organizations. Reliable financial information is essential to management efforts to maximize financial performance. To ensure consistency, an understanding of GAAP and the basic accounting concepts of a chart of accounts, double entry, debits and credits, assets, liabilities and owner's equity, accrual versus cash method of accounting, and revenues and expenses were defined. The accounting conventions of fund accounting and allowances for contractual deductions were also introduced as they are commonly seen in HCOs' financial documents. The standard financial reports (ie, balance sheet, income statement, cash flow statement, a retained earnings statement) were introduced and used to present the financial status of an entity for the FY ending September 30, 20XX. In assessing financial reports, common sizing, comparing, and using financial ratios were discussed that help in understanding the variances seen within and between financial reports and budgets as well as to understand the financial health of an organization. The monitoring and investigation of variances from what was expected or

Chapter 2 / Accounting and Finance

budgeted is an important duty in financial management. Revenue management, including the setting of fees and coding for services rendered, is vital to the communication process with payers of health care services. Likewise, expense management is important in maximizing net income, a goal of all businesses.

REFERENCES

1. Financial Accounting Standards Board. What is GAAP. Accessed April 1, 2024. https://accountingfoundation.org/accounting-and-standards/about-gaap
2. Finkler S, Kovner C, Jones C. *Financial Management for Nurse Managers and Executives*. 3rd ed. Saunders Elsevier; 2007.
3. Cleverley W, Cameron A. *Essentials of Health Care Finance*. 5th ed. Aspen Publication; 2002.
4. Gans D, Piland N, Honore P. Developing a chart of accounts: historical perspective of the Medical Group Management Association. *J Public Health Manag Pract*. 2007;13:130-132.
5. Weltman B. *The Big Idea Book for New Business Owners*. Macmillan Spectrum; 1997.
6. Berman H, Kukla S, Weeks L. *The Financial Management of Hospitals*. 8th ed. Health Administration Press; 1994.
7. Financial Accounting Standards Board. Accounting Standards. Accessed April 1, 2024. https://accountingfoundation.org/accounting-and-standards/accounting-standards
8. Drnach M. The basics of billing. In: Drnach M, ed. *The Clinical Practice of Pediatric Physical Therapy. From the NICU to Independent Living*. Lippincott Williams and Wilkins; 2008.
9. Dillon R, LaMont R. Financial statement analysis. A key to practice diagnosis and prognosis. *Clin Manag*. 1983;35:36-39.
10. Wallace W. *Financial Accounting*. South-Western Publishing; 1990.
11. Skula R, Psetian J. A comparative analysis of revenues and cost-management strategies for not-for-profit and for-profit hospitals. *Hosp Health Serv Admin*. 1997;42:117-134.
12. Case J. *Open Book Management. The Coming Business Revolution*. Harper Business; 1995:19-36.
13. Centers for Medicare and Medicaid Services. What are the value-based programs? Updated March 31, 2022. Accessed August 4, 2022. https://www.cms.gov/Medicare/Quality-Initiatives-Patient-Assessment-Instruments/Value-Based-Programs/Value-Based-Programs
14. Tammany J, O'Connell J, Allen B, Brismee M. Are productivity goals in rehabilitation associate with unethical behaviors? *Arch Rehabil Res Clin Transl*. 2019;1:1-9.
15. American Physical Therapy Association. Productivity standards in the physical therapy workforce. HOD P09-21-23-13. Published December 14, 2021. Accessed July 12, 2022. https://www.apta.org/apta-and-you/leadership-and-governance/policies/productivity-standards-physical-therapy-workforce
16. Hull B, Thut C. Productivity vs. value. Why we need to change the discussion, and how YOU can! American Physical Therapy Association. Learning Center. Published February 2020. Accessed July 12, 2022.. https://learningcenter.apta.org/
17. Garrison R. *Managerial Accounting: Concepts for Planning, Control, Decision-making*. Rev. ed. Business Publications; 1979.
18. Office of the Assistant Secretary for Planning and Evaluation. Prior HHS poverty guidelines and federal register references. Department of Health and Human Services. Accessed August 11, 2022. https://aspe.hhs.gov/topics/poverty-economic-mobility/poverty-guidelines/prior-hhs-poverty-guidelines-federal-register-references
19. American Physical Therapy Association. Code of ethics for physical therapist. Updated August 12, 2020. Accessed August 11, 2022. https://www.apta.org/apta-and-you/leadership-and-governance/policies/code-of-ethics-for-the-physical-therapist
20. American Physical Therapy Association. Pro bono services: considerations for physical therapist practice. Published August 17, 2020. Accessed August 11, 2022. https://www.apta.org/your-practice/practice-models-and-settings/pro-bono/pro-bono-services-considerations-for-physical-therapist-practice
21. American Physical Therapy Association. Guidelines: pro bono physical therapist services and organization support. Updated August 30, 2018. Accessed August 11, 2022. https://www.apta.org/apta-and-you/leadership-and-governance/policies/pro-bono-physical-therapist-services-and-organization-support
22. Scott R. For the public good. Physical therapy magazine. *Am Phys Ther Assoc*. 1993;82:82-85.
23. Nosse J, Friberg D. *Managerial and Supervisory Principles for Physical Therapists*. 3rd ed. Lippincott Williams and Wilkins; 2010.

CHAPTER 3

The History of Health Care in the United States
From Service to Business

MARK DRNACH

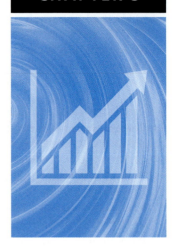

Learning Objectives

The reader will

1. Summarize the history and development of the health care system in the United States and identify how that history influences the development of the medical and physical therapy professions.
2. Identify the major contributors to the development of the treatment framework provided by physical therapists.
3. Describe the view of the patient from a recipient to a participant.
4. Describe the main elements of specific federal and state laws that impacted the growth and development of physical therapy services from the hospital to the school and people's homes.
5. Assess the impact of the biomedical and biopsychosocial models of care and the concept of value-based care on the future skills and behaviors of a business owner and health care provider.

Is health care in the United States a public service or a business or a mixture of both? To better understand the question, a private practitioner of health care, or an employee, would benefit from understanding the history that has created such an environment that started primarily as a service and that has developed into a business, with service components. The current health care environment is best described as changing, especially in this era of technologic development and global access to information. This chapter will present information on some of the key issues that have influenced the development of health care (specifically medicine and physical therapy) in the United States and how the practice of providing health care services has grown beyond the walls of the hospital setting where it began, into the schools and homes where people actively participate in their health care today. Several key factors that have influenced the development and delivery of health care include scientific advancements, epidemics, wars, technology, and federal legislation that have shaped the health care system, especially physical therapy. By understanding the influences of the past, a provider can have a better understanding of the multiple factors that influenced the current system today and participate in further developing a more efficient, effective, and fair system for the future. In order to be successful in such a dynamic environment, a health care practitioner must have clinical expertise, a business acumen, and effective communication skills to contribute to the change process. These attributes and skills will make the practitioner a more knowledgeable and effective participant in the conversation.

Chapter 3 / The History of Health Care in the United States

Early Development of the Hospital, Physician, and Physical Therapist

In the 1700s and 1800s, hospitals in the United States were charitable organizations that were focused on caring for the physically sick as well as protecting the public from those who had either physical or mental illnesses. Individuals with financial means obtained the services of a physician or nurse in their homes. Families without financial resources or the ability to care for their family members often sent them to almshouses for the poor or hospitals where they were isolated from the public, with visitations restricted. This may have helped to curb the spread of disease in the general public but not in the hospital building.[1] Hospitals in the 1800s were small and overcrowded and provided little health care. Women in religious orders saw the need and the opportunity to provide care to the sick and spiritual guidance to patients in these facilities, and thus began the relationship between the Catholic and Protestant religions and hospitals in the United States. Physicians saw the social importance of the separation and isolation of people who were physically and/or mentally ill and also the opportunity to study, teach, and practice skills on a population brought together in one place: the hospital. This altruistic service had a primary health care focus on aiding society and the patients. It went through a dramatic change owing to the necessities of the Civil War.

The Civil War in the 1860s helped to advance the science of medicine and the delivery of health care. The need for an increase in care and services for the wounded men saw the development of the ward system, where patients with similar health problems were grouped together, allowing for more specific examinations and the efficient delivery of specific treatments.[2] The need to remove wounded men from the battlefield and transport them to a hospital saw the development of the ambulance system and the establishment of large general hospitals in urban areas where a large number of the wounded could receive care.[3] Advancements in the use of anesthesia, typically chloroform, owing to its quick effect, nonflammable nature, and its effectiveness when applied in small amounts through a conical apparatus, led to the development of the first medicine inhaler.[4] Anesthesia also allowed for a more humane surgical amputation of a limb, which accounted for three out of every four surgeries that were performed.[3] At this time, this frequent surgery led to the development of prosthetic devices for the residual lower limb, which enabled the wounded soldier to stand upright and walk. The lack of able-bodied male nurses to care for the growing number of injured soldiers led to the recruitment of women to assist in their care. These female nurses not only provided physical assistance to the wounded but also helped in their mental health by writing letters, praying with them, and reading to them.[5] In addition, the female nurses carried out domestic chores in the hospitals, washing patients, cleaning, preparing food, and managing the operation of the hospital's supplies and kitchen functions, assisting with the growing need for hospital administration. By the end of the war, there were over 400 hospitals established in the United States, most of which were located in large cities, and the relationship between physician, nurse, and hospital was solidified.

The Civil War had a significant impact on the development of hospitals and the role of physicians and nurses, but it was the epidemic of infantile paralysis or poliomyelitis (polio) in the late 1800s and early 1900s, affecting children in the New England States for the first time in 1894, that was one of the events that led to the establishment of the profession of physical therapy in the United States.[6] The application of physical modalities and therapeutic procedures was incorporated into the medical management of children who contracted this disease, which then consisted mainly of bed rest and immoblization.[6] The earliest providers of these interventions were teachers of physical education, gymnastics, or corrective exercise, referred to as reconstruction aides, who, in collaboration with the physician, provided interventions that included massage, muscle training, and corrective exercise.[7] The growing utilization of health care practitioners, especially physicians and reconstruction aides (later to become physical therapists), highlighted the need for standardizations in care and provider education.

In the early part of the 20th century, the Carnegie Foundation funded a study of the schools of medicine in the United States to gather information on the education and structure of the schools throughout the country. The result of this study, in 1910, by Abraham Flexner, led to the publication of the landmark report referred to as the Flexner Report.[8] It transformed the nature and process of medical education, bringing standardization in education and the establishment of the biomedical model (eg, Nagi Model) as the gold standard of medical training.[9] The success of this reorganization resulted in the numerous advancements in the science and delivery of medicine that propelled the United States to the forefront of medical practice. Unintentionally, it may also have contributed to an imbalance between the drive for research and advancements in scientific knowledge over that of patient care.[9]

In 1917, the establishment of the Division of Special Hospitals and Physical Reconstruction in the Office of the Surgeon General of the US Army Medical Corps. provided a standard education for the preparation of reconstruction aides.[10] These efforts to train an increasing number of women to aid in rehabilitation were the result of an increasing need for reconstruction aides for the rehabilitation of people with polio and men wounded and returning home from World War I (1914-1918). By 1919, 45 hospitals in the country employed more than 700 reconstruction aides.[11] In 1921, the American Women's Physical Therapeutic Association was founded, with Mary McMillan as its president. The purpose of the organization was to establish a professional and scientific standard for those engaged in the profession of physical therapeutics.[12] In 1922, the name was changed to the American Physiotherapy Association (APA) in recognition of the men who also practiced physiotherapy.

Hospitals before the 1920s had operated without much money besides that donated by wealthy benefactors who provided the capital. Physicians donated their time, and the costs for nurses and staff tended to be low.[2] With the establishment of requirements in education and professional standards, hospitals required additional revenue to help pay for surgeons, physician, nurses, and other professional staff. That revenue came from patients who could afford the cost of the care. Baylor University Hospital in Dallas, Texas, in order to make health care more affordable to members of the local community and those who struggled to pay for care, offered a nonprofit plan for prepaid hospital coverage. This plan required a person to pay 50 cents per month, or 6 dollars a year, for up to 21 days of hospital care per year, if needed.[13] The program was a success and led to the creation of The Blue Cross Blue Shield Association, currently one of the largest health care insurance companies in the country. The purpose of these early insurance plans was not purely altruistic but a way to make money for hospitals, which at that time were struggling financially.

In the 1930s, in order to more closely align with the medical profession and make a clear distinction between the profession of physiotherapy and other professions such as nursing, occupational therapy, or chiropractic medicine, the APA agreed to allow the American Medical Association's Council on Medical Education to accredit physiotherapy schools.

---

reconstruction aides – the earliest providers of what has become to be known as *physical therapy* in the United States

biomedical model – a treatment approach that has a focus on pathology as the source of disability

Chapter 3 / The History of Health Care in the United States

In the agreement, the APA also consented to the title of *physiotherapist technician* and the requirement to work only under the direct supervision of the physician.[14] In hindsight, this may seem like an inappropriate move for professional autonomy, but in the context of an emerging profession during the Great Depression of the 1930s, this was a move toward professional legitimacy and survival. It also put the practice of physiotherapy under the direction of the physician and the biomedical model of care.

The continuing polio epidemic and the outbreak of World War II in the 1940s placed further demands on the limited number of qualified physiotherapy technicians and facilitated a period of major growth in the profession. It was during this period that physical therapy's importance was further recognized by the public and medical professionals, solidifying the importance of physical therapy in the rehabilitation of individuals in the hospital.[7] This era also saw a change in the medical specialty that focused on physical therapeutics and rehabilitation. A physician who specialized in this area used the title of *physical therapy physician*. This medical specialty officially became known as physical medicine, with the physician adopting the title of **physiatrist**, a physician who specializes in physical medicine (and rehabilitation, added in 1955).[15] This made the title of physiotherapy technician unnecessary, and practitioners adopted the title of *physical therapist*. In 1946, the Association changed its name to the American Physical Therapy Association (APTA).

Another important factor that played a role in shaping the delivery of health care is the treatment-oriented approach to illness reflective of the biomedical model of health. In the United States, the development of health care was influenced by the attitude that the body is a machine that can be fixed. Treatment is provided with the aim of curing the person of an illness or disease. This attitude is reflected in the sophisticated technology developed to maintain or prolong the life of a patient more than to help them live with a long-term illness or disabilities.[1] This influence can be seen today in the intensive care provided to the infant who is born prematurely or the elderly person whose life is extended by the use of mechanical ventilation or cardiopulmonary machines. The sophistication of knowledge and the development of technology gained through years of research have produced medical interventions that would have astounded the physicians during the Civil War era. This emphasis fostered the growth and development of the world's most sophisticated and technologically advanced health care system, which celebrates the often heroic and costly medical procedures to save or extend life, but has generally downplayed the less heroic preventive procedures that can improve the quality of life for many people in society (eg, public health services). This balance between advancements in knowledge through research and patient care could have been pursued with equal benefits for both sides, but, unfortunately, the science of medicine became more preeminent than the active interaction and care of the patient.[9]

Early Developments in Physical Therapy Treatment

The polio epidemic reached its peak in the United States in the early 1950s. In 1953, Jonas Salk, MD, discovered a vaccination that would prevent poliomyelitis. His discovery, known as the Salk vaccine, went on to virtually eradicate the disease in the United States. Physical therapists continued to provide interventions to individuals who were paralyzed by the disease and also addressed other movement disabling conditions such as cerebral palsy. During this time, the practice of physical therapy took on an additional perspective in the treatment of patients with neuromuscular diseases. Margaret Rood, a physical therapist and an occupational therapist, had a major influence on the treatment approach to patients

physiatrist – a physician who specializes in physical medicine and rehabilitation

with central nervous system (CNS) disorders. Her rehabilitation approach focused more on the neurophysiologic bases than the more traditional orthopedic approach.[16] The work of Margaret Knott and Dorothy Voss also emerged in the 1950s. Their developmentally based intervention for movement, Proprioceptive Neuromuscular Facilitation (PNF), became another intervention provided by the physical therapist along with the works of Signe Brunnstrom, in the treatment of hemiplegia, and Dr Karl and Berta Bobath, with their specialized handling techniques for children with cerebral palsy.[17-19] In the 1950s and 1960s, the traditional interventions provided by physical therapists were broadened to include a more neurophysiologic and developmental approach to the treatment of movement disorders, based on the understanding of the CNS at that time. This understanding included a direct relationship between the neurologic maturation of the CNS and motor behaviors expressed in a developmental sequence, where sensory input preceded motor output, and the presence of a hierarchical relationship of the CNS structures, where the cortex ultimately controlled complex movements.[20] These contributions provided the foundation of how physical therapy would be provided to people with movement disorders for decades. The profession of physical therapy was expanding its repertoire of interventions to address the changing needs of the patient population and the setting where they sought help: the hospital.

In the 1970s and 1980s, physical therapists and the newly created physical therapist assistants (established in 1969) were using a combination of neurophysiologic techniques to solve motor problems and to address the impairments of patients with neuromuscular diseases.[20] The basis of the interventions continued to rest on the understanding of the CNS and its influence on motor behavior. During the 1960s through the 1990s (and continuing today), research advanced the understanding of human movement, providing insight into the heterarchical relationship (instead of hierarchical) of cortical and subcortical structures of the CNS. The dynamic systems theory of motor development, along with the theories of motor control and motor learning, expanded the understanding of movement and influenced how physical therapists addressed movement impairments. The acquisition of a motor behavior and skill was seen not so much as a linear process that was closely associated with neural maturation but as a dynamic process in which new behaviors emerge as old behaviors lost their stability or primary influence as a result of a change in one of the many subsystems that impact movement (eg, cognitive, musculoskeletal, sensory, neuromuscular).[21] These theories view the patient not as a passive recipient of therapeutic interventions but as an active problem solver whose motor behavior is goal directed and whose knowledge of performance and results aids in motor learning. To integrate this understanding into practice, the physical therapist would have to modify the interventions, structure meaningful activities with active patient participation in the treatment session. This approach would be beneficial in the expanding settings, outside the walls of the hospital, where the physical therapist will practice.

Providing health care services to patients also required a shift in the paradigm of how the provider views a patient and in the expectations that the provider has for the patient's participation in the process of recovery. In the 1950s, Talcott Parson, a sociologist, suggested that people in Western countries demonstrated predictable behaviors when they are ill.[22] Parson noted that a society makes certain assumptions (known as Parson's assumptions) about a person who is ill. First, the person who is ill or sick is not solely responsible for their condition, and it is not within their power to get better. Second, being ill exempts the person from normal personal and social obligations in proportion to the severity of the illness. These two assumptions can be considered the *rights* of the person who is ill.

Parson's assumptions – one view of the rights and responsibilities of a person who is ill

Chapter 3 / The History of Health Care in the United States

There are also patient expectations or *responsibilities*. First, being sick is undesirable, and a person who is ill should take appropriate actions and enlist the aid of competent people (ie, health care professional) to aid in recovery. Second, the person is obligated to comply with the treatment and advice provided by the health care professional (Box 3.1). It is in this paternalistic environment that the biomedical model of service delivery has evolved. The patient is, by definition, the person who is ill (or the child with polio or the wounded veteran) and seeks out the consult of a physician, who writes a prescription for physical therapy to address the patient's problem. It views the patient as the recipient of care. This model of service is practiced today in states that require a referral by a physician in order for a patient to receive treatment from a physical therapist. It is practiced in many hospital settings and outpatient clinics and is reinforced by third-party payment systems that require a referral from a physician as a requirement for receiving payment for treatment.

The growth and development of medicine and physical therapy, provided primarily in hospitals, brought about other issues that would impact the delivery of health care services and shift the focus from a paternalistic view to a partnership. In the 1970s, there was a growing awareness of how society imparts limitations, intentionally or unintentionally, on people who have a disability.[23] This awareness broadened the biomedical model of care to include more of the factors that influence a person's health in addition to the pathology. In 2001, the World Health Organization published the *International Classification of Functioning, Disability and Health* (ICF).[24] This biopsychosocial model of health includes not only the status of the person's body structure and functions but also the performance of daily activities and meaningful participation that fulfill the person's desired role in society. It recognizes the environmental and personal factors that impact a person's health and requires an understanding of several other internal and external factors. These factors can be either barriers to or facilitators of the patient's full participation in society. It views the patient as a participant in their health. In 2012, the APTA adopted the language of the ICF.[25] The profession expanded its view on health and embraced a more comprehensive view to better understand and help people who seek physical therapy services.

With the increasing utilization of hospitals came the need to broaden the understanding of other factors that impact a patient's health. Factors such as infection control, to curb the spread of diseases *within* the hospital building, the need to protect information about patients who were admitted to the hospital, and the need to provide a certain level of efficient care and effective education to all who received a service from the hospital also broadened the view and responsibilities of the provider. These identified factors, as well as others, reflect the growing influence of external agencies and legislation on the delivery of services

---

BOX 3.1 • Parson's Assumptions[22]

A person who is ill:

1. Does not desire to be ill and should be provided some level of care in order to recover.
2. Is exempt from normal social roles, such as participation in work or household chores.
3. Should seek the assistance of a qualified health professional, such as a physician.
4. Should comply with the health professional's recommendations.

Parsons T. *The Social System*. Free Press; 1951.

---

biopsychosocial model – a view of health that has a broader focus on the internal and external factors that are a source of disability in the hospital and other settings. Ironically, it was a polio survivor, President Franklin D. Roosevelt, who in 1935, signed the *Social Security Act* into law, one of the most significant pieces of social legislation passed by the US Congress. It, along with other federal laws that followed, would shape the delivery and payment for health care services in the United States.

Federal and State Laws

The Social Security Act of 1935 established a system of old-age benefits for workers, benefits for workers of industrial accidents, unemployment insurance, and aid for dependent mothers and children, persons who are blind, and persons with disabilities.[26] The law laid the foundation for several health and public welfare programs in subsequent years, including disability insurance, supplemental security income, vocational rehabilitation, and, most notably, with the reauthorization and passage of the *Social Security Act of 1965*, the programs of Medicare and Medicaid. These programs involve the federal and state governments as payers for health care services for the elderly and poor. Medicare is the largest source of federal funding for medical services for people over 65 years of age and for certain individuals with permanent disabilities. Medicaid is the largest source of funding for basic medical services for the poor. The Medicaid program is a joint federal and state program, administered by the state, which can determine eligibility requirements, covered benefits, and fee schedules. In addition to Medicare and Medicaid, the Social Security Act also included supplemental security income (SSI), which provided a fixed monthly payment to eligible children and individuals over the age of 65 years, who were disabled, blind, or had limited resources.[27] Medicare, notably, also included financial supplements for graduate medical student education (GME) when training in the hospital. The extra payments from Medicare for GME have helped many teaching hospitals avoid significant financial stress and have allowed them to continue providing care to Medicare beneficiaries.[28]

The law also includes physical therapy as an entitled service, one required by law, for beneficiaries of Medicare and/or Medicaid, significantly influencing the demand for physical therapy services.

Another piece of federal legislation that significantly influenced the demand for physical therapy services was introduced in 1946, with the passage of the *Hill-Burton Hospital Construction Act*. This legislation had a major influence on the expansion of the hospital industry and the physical therapy departments that they housed. It required hospitals with over 100 beds to also have a physical therapy department, which had a major influence on how services were provided to patients. The 1950s saw additional legislative influences with the passage of physical therapy licensure laws in many states. By 1959, 45 states had a physical therapy practice act.[29] Today each state has a Physical Therapy Practice Act, which is a state law intended to protect the public from impostors or fraudulent billing practices when the services are not rendered by a physical therapist or physical therapist assistant. Many state practice acts provide information regarding the practice of physical therapy and the relationship to physician oversight. All states have some form of

Social Security Act – the most significant piece of social legislation passed by the US Congress that gave rise to the programs of Medicare and Medicaid

entitled service – a service granted by the government to qualified individuals

Physical Therapy Practice Act – a state law intended to protect the public from impostors or illegal practices by a PT

Chapter 3 / The History of Health Care in the United States

direct access to physical therapy: the ability to access physical therapy services without a physician's referral. This access can vary from unrestricted direct access to restricted direct access with the need for a referral to provide treatment after a stated number of days or period of time.

The practice of physical therapy outside the hospital and into the public educational environment was more clearly defined in 1975 with the passage of Public Law 94-142: The Education for All Handicapped Children Act, currently titled the *Individuals with Disabilities Education Act* (IDEA). This law provides for a "free and appropriate public education" (FAPE) for all children with disabilities, beginning whenever the individual state provides public education to children who are not disabled (age 5 or 6 years depending on the state). Contained in PL 94-142 are several provisions commonly encountered in the special education classroom today, including the Individualized Education Program (IEP), the contract between parents and the school district that directs the delivery of services to the eligible student. Services related to a student's education include physical therapy, again adding to the demand for such professionals to provide this service. Several states require a physical therapist to obtain a physician's referral in order to provide services owing to the requirements of the states' physical therapy practice act and, if the student's health insurance (which may be billed) requires it, continue to make the need for physician involvement necessary when physical therapy services are utilized.

As with many other federal laws, periodic reauthorization is required to ensure continued appropriations and to provide an opportunity to reevaluate the components of the law for necessary updates, clarifications, or deletions. PL 94-142 was reauthorized with amendments in 1986 as the *Education of the Handicapped Act Amendments* or PL 99-457, which contained a significant update, extending educational services to children age 3 to 5 years. Part H of this law (currently Part C of the Individuals with Disabilities Education Improvement Act. PL 108-446) included the provision of early intervention services to eligible families or children, from birth to 3 years of age. (Some states provide these services until the child is eligible for kindergarten.) This law mandates a model of service delivery with an emphasis on family-centered services in the natural setting and includes physical therapy as an early intervention service, increasing demand once again. The program of early intervention is governed by the Individualized Family Service Plan (IFSP). These federal laws had, and continue to have, a significant impact on the demand for physical therapy services in the hospital settings and outside the hospital setting in nursing homes, home health agencies, schools, and people's homes under IDEA, Part C.

There are other laws that indirectly impacted the demand for medical and physical therapy services. These include state programs and laws for workers' compensation and vocational rehabilitation. *Workers' compensation* was one of the first laws enacted that addressed work and disability. It is the US social insurance system for industrial and work-related injuries.[30] Workers' compensation is regulated at the state level and requires the employer to pay benefits and furnish care to job-related injuries sustained by the employees, regardless of fault. This may include physical therapy services. Workers' compensation laws were enacted to make litigation less costly and to eliminate the need for injured workers to prove that their injuries were the employer's fault. These programs were being adopted in the early 1900s at a time when the federal government considered social insurance and welfare to be the responsibility of the states.

direct access – state legislation that permits access to physical therapy services without a physician's referral

The concept spread rapidly throughout the country, and by 1921, only six states had yet to enact workers' compensation legislation.[30] Persons who are disabled on the job receive benefits depending on the resulting level of disability. The levels or categories of disability include permanent total disability, permanent partial disability, and temporary total disability.[30] Each category has its own amount of compensation awarded and a specified length of benefit. Each state differs in terms of the percentage of the workers' wage it will award and how long it will award the benefit. For example, for a permanent total disability, the percentage of the worker's wage ranges from 60% to 80%. The length of the permanent total disability benefits can vary from months, for the duration of the disability, or until death. Those individuals who are disabled on the job and try to get another somewhere else are protected from discrimination under the *Americans with Disabilities Act* (see Chapter 5). Workers' compensation provides financial benefits for reasonable medical care related to the injury, replacement of lost wages, and pays for vocational rehabilitation if the worker cannot return to the job they had prior to the injury.[30]

Vocational rehabilitation refers to programs conducted by State Vocational Rehabilitation agencies operating under the *Rehabilitation Act of 1973*. Vocational Rehabilitation programs provide or arrange for a wide array of training, educational, medical, and other services individualized to the needs of people with disabilities. The services are intended to help people with disabilities acquire, reacquire, and maintain gainful employment. Services may include restoration of physical functioning, or mental functioning; academic, business, or vocational training; personal or vocational adjustment training; employment counseling; and job placement and referral.[31] Vocational rehabilitation programs are eligibility programs, not entitlements. The person must have a physical or mental disability, the disability must substantially impair the person's ability to work, and a reasonable expectation must exist that the provision of services will make the person employable.

Federal and state legislation has expanded the market for medical and physical therapy services either directly, by mandating such services by law for eligible people, or indirectly, by requiring programs to help people return to work. But the government does not provide the service or deliver the public good. They are the payer of the service and require adherence to specific guidelines for payment. The service is provided by the health care professional, who either owns a practice or works for an employer, who does business in a relatively free-market capitalistic system (see Chapter 1). This difference between the payer (government) and the provider (business), in this type of market, has led to the creation of complicated payment guidelines and reporting mechanisms.[32]

A Call to Change

One hundred years after the publication of the Flexner Report, a study published in 2010 by the Commission on the Education of Health Professionals for the 21st century, chaired by Julio Frenk, shed light on the disparity and shortcomings of health education in an interdependent world.[33] The study's finding, published in the journal *Lancet*, identified specific systemic shortcomings, including the following:

- There is a mismatch between the supply of and demand for physicians and nurses by geographic regions.
- Health professional leaders have insufficiently coordinated the way they work.

vocational rehabilitation – programs conducted by State Vocational Rehabilitation agencies that provide training, educational, medical, and other services individualized to the needs of people with disabilities

- Patient-centered, interprofessional, team-based approach to health care delivery has lacked the leadership to implement systemically.
- The global dimensions of health (eg, leadership, management, policy, and communication skills) are often neglected.[34]

As stated by the authors, "reform must begin with a change in the mindset that acknowledges challenges and seeks to solve them. No different than a century ago, educational reform is a long and difficult process [that] demands leadership and requires changing perspectives, work styles, and good relationships between all stakeholders." "Instructional reforms should . . . prepare students for the realities of teamwork, to develop flexible career paths that are based on the spirit and duty of a new professionalism."[33] These educational reforms have to be supported by clinical practice that reflects a patient-centered approach to care in the development and implementation of treatment plans, an equitable distribution of services both inside the clinic and in the community, an embedded system of coordination of care among all providers associated with the patient under care, and effective leaders. Leaders must have the skills to effectively manage and communicate the necessary aspects of identifying, developing, providing, and financially sustaining optimal health care services that are needed by patients, to adhere to government guidelines, and to produce positive health outcomes (Figure 3.1).

These attributes of the health care educator and provider are necessary to produce *value-based outcomes* that are required by Medicare in certain settings and becoming more emphasized in clinical practice (Chapter 4). In 2010, President Obama signed into law the *Patient Protection and Affordable Care Act* (ACA). The ACA has the primary goal of promoting the value of health care services to patients by incentivizing health care providers and hospitals to coordinate clinically efficient patient care and produce value-based

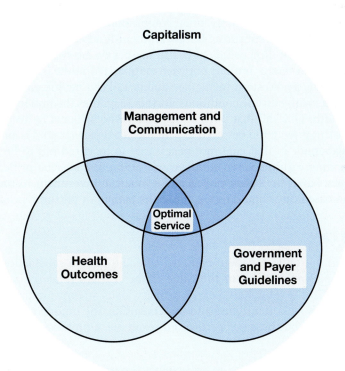

Figure 3.1 The Balancing Act of health care leaders.

outcomes.[35] This is a significant shift from a fee-for-service payment model that has predominated the health care industry for decades to a value-based outcome model, which is outcome driven instead of volume driven. The future entrepreneur in health care will have to understand how to develop and produce value-based outcomes, which include an understanding of the basic business structure and functions in this industry.

From Paternalism to Partnership

Throughout the last century, the professions of medicine and physical therapy have made advances in their knowledge and practice, owing in part to catastrophic events such as wars and epidemics, and have grown and benefited from these experiences. The drive for value-based care and outcomes, an increased need for collaboration and effective communication, and the influence of cost in health care, should not be discouraging. The altruistic and pragmatic decision-making natures of these professions have served them well and provided a base for the cultural pivots that have brought health care to the position it is in today. It is important for health care professional to engage in the conversation on change to influence the direction of health care. Discussions on access, cost, and quality of health care, justification of the effectiveness of the care provided, the promotion of patient satisfaction, and the financial survival of a practice in today's health care market, would greatly benefit from the insights and experience of a health care provider.[36] These topics are not new to the health care industry. President Franklin Roosevelt's development of Warm Springs in Georgia in the 1920s, for the treatment of people with polio, addressed the social dimension of disability as well as the medical and rehabilitative needs of the individual receiving treatment.[37] It was a view beyond the biomedical model. The financial cost of taking care of the convalescing wounded soldiers after the Civil War became a concern of the federal government, which began to emphasize the need for the wounded men to be rehabilitated and become productive tax-paying citizens. The call for the reform of the pension system would set in motion the eventual institutionalization of physical and vocational rehabilitation programs as a substitute for government-funded pensions.[38] This awareness of the financial and social dimensions of health has always been an understanding in disability or illness management, but has not been emphasized in the clinical management of the patient as it is today. Western medicine's ability to keep people alive and functioning longer, and at times with chronic conditions, further magnifies the importance of the social dimension of health. This shift has moved the patient who is ill and in need of professional care by a benevolent provider to be cured to a multifaceted partner who is an active decision maker and collaborator in that care, not necessarily to be cured but to be relatively pain free and functioning within society. And because of the cost sharing in health care today (Chapter 4), they have purchasing power and a financial investment in the care they are provided. Value-based care should be a value to the patient or person receiving that care.

Value-Based Care

Value is reflected not only in patient-centered care and patient satisfaction with the care provided but, more importantly, in the value of the services rendered to produce better health outcomes. This is value-based care's primary focus, to improve patients' health outcomes.[39] This begins with identifying and understanding the unique needs of the patients that are served by the business or practice. For example, a physical therapy practice may

value-based care – a collaborative, interdisciplinary approach to patient care with a primary focus on producing good health outcomes

Chapter 3 / The History of Health Care in the United States

start by identifying a significant number of patients who are middle-aged working adults with complaints of recurrent low back pain, who must return to work, are prescribed a few medications, mainly for control of hypertension and cholesterol, purchase over the counter pain and anti-inflammation medications, live with a significant other, and have employer-sponsored health insurance with a high deductible (Chapter 4). A team of professionals then come together to form a partnership to design and deliver a comprehensive program to efficiently address the needs of the patient. These professionals, in the example provided, could include two or more professionals, such as a physical therapist, physician, pharmacist, occupational therapist, employer, nutritionist, and social worker. The physical therapist could address the musculoskeletal and biomechanical factors associated with the patient's back pain and provide appropriate therapeutic exercises. The physician could manage the patient's medication and collaborate with the physical therapist to ensure that appropriate interventions are being provided for the identified underlying impairment (eg, mechanical derangement as opposed to a kidney disorder). The pharmacist could be involved to ensure that all of the medications, prescribed and purchased over the counter, are appropriate and managed correctly by the patient to address the current health issues. The occupational therapist could assist the patient in learning how to perform activities of daily living to decrease the stress and repetitive movements of the lower back through compensatory movement strategies or the use of an assistive device. The employer can provide input on the biomechanics of the job duties of the patient and collaborate on the appropriate modifications or accommodations that are possible at the place of employment in order to facilitate a return to work and to decrease risk of future injury. The nutritionist could provide education on the management of body weight, hypertension, and cholesterol through a diet and on how certain foods affect inflammation and pain. The social worker could be involved to address any barriers to accessing health care services or managing any out-of-pocket expenses. This interdisciplinary partnership uses an agreed upon health outcome measure and identification of the cost of care for ongoing improvements in patient outcomes.[39] One example of a standard set of value-based outcomes for adults, identified by Gangannagaripalli et al, would include the PROMIS Scale v1.2, Global Health (10 items), WHO Wellbeing Index (5 items), and the WHO Disability Assessment Schedule 2.0 (12 items).[40-43] Anyone, or all, of these assessments would be done annually and the data used to evaluate and identify ways to improve patients' overall health outcomes (Box 3.2).

By organizing partnerships to provide care to individuals with similar needs, the efficient and effective delivery of care that produces a better health outcome for the select patients is the responsibility of the interdisciplinary team rather than the health insurance administrator.[39] This is a shift in the paradigm for many health care professionals, which typically focused on the skills of the provider of care instead of the needs of a patient population. The physical therapist business owner who practices as a generalist will see any patient that comes to the practice for care. This can create inefficiencies when managing

BOX 3.2 • Building a Value-Based Outcome Program

1. Identify the unique needs of the patients served by the practice.
2. Develop partnerships with professionals who can impact the outcomes of the identified patient population. (This could range from 2 to 10, depending on the needs of the patient population and availability.)
3. Identify an appropriate health outcome that will be used, including a cost report.
4. Agree on a mode and frequency of meetings to manage the patients' care.
5. Use the outcome data to create a periodic report on the outcomes, including ways to improve.

patients to improve their outcomes, when other factors impact health outcomes and those resources are not readily available (ie, not in the partnership).

This example may sound simplistic, considering that, in reality, it can be challenging to form partnerships in the current environment of health care, find the time to communicate and manage the partnerships, and agree on a set of outcome measures that are practical in clinical practice and that provide helpful information. This is the crossroads. These are the decisions health care providers have to make, and they need to be courageous and willing to make these changes to improve the health and outcomes of the people served. It was done in the past and can be done now.

Summary

Health care in the United States is a unique mixture of a public service and business that operates in a relatively free market but with significant governmental influence to provide some level of care to certain groups of citizens (eg, the elderly and poor). It has grown from an altruistic service provided to the wounded and ill in small hospitals to a complex and community integrated system of hospitals, ambulatory clinics, and home care services that make health and wellness services available to all citizens in a variety of settings. Health care professionals throughout US history have responded to the needs of people as a result of wars and epidemics, by developing and delivering services that met those needs. The value of restoring a person to function as an active, tax-paying member of society has been an important aspect of health care. As health care providers broaden their view of patients from a biomedical to a biopsychosocial model, the importance of taking into consideration the additional internal and external factors will hopefully impact the outcome of those services on improving a patient's health. Historically, a fee-for-service industry, health care has been grown in its value and been incorporated into several state and federal laws that mandate guidelines on the provision of services for payment by the state and/or federal government. This broadening of governmental influence is a challenge in a capitalistic free-market system where the provider participates in the exchange of the good but the government pays for the services provided. That influence, and the influence of third-party payers, challenges the practitioner's participation in a competitive market where the business has to balance compliance with government and third-party payment structures with the demands and needs of the market. The health care practitioner is caught in the middle. To be successful, they must have the clinical expertise found through scientific inquiry; knowledge of the basic aspects of business, effective communication skills; and interprofessional skills to navigate toward the production and recognition of value-based care.

REFERENCES

1. Sultz H, Young K. *Health Care USA. Understanding Its Organization and Delivery.* 9th ed. Jones and Bartlett; 2018.
2. The Safety Net. A history of public hospitals in the United States from city almshouse to medical innovator—two centuries of triumph and trial. In: Hogge A, ed. *A Public Trust: Two Centuries of Care in America's Public Hospitals.* Vol 20, No 1. National Associations of Public Hospitals and Health Systems; 2006. Accessed October 30, 2023. https://essentialhospitals.org/wp-content/uploads/2014/01/TSN.pdf
3. Reilly RF. Medical and surgical care during the American Civil War, 1861-1865. *Proc (Bayl Univ Med Cent).* 2016;29(2):138-142. doi:10.1080/08998280.2016.11929390
4. Farelly E. Medical advances of the American Civil War we still use today. War History Online. Published February 14, 2019. Accessed November 2, 2023. https://www.warhistoryonline.com/history/medical-advances-civil-war.html
5. Gibbons Backus P. Female nurses during the Civil War. Angels of the battlefield. Published October 20, 2020. Updated June 1, 2021. Accessed November 2, 2023. https://www.battlefields.org/learn/articles/female-nurses-during-civil-war
6. Scott R. *Foundations of Physical Therapy. A 21st Century-Focused View of the Profession.* McGraw-Hill; 2002:1.

Chapter 3 / The History of Health Care in the United States

7. Rogers N. Polio and its role in shaping American physical therapy. *Phys Ther.* 2021;101(6):pzab126. doi:10.1093/ptj/pzab126

8. Flexner A. Medical education in the United States and Canada. *Science.* 1910;32:41-50. doi:10.1126/science.32.810.41

9. Duffy TP. The Flexner report—100 years later. *Yale J Biol Med.* 2011;84(3):269-276.

10. Pinkston D. Evolution of the practice of physical therapy in the United States. In: Scully RM, Barnes MR, eds. *Physical Therapy.* Lippincott Williams and Wilkins; 1989.

11. United States Army Medical Services. *Medical Department of the United States Army in the World War. The Surgeon General's Office.* Government Printing Office; 1923.

12. Murphy W. *Healing the Generations: A History of Physical Therapy and the American Physical Therapy Association.* Greenwich Publishing Group Inc.; 1995.

13. Blue Cross Blue Shield. An industry pioneer. Accessed November 7, 2023. https://www.bcbs.com/about-us/industry-pioneer

14. Linker B. Strength and science. Gender, physiotherapy, and medicine in early-twentieth-century America. *J Womens Hist.* 2005; 17:105-132.

15. Sandel E. The early history of physical medicine and rehabilitation in the United States. PM&R Knowledge NOW. Updated December 17, 2019. Accessed November 9, 2023. https://now.aapmr.org/the-history-of-the-specialty-of-physical-medicine-and-rehabilitation/

16. Rood MS. Neurophysiological reactions as a basis for physical therapy. *Phys Ther Rev.* 1954;34:444-449.

17. Knott M, Voss DE. *Proprioceptive Neuromuscular Facilitation.* Harper and Row, Publishers Inc.; 1956.

18. Brunnstrom S. Associated reactions of the upper extremity in adult patients with hemiplegia. *Phys Ther Rev.* 1956;36:225-236

19. Bobath B. Treatment principles and planning in cerebral palsy. *Physiotherapy.* 1963;49:122-124.

20. Stuberg W, Harbourne R. Theoretical practice in pediatric physical therapy: past, present, and future considerations. *Pediatr Phys Ther.* 1994;6:119-125.

21. Kamm K, Thelen E, Jensen J. A dynamical systems approach to motor development. *Phys Ther.* 1990; 70:763-774.

22. Parsons, T. *The Social System.* Free Press; 1951.

23. Retief M, Letsosa R. Models of disability: a brief overview. *Hts Theol Stud.* 2018;74:a4738.

24. World Health Organization. *International Classification of Functioning, Disability and Health: ICF.* World Health Organization; 2001.

25. American Physical Therapy Association. Endorsement of International Classification of Functioning, Disability and Health (ICF). HOD P06-08-11-04 [Position]. Updated August 07, 2012.

26. National Archives. Milestone documents. The Social Security Act of 1935. Updated February 8, 2022. Accessed November 12, 2023. https://www.archives.gov/milestone-documents/social-security-act

27. United States Social Security Administration. Social Security online. Supplemental Security Income overview. 2023. Accessed November 12, 2023. https://www.ssa.gov/ssi/text-over-ussi.htm

28. Institute of Medicine (US) Committee on Implementing a National Graduate Medical Education Trust Fund. *On Implementing a National Graduate Medical Education Trust Fund.* National Academies Press (US); 1997. Appendix B, History and Current Status of Medicare Graduate Medical Education Funding. Accessed on November 11, 2023. https://www.ncbi.nlm.nih.gov/books/NBK233563/

29. Murphy W. *Healing the Generations: A History of Physical Therapy and the American Physical Therapy Association.* Greenwich Publishing Group Inc.; 1995.

30. Clayton A. Worker's compensation: a background for Social Security professionals. *Soc Secur Bull.* 2003; 65(4):7-15..

31. US Equal Employment Opportunity Commission. Rehabilitation Act of 1973 (PL 93-112). Section 103. Accessed November 16, 2023. https://www.eeoc.gov/rehabilitation-act-1973-original-text

32. Jones WJ. The "business"—or "public service"—of healthcare. *J Healthc Manag.* 2000;45(5):290-293.

33. Frenk J, Chen L, Bhutta ZA, et al. Health professionals for a new century: transforming education to strengthen health systems in an interdependent world. *Lancet.* 2010;376(9756):1923-1958. doi:10.1016/S0140-6736(10)61854-5

34. Horton R. A new epoch for health professionals' education. *Lancet.* 2010;376(9756):1875-1877. doi:10.1016/S0140-6736(10)62008-9

35. Moy HP, Giardino AP, Varacallo M. Accountable care organization. In: *StatPearls.* StatPearls Publishing; 2023. Updated July 25, 2023. https://www.ncbi.nlm.nih.gov/books/NBK448136/

36. Nicholls DA. Fragility and back pain: lessons from the frontiers of biopsychosocial practice. *Phys Ther.* 2023;103(6):pzad040. doi:10.1093/ptj/pzad040

37. Wilson DJ. Polio paradise? Franklin D. Roosevelt's warm springs, physical therapy, and disability culture. *Phys Ther.* 2021;101(10):pzab214. doi:10.1093/ptj/pzab214

38. Linker B. *War's Waste: Rehabilitation in World War I America.* University of Chicago Press; 2011.

39. Teisberg E, Wallace S, O'Hara S. Defining and implementing value-based health care: a strategic framework. *Acad Med.* 2020;95(5):682-685. doi:10.1097/ACM.0000000000003122

40. Gangannagaripalli J, Albagli A, Myers SN, et al. A standard set of value-based patient-centered outcomes and measures of overall health in adults. *Patient.* 2022;15:341-351. doi:10.1007/s40271-021-00554-8
41. Gershon RC, Rothrock N, Hanrahan R, Bass M, Cella D. The use of PROMIS and assessment center to deliver patient-reported outcome measures in clinical research. *J Appl Meas.* 2010;11(3):304. https://www.codetechnology.com/promis-global-10/
42. Bech P. Measuring the dimension of Psychological General Well-Being by the WHO-5 119. *QoL Newslett.* 2004; 32:15-16. https://ogg.osu.edu/media/documents/MB%20Stream/who5.pdf
43. Üstün TB, Kostanjsek N, Chatterji S, Rehm J. *Measuring Health and Disability: Manual for WHO Disability Assessment Schedule WHODAS 2.0.* World Health Organization; 2010:90. Accessed November 25, 2023. https://www.who.int/classifications/icf/whodasii/en/

CHAPTER 4

The Influencer in Health Care
Health Insurance

MARK DRNACH

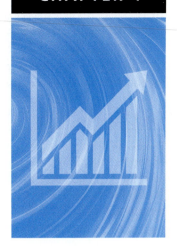

Learning Objectives

The reader will

1. Describe the basic structure and components of health care insurance in the United States.
2. Distinguish between the different federal government programs of Medicare, Medicaid, and the Affordable Care Act as they apply to the coverage of health insurance for specific populations.
3. Examine the aspects of managed care, and understand how they impact the delivery of services.
4. Classify the components of the major models of disability and health, and appreciate how they can impact a provider's view of the patient.
5. Break down the steps in clinical decision-making, and appreciate the process of reflective practice.
6. Describe the contributors to the determination of frequency and duration of rehabilitation services.
7. Recognize how clinical documentation is used to show the patient's response to care and justification for the services provided.

Health care is expensive, costing the average US citizen over 10,000 dollars annually and making up over 17% of the gross domestic product (GDP. See Chapter 1).[1] The cost of hospital care, physician services, and clinical services makes up over 50% of the total cost associated with health care.[1] Paying for these services can be a financial challenge for many people, especially those with limited resources or those who operate on a fixed income. Medical debt, or outstanding payment for medical bills, is a major source of debt in the United States and is associated with a decreased utilization of subsequent health care as a way to manage that debt.[2,3] People are more likely to have problems paying their medical bills if they are uninsured, have a low family income level (less than the federal poverty level) or reside in a non-Medicaid expansion state.[4] People who have the option to purchase or participate in health care insurance programs may do so, either by choice or by necessity, or opt not to participate. If they choose to participate, then they agree to the terms of the contract, including which services are covered, which services are not, and the limitations that are placed on the number of services or visits available under that contract. It can be a challenge for the health care provider to incorporate those insurance parameters into a plan of care if and when those parameters impact the professional's clinical choices and if the patient expects more than the insurance contract allows. Working within this three-party payment system, where the patients are the first party responsible for payment for the services; the providers the second party; who decide how much to charge for the services or pay for the service themselves (pro bono); and the third party, or insurance company, who agrees to pay for certain services covered under their agreement with the patient, can at times feel like a juggling act. This chapter provides a simple framework for working in that system and keeping all the balls in the air.

Components of Health Insurance

People, in order to decrease the significant financial burden that may accompany an injury or illness, will join other people to form a group (ie, risk pool) and provide money (ie, premiums) to an account (ie, insurance account) that will lessen the financial burden of paying for the cost of health care (ie, benefit) that may be needed in the event of an illness or injury. Risk pooling is a common practice in the insurance industry (health, property, house, flood, automobile, etc) as a form of risk management. In the health care industry, by pooling a large group of individuals together, the low cost of providing health care to healthy individuals, who require little to no major health care intervention, offsets the cost of providing a higher cost of care for those individuals who require major health care intervention. Participating in a risk pool is often done with colleagues at the place of employment (employer-sponsored health care insurance), through the federal government (Medicare, Medicaid), by joining a risk group in the marketplace made available through the Patient Protection and Affordable Care Act (ACA) or by opting to not participate in any risk group (ie, have no health insurance and pay for it directly, if and when it is required). The individuals who are participating in the risk pool/health insurance program are referred to as beneficiaries. A beneficiary is the person who benefits from the insurance that will pay for part or all of the identified covered health care services. These benefits, or covered services, are listed in the insurance agreement/plan along with those services that are not covered or limited. Health insurance companies work with health providers, such as hospitals, physicians, and ambulatory care centers (called the *network*) and establish payments for a set group of services that will be included in the plan. The beneficiary agrees to pay a premium, which is a set amount of money, typically paid monthly, for a set number of services in a given time period, typically 1 year. The cost of the monthly premium is often a significant consideration for the purchaser of health insurance, but the lowest monthly premium may not be the best option to meet an individual's health care needs. A higher premium with a lower deductible may save more money, depending on the individual's needs and circumstances. Also, the inclusion of specific services, service providers, and a certain number of service visits is important to consider. The deductible is the amount of money a person will have to pay for health care services before the insurance will start paying for part or for all of the cost of the services provided. This deductible amount was agreed on at the signing of the insurance contract. Many insurance plans pay for preventive services like annual checkups and screenings before the deductible is met. Some plans have separate deductibles for different services, such as medications or equipment. Family plans often have both individual deductions, which apply to each person in the family plan, and a family deductible, which applies to all the family members in the plan.[5]

risk pooling – a common practice in the insurance industry as a form of risk management

beneficiary – person who benefits from the insurance

premium – a set amount of money, typically paid monthly, for an insurance policy

deductible – the amount of money a person will have to pay for health care services before the insurance will start paying for part or for all of the cost of the services provided

Chapter 4 / The Influencer in Health Care

Generally, plans with lower monthly premiums have higher deductibles, and plans with higher monthly premiums have lower deductibles.

Health plans also have copayments for services, commonly referred to as copays. This is a form of cost sharing in which the beneficiary is responsible for paying a certain fixed amount, based on the plan and the service received, at the time that a service is provided. Copays are usually associated with physician visits and prescription drug purchases, but not all services require a copay (eg, preventive services). The amount a beneficiary pays in copays for medical services typically does not count toward the beneficiary's deductible threshold. As a general rule, insurance plans with a lower monthly premium will have higher copay requirements, and plans with higher monthly premiums will have lower copay requirements.

Copays should not be confused with coinsurance. Coinsurance is another form of cost sharing where the beneficiary is responsible for part of the payment for services provided once the deductible has been met. Instead of a fixed amount, as with copays, coinsurance is based on a percentage of the cost. If the insurance plan has an 80/20 coinsurance clause, the insurance will pay for 80% of the cost for services received, once the deductible has been met, and the beneficiary will be responsible for the remaining 20% of the cost. This allocation may also be applied if the beneficiary received services from a provider who is *out of the network*.

Health insurance plans also have an out-of-pocket maximum amount of money that the beneficiary is responsible for in a given calendar year. This is the total amount of additional money paid for health services that the beneficiary is responsible for paying before the insurance will pay for 100% of the cost of services received. Deductibles, copays, and coinsurance payments factor into this amount. Basically, there are two cost sharing thresholds that the beneficiary has to reach before the insurance company pays 100% of the costs of health care services. The first threshold is the deductible. Once the deductible amount has been reached, the beneficiary will have to pay the coinsurance (eg, 80/20) until the maximum out-of-pocket threshold is reached. At this point, the insurance company will pay for any additional costs associated with the covered services of the insurance plan.

Health insurance plans typically run on the calendar year. This means that health care costs for the beneficiary will be higher at the beginning of the calendar year until the deductible limit is reached. At that point, the beneficiary and the insurance company share the cost of covered services until the out-of-pocket maximum is reached. At that point, the health care company will assume 100% of the cost of the covered services. Once the new year is reached, the amounts paid reset to zero. Health insurance plans help to protect the beneficiary from the high cost of medical expenses and provide financial access to certain essential health services; however, plans can vary in the specific services, and the amount of those services, that they cover. It is the responsibility of the purchaser to read and understand exactly what is in the health insurance plan before agreeing to purchase the health insurance (Box 4.1). The purchaser of the health insurance plan should review the plan and make sure that any desired provider or service is included in the plan, especially if specialists are needed in the management of a person's health. Ensuring that the appropriate providers are included in a plan or network and that the number of services or

copayment – a form of cost sharing in which the beneficiary is responsible for paying a certain fixed amount at the time that a service is provided

coinsurance – a form of cost sharing where the beneficiary is responsible for a percentage of the payment for services provided once the deductible has been met

out-of-pocket maximum – the amount of money that a beneficiary is responsible for in a given calendar year

BOX 4.1 • Basic Questions to Consider When Purchasing Health Insurance

1. Who is the beneficiary?
2. What are the beneficiary's specific health needs at this time and in the next calendar year?
3. Are the covered services, providers in the network, and medications desired or needed by the beneficiary?
4. Are the service limits acceptable?
5. Will the premium payment work in the monthly budget?
6. How much is the deductible, and can the expense be managed?
7. How much is the copay and what is the estimated cost per year?
8. What is the percentage (eg, 80/20) and estimated amount of the coinsurance per year?
9. What is the total out-of-pocket limit? If needed, how will this be paid?

visits covered is acceptable to the purchaser can lead to a more informed decision on the appropriateness of the plan for the individual's current or anticipated health care needs.

Not all individuals have options when it comes to health insurance coverage. Many unemployed persons do not have the option of employer-based insurance plans and even when they do, may opt not to purchase health insurance owing to the high cost.[6] Low-income individuals may not be eligible for Medicaid in their state, and those who could purchase health insurance through the marketplace may not be able to afford it or have access to limited plans that fit their individual needs.

Types of Health Insurance

Health insurance plays a significant role in the US health care system. There are basically two types of health insurance, *government insurance* such as Medicare and Medicaid, which are run by the federal and state governments, respectively, and *private insurance*, from companies such as Blue Cross/Blue Shield, which individuals can either self-purchase or participate in through their employers (ie, employer-sponsored plans). Private insurance programs are not run by the government, but both government and private insurance programs have certain structures from which they manage the utilization and payment of services provided. Historically, this has been done through a fee-for-service payment structure. The health insurance company would pay health care providers their fees, typically agreed on by the providers and insurance company, based on the services that were covered and provided to the patients. These services included the cost of the patient visit/encounter and the cost of any tests that were ordered in the course of the examination, diagnosis, and treatment. The services were billed separately, or unbundled, with a resultant focus on volume of care to address financial gains or needs. In the early 1970s, there was a growing concern about the rising cost and quality of health care in the United States as well as the distribution of and access to services in many geographic regions.[7] Responding to public demand, the Nixon Administration began exploring other more efficient modes of delivery to manage health care in the country. The result was the creation of the *Health Maintenance Organization Act of 1973*, which established a federal program to develop alternatives to the traditional forms of health care delivery and financing and

fee-for-service payment – payments made to health care providers based on the individual services that were covered and provided to patients

unbundled – a term used to describe insurance payments made for individual services

Chapter 4 / The Influencer in Health Care

69

to promote the development and use of health maintenance organizations (HMO).[8] An HMO is a form of a managed care organization (MCO) that combines the provider and insurer into one entity to manage patient care. The management of care in this system is population based rather than individually based. This enables the HMO to determine the projected use of health services by examining the demographics of the beneficiaries and the anticipated utilization of services. This information is then factored into the premium level charged to the beneficiaries and creates a form of financial risk sharing with the beneficiary by including copayments and deductibles.[9] Initially, the premium for an HMO insurance plan was cheaper than other plans, leading more people to choose this option. Patients with an HMO must have a primary care provider (PCP) and require a referral from their PCP to seek the services of a specialist.[10] HMOs also control costs by including certain providers within their network, having specific services that would be covered and specific limits on those services, and covering the cost of preventive services to help prevent the onset of more chronic conditions resulting in more costly care. Payments for services are also bundled together as one payment instead for each individual treatment, test, or procedure.[11] Bundling of payments is an attempt to reward providers for coordinating care, preventing complications from developing and errors from occurring, and reducing unnecessary or duplicative tests or treatments.[10,11] HMOs also introduced the concept of preauthorization to the health care system and emphasized utilization review of the services provided, which led to a shift from inpatient care (decreasing the length of stay) to outpatient and home care settings. This management of patient care was intended to decrease costs, broaden access, and improve quality, but the cost of health care continued to rise.[12]

The organizational forms of MCOs continued to evolve in response to the market forces such as employer preferences, beneficiary demands, and government agencies' requirements. A *preferred provider organization* (PPO) is one type of MCO and currently the most common type of health plan.[13] A PPO includes a network of practitioners (or *preferred* providers) that offer more flexibility in choices for the beneficiary than does a typical HMO. Generally, there is no requirement for a referral by a PCP to see a specialist, but the PPO still provides financial incentives for utilizing practitioners within the network.[14] A *point-of-service* plan (POS) is the least common type of health plan, combines the features of an HMO and a PPO, such as using a network of providers who are reimbursed a set amount for services provided, but require a PCP who controls access to specialists.[13] POS plans are provided at a lower copay cost but with fewer in-network choices for the beneficiaries, unless they choose to go out-of-network and pay more in copays and deductibles for the services offered.[14] Compared with fee-for-service plans, managed care plans have produced a decrease in the utilization of inpatient procedures, an increase in the use of preventive services, and more cost-effective hospital care.[15]

With the development of private insurance and employer-based plans, it became evident early on that these plans exclude the poor and the elderly who are unemployed or who cannot afford the cost of health insurance. In 1965, the United States Congress passed the amendments to the Social Security Act and created Title XVIII (Medicare) and Title XIX (Medicaid).[16] This historical legislation introduced government health insurance for the elderly and the poor, respectively. Originally intended to cover hospital costs (Medicare Part A) and medical services, including office visits (Medicare Part B), it has expanded

---

health maintenance organization – an organization that combines the provider and the insurer into one entity to manage patient care. The management of care in this system is population based rather than individually based.

bundled – a term used to describe insurance payments made for a collection of services

Table 4.1 The Parts of Medicare

Medicare	Covered	Funded
Part A	Inpatient hospital care Limited skilled nursing facility care Home health care related to hospitalization Hospice care	Mandatory payroll tax
Part B	Physician services Outpatient hospital services End-stage renal disease services Medical equipment	Premiums paid by beneficiaries
Part C	Medicare Advantage Managed care for Part A and B Private insurance companies administer the Medicare contract. May cover additional services not covered by Part A and B such as dental or eye care	Premiums paid by beneficiaries
Part D	Outpatient prescription drug coverage provided through private health plans that contract with the federal government. Federal government may set limits on drug costs.	Premiums paid by beneficiaries

to include a managed care option (Medicare Part C) and coverage for prescription drugs (Medicare Part D). Private insurance plans were adopted by Medicare Part C, or Medicare Advantage, with the aim of providing beneficiaries with options beyond those offered in Parts A and B and to attempt to produce the cost savings that were achieved with private insurance plans.[17] Yet Medicare was never intended to pay for any and all health services. Similarly to private insurance, Medicare beneficiaries are expected to share in the cost of services through deductibles, and coinsurance, and, therefore, the coverage they have depends on their choice and financial situation (Table 4.1).

The Medicaid program (Title XIX) is a joint federal and state program, administered by the state, which can determine eligibility requirements, covered benefits, and fee schedules. In order to participate, federal law requires states to cover certain groups of individuals that include families with low incomes (ie, financial eligibility), qualified pregnant women and children, individuals who receive Supplemental Security Income (SSI), or people with a disability as defined by the Social Security Administration (ie, functional eligibility), to name a few (Box 4.2). Services offered by Medicaid are extensive and usually free. States are allowed to provide a variety of services, but the federal government requires each state to make available certain basic services (Box 4.3).

BOX 4.2 • Social Security Administration's Definition of Disability

The Social Security Act defines disability (for adults) as "inability to engage in any substantial gainful activity by reason of any medically determinable physical or mental impairment which can be expected to result in death or which has lasted or expected to last for a continuous period of not less than 12 months" (Section 223 [d][1]). Amendments to the Act in 1967 further specified that an individual's physical and mental impairment(s) must be "... of such severity that he is not only unable to do his previous work but cannot, considering his age, education, and work experience, engage in any other kind of substantial gainful work which exists in the national economy, regardless of whether such work exists in the immediate area in which he lives, or whether a specific job vacancy exists for him, or whether he would be hired if he applied for work" (Section 223 and 1614 of the Act).

BOX 4.3 • Medicaid Mandatory Services

Inpatient hospital services
Outpatient hospital services
EPSDT: Early and Periodic Screening, Diagnostic, and Treatment Services
Nursing Facility Services
Home health services
Physician services
Rural health clinic services
Federally qualified health center services
Laboratory and x-ray services
Family planning services
Nurse Midwife services
Certified Pediatric and Family Nurse Practitioner services
Freestanding Birth Center services (when licensed or otherwise recognized by the state)
Transportation to medical care
Tobacco cessation counseling for pregnant women

Medicaid.gov. Mandatory & optional Medicaid benefits. Accessed October 10, 2023. https://www.medicaid.gov/medicaid/benefits/mandatory-optional-medicaid-benefits/index.html

Medicaid directs the highest percentage of its expenditures to long-term services and supports, which include (1) other health, residential, and personal care; (2) nursing care facilities and continuing care retirement communities; and (3) home health care.[18] Because of the demonstrations of cost savings of MCOs, managed care has become more attractive to government agencies. Managed care has now replaced fee-for-service as the predominant payment model in Medicaid.[19]

Private insurance and employer-based plans excluded not only the poor and the elderly but also other entities such as small businesses, farmers, and people who are self-employed. These entities could not participate in or create a risk pool large enough to offset the cost of health care while keeping premiums at a reasonable level. Therefore, many were uninsured, and the uninsured cost the health care system money. In 2010, President Obama signed into law the Patient Protection and Affordable Care Act (ACA).[20] This Act created a federally facilitated marketplace where qualified individuals (those who do not have access to employer-sponsored or government plans) could participate in a large risk pool (offered by participating health insurance companies participating in the marketplace), compare the covered services provided by health plans, and obtain affordable health care insurance. The ACA also notably expands Medicaid coverage in those states that choose to participate in the expansion, prohibits an insurance company from refusing individuals with preexisting conditions from obtaining health insurance or charging them more because of the preexisting condition, and allows children to continue on their parent's health insurance until the age of 26 years, in addition to mandating that the participating insurance companies provide specific health care servcies[21] (Box 4.4). The ACA's intent is to expand access to health insurance for millions of Americans, protect consumers from unfair insurance practices, lower cost by mandating certain preventive services, and hold insurance companies accountable for the dollars spent on health care services

Patient Protection and Affordable Care Act (ACA) – created a federally facilitated marketplace so small businesses, farmers, and those who are self-employed could afford health insurance

BOX 4.4 • Marketplace Plans: 10 Essential Benefits

1. Ambulatory patient services
2. Emergency services
3. Hospitalization
4. Pregnancy, maternity, and newborn care
5. Services for mental health and substance use disorders
6. Prescription drugs
7. Rehabilitative and habilitative services and devices
8. Laboratory services
9. Services for prevention, wellness, and chronic disease management
10. Pediatric services, including oral and vision care.

Source: HealthCare.gov. Health benefits and coverage. Accessed October 12, 2023. https://www.healthcare.gov/coverage/what-marketplace-plans-cover/

and quality improvement efforts.[21] The ACA has a primary goal of promoting the value of health care services to patients by incentivizing health care providers and hospitals to coordinate clinically efficient patient care and produce value-based outcomes.[22] Value-based outcomes are defined as the improvement in a patient's health outcome relative to the cost of providing the care.[23]

This is a significant shift from a fee-for-service payment model, which is volume driven, to a value-based outcome model, which is outcome driven.

The ACA adopted the use of accountable care organizations (ACO) in the Medicare program. An ACO is a group of physicians, hospitals, and other health care providers, who come together voluntarily to provide coordinated high-quality care to the Medicare patients they serve. Coordinated care helps ensure that patients receive timely, appropriate care, with the goal of avoiding unnecessary duplication of services and preventing medical errors.[24] When an ACO succeeds in both delivering high-quality coordinated care, as measured by benchmarks in patient experience, care coordination, safety, and prevention, and showing evidence of cost-effective care, the ACO may be eligible to share in the financial savings it achieves for the Medicare program (also known as performance payments).[25] A primary structural and conceptual difference between HMOs and ACOs is that HMOs are insurance groups that contract with providers, whereas ACOs consist of provider groups that contract with insurers.[10] The ACA also established the Centers for Medicare and Medicaid Services Innovation Center to test new payment strategies that are designed to improve patient care, lower costs, and promote patient-centered practices for people covered under Medicare, Medicaid, and/or the Children's Health Insurance Program (CHIP).[26] Subsequent federal legislation continues to emphasize cost reductions and quality initiatives, shifting the focus from payment for services provided to payment for cost-effective outcomes achieved. This has included the implementation, in 2019, of the Patient Driven Payment Model (PDPM).[27] This model, used by Medicare for patients in skilled nursing facilities under Medicare Part A, attempts to improve payment accuracy by focusing on patient characteristics and goals, rather than volume of services.[28] An important aspect of

value-based outcome – improvements in a patient's health outcome relative to the cost

accountable care organization – a group of physicians, hospitals, and other health care providers, who come together voluntarily to provide coordinated high-quality care to the Medicare patients they serve

Chapter 4 / The Influencer in Health Care

patient outcomes is patient satisfaction, which is influenced by the amount of time spent with the patient, the quality of the verbal and nonverbal communication, and the patient's opinion about the value of the health information provided and the manner in which it was delivered[29] (Chapter 8). This shift will require providers and hospitals to pay more attention to providing patient-centered care and broaden the historical definition of provider productivity and the contributors to the production of value-based outcomes.

Productivity

Productivity is a measurement of work and has historically been defined as the cost of the resources used (eg, provision of a health service) to the volume or number of billable units produced. It reflects the achievement of financial targets.

$$\text{Productivity} = \frac{\text{Output (eg, number of billable services provided)}}{\text{(Input (eg, cost of providing those services)}}$$

By increasing the number of billable units provided (the numerator), a business could increase productivity, given a fixed cost of the input (the denominator). Maximizing productivity would maximize profits and, ultimately, wages of the employees. This is one view of productivity, which focuses on volume for profit. As the health care payers shift from a volume-based payment model of productivity measurement to a value-based outcome payment model, productivity must be viewed as more than the number of billable units produced. It should capture the use of evidence-based practice, adherence to ethical principles, respecting clinical judgment, and the unique aspects of the model of care delivery in the clinical setting to optimize patient outcomes.[30,31] Value is added when providers' expertise is effectively utilized, and when time is allocated to educate the patients and caregivers, to consult with other experts and to collaborate with the medical team.[32] This reflects the productivity to achieve targeted outcomes, including, but not limited to, financial targets.

$$\text{Productivity} = \frac{\text{Output (eg, outcomes achieved)}}{\text{Input (eg, cost of the components needed to achieve those outcomes)}}$$

Broadening the definition of productivity and adding value to the factors that lead to optimal patient outcomes and patient satisfaction will clarify and promote the shift to value-based outcomes. This shift also requires providers to reflect on how they make decisions about patient care and communicate those decisions to others. Measuring health outcomes is not as complex as it may be perceived. Practitioners should understand the framework in which they make clinical decisions and focus on capturing and using data that define the health of their patients.

Clinical Decision-Making

There are several aspects of clinical decision-making that influence practitioners' behaviors and choices in the management of patients. The most essential are how practitioners view, or frame, the patients in front of them. Are they patients who need to be fixed, or understood, or both? What are the steps used to collect and evaluate the information that will satisfy a patient's primary concern or reason for seeking services? What are the barriers to and the facilitators of the achievement of the desired goals? This includes the status of the

productivity – a measurement of work

74 Section 1 / The Setup

patient, the clinical expertise of the provider, the resources and services available in the clinical setting, and the amount of funding to pay for those needed resources and services. What information is needed to guide the clinical decisions, evaluate progress, and justify the interventions provided? What outcome is to be achieved, and how will it be measured?

Frameworks

How the practitioner views the patient in front of him or her has its foundation in the Nagi Model of Disablement[33] (Figure 4.1). This model reflects a treatment approach to an identified disability with the aim of ameliorating the pathology or impairment in order to cure or lessen the disability. This construct emphasizes the factors that impact a person more from an individual perspective than from the environmental or societal aspects.[34] In this framework of moving from health to disability, normally functioning cells start to function abnormally, producing unintended results. When a threshold of abnormal activity is reached, the process can be identified as a *pathology*.

This atypical activity can be benign and not impair the body systems' functioning to the point of a measurable impairment, or it can reach a threshold of activity that does impact the body system identified as an *impairment* in structure or functioning. People can live and fulfill their role in society with impairments in body systems and structures. Examples include people with diabetes, cardiovascular disease, certain degrees of muscle weakness, or certain levels of mild cognitive impairments. It is when these impairments reach a certain threshold that the person's ability to function is impacted, and they are then classified as *functional limitations*. And when these functional limitations reach a certain threshold where they significantly impact a person's ability to function in day-to-day activities, the person is said to be disabled or to be having a *disability*. This framework or view emphasizes treatment of the pathology, which can be done through the application of chemicals (eg, medications, radiation) that alter the cells' functioning, or surgical removal of the abnormal pathology. It is a very treatment-centered approach, in which the body is viewed as a machine to be fixed. Medical care is viewed as the main issue related to disability, and, at a political level, emphasizes the need for health care policy reform or legislation that provides access to health care services, such as the ACA, Medicare, and Medicaid. These programs provide health insurance coverage for eligible citizens.

The World Health Organization's (WHO) International Classification of Functioning, Disability, and Health (ICF) is an integration of a medical and social model of disablement (Figure 4.2). It is a framework for measuring health and disability at the individual and population levels.[35] At the individual level, the ICF model shifts the focus of the consequences of the pathology to the components of a person's health. As a clinical framework, the ICF has applications in the development of a more detailed description of a person and

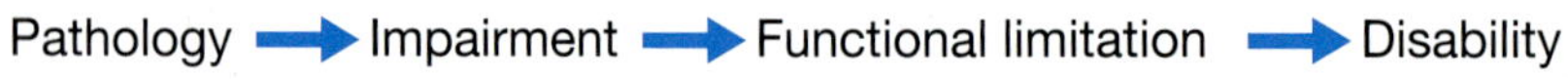

Pathology ➡ Impairment ➡ Functional limitation ➡ Disability

Figure 4.1 **The Nagi model of disablement**. (From Nagi S. Some conceptual issues in disability and rehabilitation. In: Sussman M, ed. *Sociology and Rehabilitation*. American Sociological Association; 1965: 100-113.)

Nagi Model of Disablement – a historical model that reflects a treatment approach to an identified disability with the aim of ameliorating the pathology or impairment in order to cure or lessen the disability

International Classification of Functioning, Disability, and Health (ICF) – a biosocial model of a person's health and the many internal and external factors that contribute to it

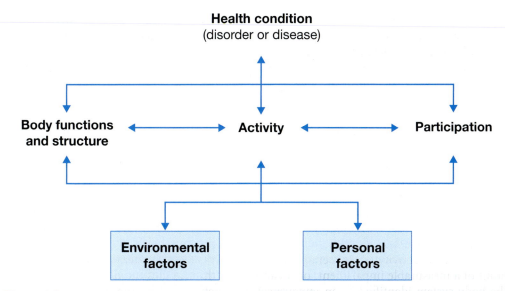

Figure 4.2 The ICF model of health. (Reprinted with permission from World Health Organization. The international classification of functioning, disability and health (ICF). World Health Organization; 2001. https://www.who.int/classifications/icf/en/.)

the factors that contribute to their health.[36] As a biosocial model of disability, the ICF views disability not as an attribute of an individual alone but as a collection of conditions, many of which are created by society and act as barriers to the individual's full participation in society. Social reform is viewed as the main issue related to disability and, at a political level, the need for legislation that addresses barriers to participation, such as the Americans with Disabilities Act and the Individuals with Disabilities Education Act. The contextual factors represented in the ICF model include environmental factors (eg, services, systems, and policies that impact the person) and personal factors (eg, gender, fitness level, and habits that impact the person). Both can have a positive or negative impact on a person's body function, structures, activities, and/or participation. It also emphasizes other factors that influence a person's health. The contextual factors also emphasize other influences of a person's health, such as the availability and choice of health care insurance. These contextual factors are taken into consideration when creating an appropriate treatment plan for a specific health condition, one that understands the many external factors that impact a person's health and the resources available to that person in addition to the underlying pathology.

When a health provider decides to address a certain condition in a patient but is limited by external factors, such as insurance service coverage limitations, the patient's ability to consistently obtain transportation for treatment, or the lack of specific services in certain geographic areas or clinical settings, a conflict may arise. The ethical dilemma created depends on the participants' point of view. One view values freedom, independence, and personal responsibility, whereas the other view values community, social justice, and equality.[37] Most people (>90%) in the United States have health insurance.[38] Some believe that people have the freedom and responsibility to choose a health plan that is appropriate for them, but that choice is often influenced by the cost. People will choose a plan that they can afford without giving much thought to the services that are provided, outside the basic services of prevention, hospital, and physician care. It is their right and their responsibility to follow through with the plan of care. Others believe that society has a moral obligation to address the social determinants of health (see Chapter 11) that impact people's health to the degree that the current health care systems cannot adequately address. Most hospitals and physician offices are repair shops, trying to correct the damage caused by these social determinants of health.[39] Health care is a human right, and addressing the societal factors that impact people's health, such as access to health care, early childhood education, transportation, the availability of healthy foods, and improved air and water quality, would significantly improve the health of the people in society. Without understanding and respecting these different points of view, interprofessional and interpersonal communication and collaboration can be impaired and can negatively impact the efficient management of the patient. Understanding the framework in which the provider and the patient view health or disability and the ethical point of view adopted by each can influence the patient's expectations of the services provided and the provider's clinical decision-making process.

The Steps in Clinical Decision-Making

Work by Rothstein and Echternach described the steps in clinical decision-making in a Hypothesis-Oriented Algorithm for Clinicians (HOAC II)[40] (Box 4.5). Part 1 of this process recognizes that patients identify their goals prior to the initial visit to the health care provider. People seek health care services to feel better, discover the reason for their ailment, obtain information on how to remain healthy, or manage a chronic illness. These are labeled as patient-identified problems or goals. This important aspect of the clinical decision-making, to identify the patient's goals, is a key component of the patient-centered care and can guide the subsequent examination process. Once initial data are gathered from the examination process, the provider can use the information gained to create a nonpatient identified problem list, the problems that the provider concludes from the presenting patient symptoms and clinical examination findings. At this point, a possible reason for the existence of the patient's problem can be hypothesized. This hypothesis helps the provider to make a decision on the patient's goals. Are they achievable? What specific interventions and dosage are needed? Is a referral to, or consultation with, another provider appropriate?

BOX 4.5 • Brief Outline of Hypothesis-Oriented Algorithm for Clinicians II

Part I
 Collect initial data.
 Obtain patient-identified problem.
 Formulate an examination strategy.
 Conduct the examination and analyze the data.
 Add nonpatient identified problems found during the examination.
 Generate a hypothesis as to why the problem exists and what would happen if no intervention were provided.
 Refine the problem list.
 Establish goals for each problem.
 Plan intervention strategy.
 Implement plan.
Part II
 Reassessment/Reflection
 Have the goals been met?
 How has the patient responded to the interventions?
 Is it reasonable to expect to see the desired change?
 Have additional problems occurred?

Adapted from Rothstein JM, Echternach JL, Riddle DL. The hypothesis-oriented algorithm for clinicians II (HOAC II): a guide for patient management. *Phys Ther.* 2003;83(5):455-470.

Chapter 4 / The Influencer in Health Care

What anticipated problems may arise if no interventions are provided or delayed? The next step is to create a specific treatment plan. This plan begins as a cognitive process that includes the expertise and experience of the practitioner, the purpose of the clinical setting, and the patient's goals and ability to participate in the plan. All three of these factors are significant contributors to the patient's desired outcome. A limitation in any one of these factors will impact the plan of care. Can the plan be addressed by the expertise of the practitioner? Is the patient in a clinical setting that is appropriate to address these issues? And does a patient have the ability to participate in the program, including financial resources, to support the plan of care? This final factor, having access to financial resources, is currently a major driver and can take precedence in the decision-making process. Although it is a significant factor, it should not replace the clinical expertise that develops the plan of care but can shape the implementation of the plan. In the implementation phase, the practitioner has to decide how much of the intervention to provide (ie, the dosage), identify the appropriate person to deliver the intervention (eg, a professional assistant, caregiver, the patient), and determine the external factors that impact that implementation, including payment for the services and the availability of willing and capable caregivers or providers to provide the interventions to produce the intended outcomes. Any barrier to the originally conceived plan may alter the achievement of the goals or outcome originally intended. In the acute care setting, the patient may not be able to tolerate the dosage of the interventions provided, and, therefore, the plan will have to be adjusted. In the outpatient setting, the patient may not be able to attend all the prescribed treatment sessions, owing to personal factors such as fluctuating health status, transportation issues, or the number of treatment sessions allowed by the chosen third-party payer. These issues factor into the reassessment and subsequent reflective practice in Part 2 of the HOAC II.[37]

Similarly to the HOAC II, Kenyon developed a Hypothesis-Oriented Pediatric Focused Algorithm for clinical decision making[41] (Box 4.6). This algorithm is similar to the one developed by Rothstein and Echternach but includes the recognition of a mental image of the patient that the practitioner sees prior to the patient encounter. This image may impact the practitioner's clinical decision-making options and course of action. For example, if a patient with a complaint of low back pain is scheduled, the practitioner may have a mental image of a middle-aged person who performs physical labor and has symptoms consistent with an L4-L5 dysfunction of the spine. From that image, the questions that will be asked

---

BOX 4.6 • Brief Outline of Kenyon's Pediatric Focused Algorithm

Initial hypothesis. Creating a mental image
Initial data collection
Generate a problem statement
Hypothesize goals
Examination planning
Examination
Evaluation
Diagnosis and prognosis
General intervention planning
Intervention session planning
Reflection
Formal reexamination

Adapted from Kenyon LK. The hypothesis-oriented pediatric focused algorithm: a framework for clinical reasoning in pediatric physical therapist practice. *Phys Ther.* 2013;93(3):413-420.

in the history, the clinical tests and measures used in the examination, and the treatment plan can be anticipated but not established. Both algorithms capture the importance of reflective practice: to cognitively review the patient encounter and decide whether and how the treatment might be improved to better align with the desired outcomes. It is also important to reflect on the ethical aspects of care. The purpose of this process is to review the management of the patient and the patient encounters and to identify the applicable elements of ethical practice associated with the plan and patient interactions. These ethical issues may include justice (fairness, treating people equally), fidelity (keeping information confidential), autonomy (obtaining informed consent), or beneficence (acting in the patient's best interest). It is through this reflective process that a practitioner becomes a better provider of care, especially in an environment with other personal and external factors to consider. One such factor is the number of visits that are allowed by the third-party payer or the patient (when self-pay or by desire). This can be perceived as a barrier if the payer allows only a specific number of visits (or frequency) for a specific condition.

Frequency and Duration of Services

Health care practitioners in rehabilitation, including physicians, are frequently presented with the question of how much therapy is needed for a patient and how long it will be provided.[42] The ability to make a *reasonable* recommendation on the frequency and duration of treatment depends on several variables that influence the decision on how frequently and for what duration the services are recommended. These include such factors as the severity of the patient's impairments, the chosen interventions' effectiveness and appropriate dosage, the clinical setting where the services are provided, and the personal (eg, general health and habits) and external factors (access to insurance) associated with the patient[43-46] (Figure 4.3).

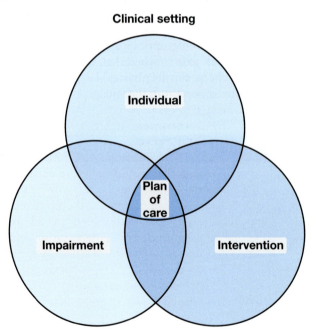

Figure 4.3 Factors that influence frequency and duration of care.

reflective practice – to cognitively review the patient encounter and decide if and how the treatment might be improved to better align with the desired outcomes

Chapter 4 / The Influencer in Health Care

In the current environment of evidence-based practice and cost control, justification of frequency and duration based solely on the available published evidence would be very limited. With multiple factors to be considered by various constituents (eg, the patient, therapists, caregivers, administrators, and third-party payers), the practitioner must work with the patient during each session to discuss, evaluate, and reflect on the patient's response to the treatment provided. This collaborative process of clinical reasoning, an aspect of reflective practice, promotes the development of expertise in clinical practice.[47] Ongoing discussions on the patient's understanding of the treatment and recovery process, current expectations, and current objective data guide the direction of the treatment plan. Are the appropriate factors in this process being considered? Are they being weighted correctly? Is the most effective intervention being provided by the most appropriate provider? Clarity and communication on the factors relating to frequency and duration decisions should aid in the process of developing an appropriate level of services to promote the optimal outcome for the patient. The process begins by identifying the needs and goals of the patient in the clinical setting where the patient receives care. The frequency and duration of treatment will be based on the clear and understandable goals and expectations set up at the initial evaluation for this specific episode of care. Agreement with the patient and family/caregivers concerning the established goals is necessary for a manageable plan of care that can be timely, and in the end, evaluated for its effectiveness in producing the desired outcome. Determining the frequency and duration of care is a dynamic process with several variables that can alter the course of treatment. These variables can include the availability of a willing and capable caregiver, the effectiveness of the available interventions on the identified impairments, financial constraints, or the availability and use of assistive technology. Identification of those variables and their influence on the outcomes is important to document and monitor during the progression in the plan of care.

If the intervention used requires frequent administration in order to effect a change, the ability and compliance of the caregiver are vital to the establishment of the frequency of visits. If muscle strengthening is the key to goal achievement and there is no willing and able caregiver, then the frequency of strengthening exercises provided by a practitioner may need to be 3 to 5 days a week in order to promote muscle strengthening. If a caregiver is willing and able, then 1 time a week may be all that is necessary to monitor and progress the program. If the caregiver is competent in the management of the condition, then 1 time a month may be all that is needed to evaluate the effectiveness of the plan of care. The ability to work as a team, including the caregiver, is an important factor in determining the frequency of intervention as well as the duration.

The duration of the episode of care is determined by a well-established plan of care that outlines the expected sequence of events that would move the patient to their established goals. The plan should include reasonable timelines for improvements that take into consideration the acuity level of the patient, the impairments, the effectiveness of the interventions, and the setting where the interventions are delivered. In addition, the plan should consider the external factors of caregiver support and the available financial resources, as well as other known barriers or facilitators to the attainment of the established goals and outcomes (See Figure 4.3). Changes in the patient or family's situation, concerns, schedules, and priorities are also important factors that can impact the duration of care. A relapse of the illness, the consistency of the caregiver, or compliance with the home program

clinical reasoning – an aspect of reflective practice when the provider works with the patient, or the patient's presenting signs and symptoms, and discusses, evaluates, and reflects on the patient's response to the treatment provided and determines the next course of action

may significantly impact the intended outcome of services. Management of the duration of the episode of care should be monitored through appropriate and objective documentation, which can be used to educate the patient, caregivers, and other team members, on the progress toward the intended goals and outcomes.

Documentation

Documentation is an essential component of health care and is a key factor in the patient management process. By definition, documentation is any entry into a patient's record that identifies that care or a service has been provided.[48] This occurs at every visit or encounter and is used to record a patient's performance during a particular treatment session and the patient's response to the interventions during an episode of care. This documentation should contain objective information regarding the effectiveness of the intervention during the session. This objective data reflects the rate of progress and goal attainment. Many of the interventions provided in health care are aimed at making quantitative and qualitative changes in the patient's health and ability to move and interact within the environment. Capturing and communicating this information is essential to the success of the plan of care, producing outcomes, and providing justification (to the patient, administrators, and payers) for the services provided.

In order to promote this success, written information should be objective, clear, concise, organized and should reflect current practice. Documentation, when used to justify an intervention or as evidence toward outcomes, requires a high standard of reliability and validity. Additionally, it has to be understood by all members of the health care team associated with the management of the patient's care. Today, it is not uncommon for health care services, in some settings, to be delivered by more than one provider. In addition, other caregivers will implement specific strategies or activities in daily routines at home or at school. In order to promote consistency, this should involve the use of understandable and agreed upon terminology, clear communication, and collaboration among all the members of the team, including the family (Box 4.7).

In today's health care environment, providers and administrators are working in an environment of regulations and the need to justify the costs of services, trying to balance cost and quality effectively. The participation of the provider is crucial in this process, providing meaningful information on the patient's current status, the projection for future visits, and the rate of progress that the patient is making in the plan of care. Utilizing what was documented is just as important as capturing information clearly and objectively.

Utilization of Daily Documentation

At each visit, documentation is required that should be organized in some consistent format. Organizing information into subjective, objective, assessment, and plan (SOAP notes) is one way of structuring that information. The SOAP note format separates the documented information into subjective information, objective information, the overall assessment of the current interventions, and a plan for the future. Documenting *subjective* information should be limited to that which is relevant to the plan of care or which could have a significant impact on the treatment plan. Key points of the subjective report are the patient's symptoms, currently and since the last visit, and the reported effectiveness of any interventions from the last visit. Remember that a symptom is defined from the patient's point of view, conveying what the patient experiences. Signs are the data collected by the

symptom – defined from the patient's point of view, what the patient experiences
signs – the data collected by the practitioner from the clinical tests and measures

Chapter 4 / The Influencer in Health Care

BOX 4.7 • Terminology

Levels of Assistance

Independent: No assistance or supervision is necessary to safely perform the activity with or without assistive devices or modifications.

Minimal: One point of contact is necessary for the safe performance of the activity, including helping with the application of the assistive device, orthotic, or prosthetic and/or the stabilization of the assistive device, or 25% effort on the caregiver's part is needed to complete the task.

Moderate: Two points of contact are necessary (by one or more people) for the safe performance of the activity, or 50% effort on the caregiver's part is needed to complete the task.

Maximal: Three points of contact are necessary (by one or more people) for the safe performance of the activity, or 75% effort on the caregiver's part is needed to complete the task.

Dependent: The patient is totally dependent and does not assist.

Adapted from Shields RK, Leo KC, Miller B, Dostal WF, Barr R. An acute care physical therapy clinical practice database for outcomes research. *Phys Ther.* 1994;74(5):463-470.

Impairment in Balance

The following definitions can be separated into static and dynamic balance. If the patient's balance is evaluated using an assistive device, it should be noted in the documentation.

The degree of impairment is based on the reported frequency of loss of balance.

Normal: Able to maintain static and dynamic positions against maximal resistance; displays age-appropriate balance reactions; independent in balance activities without limiting functional ability; able to weight shift in all directions without limitations.

Mild: Able to maintain static positions against moderate resistance; independent in dynamic balance activities but experiences an occasional loss of balance, without consequence. Loss of balance does not occur daily. May limit some functional ability; no support needed for routine activities; occasional use of an assistive device for some activities; weight shift limitations are evident.

Moderate: Requires supervision or contact guarding during static and dynamic activities secondary to daily loss of balance. Balance deficit impacts functional ability. Needs an assistive device to perform activities safely.

Severe: Requires physical assistance to maintain static and/or dynamic balance; unable to move trunk from midline without some level of assistance secondary to loss of balance.

Absent: No evidence of any balance reactions/responses in either static or dynamic positions.

Reprinted with permission from Drnach M. Physical therapy and children. In: Drnach M, ed. *The Clinical Practice of Pediatric Physical Therapy: From the NICU to Independent Living.* Wolters Kluwer Health/Lippincott Williams and Wilkins; 2008:3-30.

Impairment in Coordination

For the extremity tested: Based on the patient's age and the degree to which the impairment limits performance of the extremity in activities of daily living.

Normal: Able to demonstrate age-appropriate reciprocal movement patterns at the expected speed and rhythm; does not limit functional activities

Mild: Able to demonstrate age-appropriate reciprocal movement patterns at a decreased speed and/or rhythm; does not significantly limit daily functional activities but may alter the quality of movement.

Moderate: Able to demonstrate age-appropriate reciprocal movement patterns at a decreased speed and/or rhythm; does limit daily functional activities

Severe: Attempts to perform but cannot complete age-appropriate reciprocal movement patterns; significantly limits functional activities

Absent: No evidence of any ability to demonstrate reciprocal movement patterns

Reprinted with permission from Drnach M. Physical therapy and children. In: Drnach M, ed. *The Clinical Practice of Pediatric Physical Therapy: From the NICU to Independent Living.* Wolters Kluwer Health/Lippincott Williams and Wilkins; 2008:3-30.

practitioner from the clinical tests and measures. *Objective* information is the heart of the clinical note. Objective information should clearly demonstrate the changes in the patient's status as it relates to the established plan of care. In addition to the narrative, a flow chart could also be constructed to visually see the change in the patient's objective data over time. Flow charts without a supporting narrative do not meet the requirements of comprehensive documentation but are very helpful in monitoring the rate of patient progress or lack of progress. Monitoring a patient's performance in this manner can also alert the provider to a lack of patient response over time (eg, 2 weeks) and the need to alter or replace the intervention. *Assessment* of the patient's response to treatment should also include an assessment of the progress in the overall plan of care. Interpretations of the objective measures and the rate at which the patient is progressing should be noted. An example of an assessment: The patient has improved in her transition skills, now requiring minimum assistance to negotiate the stairs with a standard cane and assist of the handrail. She has met her goal of walking 50 feet over level surfaces with the assist of a standard cane. Her moderate impairment in upper extremity coordination remains unchanged since her initial evaluation. She has met 66% (two of three) of the goals stated in her initial evaluation.

If it is noted that the level of impairment in coordination has not improved in the last 2 weeks, this should trigger an evaluation of the effectiveness of the current interventions for this condition.

After the assessment, a *plan* should be developed to include what is expected at the next patient visit. This provides the patient and the provider with the expectations for the next session and may save time at the beginning of the next session. This is also vital for continuity when multiple providers are used in the delivery of services. By reviewing the previous session's documentation, the provider can see what was planned for the current visit. This aids in planning, ensuring that the recommendations or trials of new interventions take place as discussed, promoting an efficient delivery of services that is patient-centered instead of provider-centered. The timely delivery of services will have an impact on the outcome of the services provided.

Outcomes

The outcome or result of the provision of health care services should be viewed in the context of the established episode of care and the patient's health outcome. Were the goals identified at the initial evaluation met? If they were, is the patient now functioning at the expected level for their age and ability? Is there evidence that the patient's health has improved? Are there current medical or health issues that would limit the patient from progressing further at this point? If goals were not met, why? Were professional services or referrals to other providers appropriately utilized in this episode of care? Was the team effective? Was the insurance-approved number of visits adequate to facilitate a measurable change? These are just some reasons that may explain why a patient-centered goal was not achieved or the expected outcome not produced by the end of the episode of care. But often they are achieved. The health outcome has been met. The patient was satisfied with the services delivered. The overall percentage of goals achieved is a quick and easy assessment of the plan of care and should be determined and communicated to the patient and payer. It is one aspect of the effectiveness of the care provided.

In addition to the number of goals achieved, the use of standardized outcome measures is helpful to demonstrate the effectiveness and benefit of the services provided. In

outcome – the result of the provision of health care services viewed in the context of the established plan of care

Chapter 4 / The Influencer in Health Care

rehabilitation, there are a core set of outcome measures that have been identified by the Academy of Neurologic Physical Therapy and presented as a clinical practice guideline (CPG) to help guide the clinical decision-making and rehabilitation management of adults with neurologic conditions.[49] This CPG is applicable to all adults with a neurologic condition, from acute to chronic, who are seen in the rehabilitation setting. The identified core set are clinically applicable, requiring minimal setup and time to administer (5-20 minutes), and have strong psychometric properties (Box 4.8). They are one example of appropriate outcome measures to use in clinical practice. Additional condition-specific or setting specific standardized assessments should be used as part of the overall outcome assessment that should also include the patient's performance, satisfaction, and efficient use of financial and personnel resources. It is important as health care transitions from a volume-based payment system to a value-based system that the time needed for patient and caregiver education, professional consultation and collaboration be documented to provide evidence and support for the actions that are necessary for a successful outcome.

Communicating With the Payer

Health care insurance companies are in business to make a profit. In doing so, they charge premiums to people who purchase their insurance plans and pay participating providers who delivered those services. The money that is left after this distribution will factor into the profits of the company. Therefore, the reason for the reimbursement is vital to an insurance company's bottom line. Health insurance companies, including Medicare and Medicaid, are managing people's financial risk and, in doing so, have guidelines on what services will be paid and how they will authorize payment for those services. Payments are made for services that are deemed to be **medically necessary** to diagnose or treat an illness, injury, condition, disease, or its symptoms and that meet accepted standards of current medical practice.[50] This is captured in the documentation that is provided and codes that are used to communicate the medical diagnosis and services delivered (Chapter 8). The documentation must show a plan of care that is based on the working diagnosis and the frequency and duration of services needed for the patient to reach the agreed upon goals. Subsequent reports will show the patient's progress toward the goals identified in the plan, with any adjustments to the plan or goals justified. Audits are performed to determine that the insurance company's guidelines have been complied with, that proper

---

BOX 4.8 • A Core Set of Outcome Measures: A Clinical Practice Guideline

Berg Balance Scale
Functional Gait Assessment
Activities-specific Balance Confidence
10-Meter Walk Test
6-Minute Walk Test
5 Times Sit-to-Stand

Specifics on the core set of tests can be obtained from Moore JL, Potter K, Blankshain K, Kaplan SL, O'Dwyer LC, Sullivan JE. A core set of outcome measures for adults with neurologic conditions undergoing rehabilitation: a clinical practice guideline. *J Neurol Phys Ther*. 2018;42(3):174-220.

---

medically necessary – examinations, evaluations, and treatments in health care that meet accepted standards of current medical practice and are deemed appropriate for a specific diagnosis or disease

utilization of services (including tests and procedures performed) were performed, that the benefit of the services provided to the patient is evident, and that the services were delivered in a timely and cost-effective manner. This is done to ensure that the reimbursements for health care services, which are reasonable and necessary, are appropriate, efficient, and aligned with the insurance plan of the beneficiary.

In this collaboration, the provider should know the medical diagnosis of the patient; the clinical services that are medically necessary and available in the specific clinical setting; the amount of services that are appropriate to address the patient's goals and outcomes; and the payer guidelines for documentation, prior authorization, and other payer-specific requirements (eg, a patient with low back pain has to receive a course of physical therapy treatment before the patient will be considered for surgical intervention). This depends on clear and organized documentation that captures objective data that show the benefit of the services rendered. Third-party payers, and patients who pay cash, will want to see the benefit of their purchase. A providers' documentation must clearly show that benefit and the data used in their clinical decision-making process. Having a clear and organized system can decrease the influence of bias or personal opinion in the outcome of the service.

Having clear, objective, and succinct documentation also helps with the verbal communication to a payer or case manager when providing updates, seeking prior authorization or justification for services prescribed. The aspects of interprofessional communication, such as showing respect and providing helpful information, apply (see Box 8.5 in Chapter 8 for additional aspects). This communication can happen in face-to-face encounters or can be facilitated through the use of electronic communication, which can be of considerable benefit to the patient and the organization, improving patient outcomes, satisfaction, and continuity of care.[51-53]

Summary

Health care is expensive, and paying for these services can be a financial challenge for many people. Health insurance is one way to manage that financial risk and is purchased by most people in the United States through either private or government insurance programs. These programs aim to remain financially solvent by sharing the cost of health care through deductibles, copayments, coinsurance, selected providers within the network, established insurance guidelines, and controls on the utilization of services. Providers must be aware of these external factors that impact a person's utilization of health care services. By using a third party to pay for health care services, beneficiaries agree to the structure of the plan they purchased. These purchases are often based on cost and not on the services available for many reasons, one being the belief that the person will not need the service. People do not plan on becoming ill or requiring rehabilitation services or the services of a specialist. But when that does happen, the services, providers, and guidelines of the insurance plan become more relevant. Providers must collaborate with a team of people to develop a treatment plan that promotes the optimal health outcome for the patient. This team includes the patient, other providers, and the patient's insurance company to optimize the utilization and delivery of services toward a satisfactory outcome. This is supported by professional documentation and communication that is truthful, respectful, helpful, and timely for the benefit of the patient, the providers, and the health care system in general.

REFERENCES

1. Center for Disease Control and Prevention. *Health expenditures*. National Center for Health Statistics. Published May 17, 2023. Accessed November 2, 2023. https://www.cdc.gov/nchs/fastats/health-expenditures.htm
2. Kluender R, Mahoney N, Wong F, Yin W. Medical debt in the US, 2009-2020. *JAMA*. 2021;326(3):250-256. doi:10.1001/jama.2021.8694

Chapter 4 / The Influencer in Health Care

3. Kalousova L, Burgard SA. Debt and foregone medical care. *J Health Soc Behav.* 2013;54(2):204-220. doi:10.1177/0022146513483772
4. Cohen R, Cha A. Problems paying medical bills: United States 2021. National Health Statistics Report. No. 180. January 18, 2023.
5. HealthCare.gov. *Deductible.* Accessed September 18, 2023. https://www.healthcare.gov/glossary/deductible/
6. Tolbert J, Drake P, Damico A. Key facts about the uninsured population. KFF. Published December 19, 2022. https://www.kff.org/uninsured/issue-brief/key-facts-about-the-uninsured-population/
7. Gruber LR, Shadle M, Polich CL. From movement to industry: the growth of HMOs. *Health Aff (Millwood).* 1988;7(3):197-208. doi:10.1377/hlthaff.7.3.197
8. Health Maintenance Organization Act of 1973. Public Law 93-222. Codified as 42 U.S.C. §300e
9. Johnson J, Davey K, Grennhill R. Financing health care. In: *Sultz and Young's Health Care USA. Understanding Its Organization and Delivery.* 10th ed. Jones and Bartlett; 2023:95-139.
10. Falkson SR, Srinivasan VN. Health maintenance organization. In: *StatPearls.* StatPearls Publishing; 2023. Updated March 6, 2023. Accessed October 2, 2023. https://www.ncbi.nlm.nih.gov/books/NBK554454/
11. HealthCare.gov. Payment bundling. Accessed October 2, 2023. https://www.healthcare.gov/glossary/payment-bundling/
12. US Center for Medicare and Medicaid Services. National health expenditure summary, including shares of GDP, CY1960-2021. Updated September 6, 2023. Accessed October 3, 2023. https://www.cms.gov/data-research/statistics-trends-and-reports/national-health-expenditure-data/historical
13. KFF. 2021 employer health benefits survey. Section 5. Market share of health plans. Published November 10, 2021. Accessed October 3, 2023. https://www.kff.org/report-section/ehbs-2021-section-5-market-shares-of-health-plans/
14. Institute of Medicine (US) Committee on Quality Assurance and Accreditation Guidelines for Managed Behavioral Health Care; Edmunds M, Frank R, et al, eds. Trends in managed care. In: *Managing Managed Care: Quality Improvement in Behavioral Health.* National Academies Press (US); 1997. https://www.ncbi.nlm.nih.gov/books/NBK233217/
15. Namburi N, Tadi P. Managed care economics. In: *StatPearls.* StatPearls Publishing; 2023. Accessed January 30, 2023. https://www.ncbi.nlm.nih.gov/books/NBK556053/
16. National Archives. Medicare and Medicaid Act (1965). Published February 8, 2022. Accessed October 9, 2023. https://www.archives.gov/milestone-documents/medicare-and-medicaid-act
17. McGuire TG, Newhouse JP, Sinaiko AD. An economic history of Medicare part C. *Milbank Q.* 2011;89(2):289-332. doi:10.1111/j.1468-0009.2011.00629.x. Erratum in: *Milbank Q.* 2013;91(1):210.
18. Congressional Research Service. U.S. healthcare coverage and spending. Published February 6, 2023. Accessed October 10, 2023. https://sgp.fas.org/crs/misc/IF10830.pdf
19. US Department of Inspector General. Data brief. Nationwide, almost all Medicaid managed plans achieved their medical loss ratio targets. Published August 2021. Accessed November 2, 2023. https://oig.hhs.gov/oei/reports/OEI-03-20-00230.pdf
20. Patient Protection and Affordable Care Act of 2010. *Pub. Law* No. 111-148, 124 Stat. 119. 42 U.S.C. § 18001.
21. U.S. Department of Health and Human Services. About the Affordable Care Act. Published March 17, 2022. Accessed October 12, 2023. https://www.hhs.gov/healthcare/about-the-aca/index.html
22. Moy HP, Giardino AP, Varacallo M. Accountable care organization. In: *StatPearls.* StatPearls Publishing; 2023. Updated July 25, 2023. https://www.ncbi.nlm.nih.gov/books/NBK448136/
23. Teisberg E, Wallace S, O'Hara S. Defining and implementing value-based health care: a strategic framework. *Acad Med.* 2020;95(5):682-685. doi:10.1097/ACM.0000000000003122
24. Centers for Medicare and Medicaid Services. Accountable care organizations (ACOs): general information. Accessed October 15, 2023. https://www.cms.gov/priorities/innovation/innovation-models/ACO
25. Centers for Medicare and Medicaid Services. Shared savings programs. Published September 6, 2023. Accessed October 15, 2023. https://www.cms.gov/medicare/payment/fee-for-service-providers/shared-savings-program-ssp-acos
26. Centers for Medicare and Medicaid Services. About the CMS Innovation Center. Published September 23, 2023. Accessed October 16, 2023. https://www.cms.gov/priorities/innovation/About
27. Prusynski R. Medicare payment policy in skilled nursing facilities: lessons from a history of mixed success. *J Am Geriatr Soc.* 2021;69(12):3358-3364. doi:10.1111/jgs.17490
28. Centers for Medicare and Medicaid Services, U.S. Department of Health and Human Services. Medicare program; prospective payment system and consolidated billing for skilled nursing facilities (SNF) final rule for FY 2019, SNF value-based purchasing program, and SNF quality reporting program. Final rule. *Fed Regist.* 2018;83(153):39162-39290.
29. Moslehpour M, Shalehah A, Fadzlul Rahman F, Lin K-H. The effect of physician communication on inpatient satisfaction healthcare. 2022. Accessed November 2, 2023. http://doi.org/10.3390/healthcare10030463
30. Tammany J, O'Connell J, Allen B, Brismee M. Are productivity goals in rehabilitation associate with unethical behaviors? *Arch Rehabil Res Clin Transl.* 2019;1:1-9.

31. American Physical Therapy Association. Productivity standards in the physical therapy workforce. HOD P09-21-23-13. Published December 14, 2021. Accessed October 10, 2023. https://www.apta.org/apta-and-you/leadership-and-governance/policies/productivity-standards-physical-therapy-workforce

32. Hull B, Thut C. Productivity vs. value. Why we need to change the discussion. American Physical Therapy Association, Combined Section Meeting. Denver CO. Published February 2020. Accessed October 10, 2023. https://www.researchgate.net/publication/341385241_Productivity_Vs_Value_Why_We_Need_to_Change_the_Discussion_Presentation_Handout

33. Nagi S. Some conceptual issues in disability and rehabilitation. In: Sussman M, ed. *Sociology and Rehabilitation*. American Sociological Association; 1965:100-113.

34. Clifton D. Disablement models. In: Clifton D, ed. *Physical Rehabilitation's Role in Disability Management. Unique Perspectives for Success*. Elsevier Saunders Publishers; 2005.

35. World Health Organization. The international classification of functioning, disability and health. Published 2023. Accessed October 26, 2023. https://www.who.int/standards/classifications/international-classification-of-functioning-disability-and-health

36. Ustun TB, Chatterji S, Bickenbach J, et al. The international classification of functioning, disability and health: a new tool for understanding disability and health. *Disabil Rehabil*. 2003;25:565-571.

37. Moyers P. Implications of policy and reimbursement for interprofessional rehabilitation ethics. In: Swisher L, Royeen C, eds. *Rehabilitation Ethics for Interprofessional Practice*. Jones and Bartlett Learning; 2020:196-197.

38. Keisler-Starkey K, Bunch L. US Census Bureau. Health insurance coverage in the United States: 2020. Report number P60-274. Published September 14, 2021. Accessed October 25, 2023. https://www.census.gov/library/publications/2021/demo/p60-274.html

39. Berwick DM. The moral determinants of health. *JAMA*. 2020;324(3):225-226. doi:10.1001/jama.2020.11129

40. Rothstein JM, Echternach JL, Riddle DL. The hypothesis-oriented algorithm for clinicians II (HOAC II): a guide for patient management. *Phys Ther*. 2003;83(5):455-470.

41. Kenyon LK. The hypothesis-oriented pediatric focused algorithm: a framework for clinical reasoning in pediatric physical therapist practice. *Phys Ther*. 2013;93(3):413-420. doi:10.2522/ptj.20120080

42. Michaud L, American Academy of Pediatrics Committee on Children with Disabilities. Prescribing therapy services for children with motor disabilities. *Pediatrics*. 2004;113:1836-1838.

43. Kaminker MK, Chiarella LA, O'Neil ME, Dichter CG. Decision making for physical therapy service delivery in schools: a nationwide survey of pediatric physical therapists. *Phys Ther*. 2004;84:919-933.

44. O'Neil and Palisano. Attitudes towards family-centered care and clinical decision making in early intervention among physical therapists. *Pediatr Phys Ther*. 2000; 12:173–182.

45. Effgen S. Factors affecting the termination of physical therapy services for children in school settings. *Pediatr Phys Ther*. 2000;12:121-126.

46. Montgomery P. Frequency and duration of pediatric PT. *Phys Ther Mag*. 1994;2:42-47.

47. Jensen G, Shepard K, Gwyer J, Hack L. Expert practice in physical therapy. *Phys Ther*. 2000;80:28-43.

48. American Physical Therapy Association. Position on Authority for Physical Therapy Documentation. HOD 06-98-11-11 (Program 32) [Initial HOD 06-97-15-23].

49. Moore JL, Potter K, Blankshain K, Kaplan SL, O'Dwyer LC, Sullivan JE. A core set of outcome measures for adults with neurologic conditions undergoing rehabilitation: a clinical practice guideline. *J Neurol Phys Ther*. 2018;42(3):174-220. doi:10.1097/NPT.0000000000000229

50. HealthCare.gov. Medically necessary. Accessed October 26, 2023. https://www.healthcare.gov/glossary/medically-necessary/

51. Papermaster AE, Champion JD. Exploring the use of curbside consultations for interprofessional collaboration and clinical decision-making. *J Interprof Care*. 2021;35(3):368-375. doi:10.1080/13561820.2020.1768057

52. Anderson R. Effects of an electronic health record tool on team communication and patient mobility: a 2-year follow-up study. *Crit Care Nurse*. 2022;42(2):23-21.

53. Block L, LaVine NA, Martinez J, et al. A novel longitudinal interprofessional ambulatory training practice: the improving patient access care and cost through training (IMPACcT) clinic. *J Interprof Care*. 2021;35(3):472-475. doi:10.1080/13561820.2020.1751595

SECTION 2
The Decision

CHAPTER 5

Employment Options

MARK DRNACH

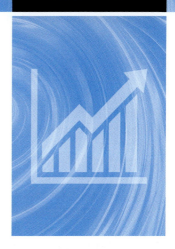

Learning Objectives

The reader will

1. Understand the basic structures of contracts for services.
2. Be familiar with employment options from independent contractor to employee of a business.
3. Identify the basic expectations for working in various settings as a physical therapist or rehabilitation provider.
4. Be able to discuss the key laws and accreditation agencies that impact the behavior of the employer and employee.

Health care providers today, especially those in the allied health professions, often have a variety of options when it comes to the practice setting in which to work. These can range from working as an independent contractor, a health care consultant, a proprietor of a business, or an employee of an entity. As the market for physical therapists becomes more competitive, owing to the increasing supply of physical therapy graduates from an increasing number of accredited programs, the practicing physical therapists will have to strategically consider the employment options that are available.[1] Health care professionals have the option of working full time for an employer and also providing part time or **PRN** (Latin for *pro re nata* or as needed) work for another employer as long as there is no conflict of interest. Generally, part-time employees do not receive the same benefits of full-time employees, and employees who are PRN typically do not receive benefits at all. This aspect of part-time and PRN employment is typically a negative factor for professionals seeking full-time employment that offers benefits. But for those seeking to supplement a full-time job salary or to provide services in a niche market of interest on a limited basis, it is a positive factor. In addition, health care professionals can create contracts with other entities to provide services as specified under the contractual arrangement, thereby becoming independent contractors or consultants. Practice owners, or proprietors of a business, can offer services to individual patients as well as a variety of entities, such as schools, skilled nursing facilities, or intermediate care facilities, through contractual agreements to outsource physical therapists or other rehabilitation providers. This type of business diversification and integration into other practice settings can be a helpful model to sustain a practice during volatile periods in a particular health care environment. And, finally, there

88

Section 2 / The Decision

is the option of working in an institution of higher education as a faculty member, either full time, part time, or on an adjunct basis, to educate future health care providers.

Understanding the basic structure of these business relationships provides health care professionals with options in delivering services in a way that meets both their professional and their personal needs.

Independent Contractor

A health care professional can become an independent contractor entering into private practice with minimal investment. An independent contractor provides services under an explicit contract to do specific tasks for a specified amount of time for a contracting company or business.[2] Independent contractors are self-employed and are not considered employees of the contracting company; therefore, they do not receive the benefits that are often part of the compensation package provided to employees (eg, health care insurance, dental and vision insurance, malpractice insurance, or income and social security tax payments). They are typically reimbursed at an hourly rate for services provided. The hourly rate is higher than the hourly rate of an employee owing to the cost savings associated with all the benefits and taxes that are commonly paid by the employer on the employee's behalf. The reimbursement rate, set by the independent contractor, should cover the self-employment tax (Social Security and Medicare tax) and other costs associated with the delivery of services, such as supplies, mileage, liability insurance, and maintenance of licensure.[3] Owing to the nature of the work arrangement, which is articulated in the explicit contract, independent contractors are not guaranteed long-term employment. There are additional factors that the Internal Revenue Service (IRS) examines to determine if an individual is an independent contractor or an employee. The general rule is that an individual is an independent contractor if the payer has the right to control or direct *only* the result of the work and not what will be done and how it will be done.[2]

The Contract

There are basically two types of contracts, implicit and explicit. An implicit, or implied, contract is created by the intent and actions of the parties involved. If a practice is in the business of providing physical therapy services and a person comes to the practice for that service and the practice agrees to provide the service, an implied contract is created by the intent and actions of the parties involved. It does not have to be explicitly created. It is implied and is legally binding. An explicit contract is a written agreement that creates a legal arrangement between two or more parties (Box 5.1). An explicit contract clearly states, in written form, basic elements of the agreement such as the identification of the contracting parties, a statement of the services that are being purchased, the term or length

PRN – pro re nata. Latin term for "as needed." As an employment status, is also called "casual."

independent contractor – a provider of services that are delivered under an explicit contract to provide services or goods for a specific amount of time for the contracting company

self-employment tax – mandatory taxes on earning that include Social Security and Medicare taxes

implicit contract – an implied contract based on the nature of the business and the intent and actions of the parties involved. It is not explicitly written

explicit contract – a written contract or agreement between parties

Chapter 5 / Employment Options

> ## BOX 5.1 • Sample of a Basic Contract to Provide Physical Therapy Services to a School
>
> ### Basic Agreement to Provide Physical Therapy Services
>
> 1. CONTRACTING PARTIES: This service contract and agreement is between _____ PT, of *city, state* and the County Board of Education ("Board") of *city, state.*
> 2. STATEMENT OF SERVICES: _____ shall provide physical therapy services to eligible students in accordance with the students Individual Educational Plan for the term of this agreement. Services shall include evaluations to determine eligibility, direct and consultative services, and staff training. The hours of services will not exceed 8 hours per week and will be delivered on Mondays and Wednesdays unless other arrangements are made with the provider.
> 3. TERMS OF AGREEMENT: The term of this agreement shall be for the duration of the 20XX-20XX academic school year, excluding the extended school year program.
> 4. TERMINATION: This contract may be terminated by either party prior to the scheduled termination date with thirty (30) days written notice to the other party. _____ or the board, may, by written notice, terminate this contract at any time due to a material breach by the other party.
> 5. CONTRACT AMOUNT AND FEES: The board agrees to reimburse _____ at the rate of _____ dollars per hour and 0.XX cents per mile traveled for services rendered during the duration of this contract.
> 6. BASIS OF FEE CALCULATION: _____ agrees to provide the board with documentation of hours worked and miles traveled. This information will be provided on a monthly basis.
> 7. PAYMENT: Payment for services provided by _____ shall be sent to _____, within thirty (30) days of invoice provided to the board.
> 8. DUTIES AND RESPONSIBILITIES: _____ is responsible for maintaining a current license to practice physical therapy in the State of XX and for carrying the appropriate professional liability insurance. Applicable documentation of services rendered will be provided by _____ and will be stored by the board. This may include the student's evaluations, treatment documentation, monthly summaries, and annual report.
> IN WITNESS WHEREOF, the parties hereto have duly executed and delivered this Agreement for the 20XX-20XX academic school year.
>
> _____   _____
> PT   Date
>
> _____   _____
> Date
> Superintendent
>
> *Note to reader: This example does not provide legal advice and should not be used as such. It is used as an explicit example of the basic components of an agreement between the contractor and contractee.*

of the agreement, how the agreement can be terminated, the fee for services, the basis of the fee calculation, payment, and other duties and responsibilities of the parties involved. It is prudent for a new independent contractor who is creating a contract for services to seek the professional advice of an attorney who specialized in contract law to ensure that the contract addresses the needs and protects the interests of the independent contractor.

A frequent question that arises with an independent contractor is how to set a fee for the services. This can be addressed simply by completing a cost analysis (Chapter 1, Cost Worksheet) to determine the actual cost associated with a full-time employee. Remember that as an independent contractor, a self-employment tax is factored into the equation. This tax rate is currently 15.3% of net revenue.[3] Taking the total cost and dividing by 2,080 hours (the number of hours in a full-time job, working 40 hours per week for

52 weeks in a year) determines the cost per hour. This would be the fee to cover the cost, but an additional amount should be added to obtain a specific profit margin or to meet the going-rate fee for physical therapy services in that geographic location (Chapter 1).

Business Structure

An independent contractor and a sole proprietor of a physical therapy practice are both self-employed. The key difference is that the independent contractor provides services to contracting entities under the structure provided by the explicit contract. A sole proprietor can also provide services to contracting entities but also provides services directly to people and bills them for the services provided. Sole proprietorship is a type of business that has not adopted a formal business structure, is not incorporated or registered with the state, and is the simplest form of a business.[4] The profits made or losses incurred are treated as the proprietor's personal income and are reported as such to the IRS. The proprietor is also liable for any debts, actions, or omissions that caused harm in the delivery of services. To protect a proprietor from personal responsibilities for debts, the proprietor can form a limited liability corporation (LLC). An LLC is a formal business structure that requires *articles of organization* to be filed with the state (Secretary of State) to legally establish the business. These articles typically include the name of the LLC, the principal agent, a statement of purpose, location, and how the business will be organized and managed. This type of business structure limits the personal liability of the owner's assets, such as a house or savings account, in the event the business fails and there are debts to pay or the business is found liable in a lawsuit and compensation for damages is awarded.[4] The owner of an LLC is considered self-employed and must pay the self-employment tax. The profits made or losses incurred are treated as the owner's personal income and are reported as such to the IRS. To be a legally separate business from the owner, the business can be incorporated. A corporation is a business structure that is recognized as a legal person separate from the owners. It requires *articles of incorporation* similar to the articles of organization, which typically include items such as identification of a board of directors, board meetings minutes, an organizational structure, and more extensive record keeping but provides the most protection from personal liability. The corporation will continue to exist even if the original member/members are no longer involved. As two separate entities, taxes are paid on the profits of the incorporated business (corporate tax), and the owner pays taxes on the salary received from the business (ie, twice taxed).[4]

Although there are options for a physical therapist to be an independent contractor or a business owner (Chapter 6), most choose to become an employee, providing services in a variety of settings.

The Employee

The three largest practice settings for physical therapists are offices of physical, occupational speech therapists and audiologists, hospitals, and home care agencies.[5] Only 3% of physical therapists are classified as self-employed workers; the rest are employees of some entity. As such, they receive a salary and benefits reflective of their clinical skills and years of

sole proprietorship – the simplest form of a business. Will include the provision of services directly to a patient or specific market

limited liability corporation – a type of business structure that limits personal liability of the owner but views the owner and the business as the same entity

corporation – a type of business structure that limits personal liability of the owner and views the owner and the business as separate entities

experience, with variations based on the practice's need, clinical setting, and geographic location. The unique feature of being an employee is that the professional becomes an agent of the employer. As such, the employee agrees to follow the established policies and procedures, job description, and service delivery expectations defined by the employer's business model, including the mission of the business, the model of service delivery, and the target market identified for its services. They are also under the employment-at-will doctrine, which states that employment can be terminated at any time by either the employee or employer for any reason or no reason, with or without notice or cause, provided that it is not for an unlawful discriminatory reason such as gender, age, nationality, race, religion, pregnancy status, or disability.[6] Such prohibitions on discriminatory actions are based on the federal Civil Rights Act of 1964 and on individual state antidiscrimination laws.[7] In most states, employment is presumed to be at-will unless agreed otherwise, in which case employment is terminable for cause (ie, a breach of a contractual agreement).[6] As an employee, the health care professional agrees to abide by the policies and procedures of the organization, represent the organization to the public in a manner that is acceptable to the practice, adhere to job description, and receives a salary and benefits that are agreed upon at the time of hire (Chapter 6). As a professional employee, payment received for work provided is exempt from overtime pay in accordance with the Fair Labor Standards Act (FLSA).[8] Exempt employees include professionals who are compensated by an annual salary, who perform work that requires advanced knowledge in a science through formal prolonged instruction and that requires a consistent exercise of discretion and judgment in their work. There are also exemptions for other types of work in executive and administrative capacities. Nonexempt employees can be workers who perform work involving repetitive operations with their hands, nonmanagement employees in production, maintenance, construction, and similar occupations such as carpenters, electricians, mechanics, plumbers, iron workers, craftsmen, operating engineers, construction workers, and other hourly laborers. Employees, independent contractors, and practice owners must have a basic understanding of the FLSA and ensure compliance with the legal requirements for a minimum wage, overtime pay, recordkeeping, and youth employment that affect employees in both the private and the government sectors.[8]

Employees and job applicants also come with a variety of background experiences, cultural perspectives, and abilities. The employer must be cognizant of an inherent bias that may be present when interviewing applicants and in dealing with current employees. The Americans with Disabilities Act of 1990 (ADA) prohibits discrimination on the basis of disability in employment, state and local government, public accommodations, commercial facilities, transportation, and telecommunications.[9] To be protected by the ADA, a person must have a disability or have a relationship or association with an individual with a disability. An individual with a disability is defined by the ADA as a person who has a

---

agent of the employer – an employee of a business who is required to comply with the business' policies and procedures, job description, and service delivery expectations defined by the owner's business model

employment-at-will – a doctrine in the United States that states that the employee's employment is at the will of the employer. Either have the right to terminate the relationship except for unlawful purposes

for cause – a reason to terminate an employment arrangement owing to a breach in the employment contract

individual with a disability – defined by the ADA as a person who has a physical or mental impairment that substantially limits one or more major life activities; or a person who has a history of such impairment or a person perceived by others to have such an impairment

BOX 5.2 • Example of Appropriate Interview Questions Based on the Job Description

Are you physically able to carry out the demands of the job? This may include lifting from the floor, lifting overhead, or carrying objects.
Are you available to work during the company's scheduled office hours?
Do you have the basic skills to access and use a computer?
Are you available to work 40 hours a week?
Are you available to work on the weekend?

US Equal Opportunity Employment Commission. Prohibited employment policies/practices. Accessed July 8, 2023. https://www.eeoc.gov/prohibited-employment-policiespractices

physical or mental impairment that substantially limits one or more major life activities, a person who has a history or record of such impairment, or a person who is perceived by others as having such impairment. The ADA does not specifically name all of the impairments that are covered.[9] Title I (Equal Opportunity Employment) requires employers with 15 or more employees to provide qualified individuals with disabilities with an equal opportunity to benefit from the full range of employment-related opportunities available to others. It prohibits discrimination in recruitment, hiring, promotions, training, pay, social activities, and other privileges of employment. This Title restricts questions that can be asked about an applicant's disability before a job offer is made, and it requires that employers make reasonable accommodation to the known physical or mental limitations of otherwise qualified individuals with disabilities, unless it results in undue hardship[9] (Box 5.2).

The US Department of Justice, Civil Rights Division, provides a free online resource to help small businesses comply with the ADA law and should be a reference for all business owners and employees.[10]

Many federal laws that affect employment begin with the first employee hired (eg, FLSA, OSHA), whereas others become applicable when a practice has 15 or more employees (eg, ADA, Title VII of the Civil Rights Act), or 20 (eg, Age Discrimination in Employment Act) or more employees (the Family Medical Leave Act requires 50 employees). It is prudent for an owner of a practice to become familiar with these federal requirements and to practice in a way that is fair and equitable to all. Obtaining the advice of a Human Resource (HR) consultant or legal consul familiar with employment law is important, especially when establishing the policies and procedures of a business or practice. Each state also has some form of statute (ie, law), sometimes referred to as an Act, which oversees the practice of physical therapy in the state, requires a license to practice, and defines how the practice of physical therapy is provided in that particular state. These statutes create and empower a state agency, commonly a state board of physical therapy (or other licensed health providers), to enforce the Act through rules and regulations that clarify the statutes' requirements in such areas as the need for a referral to provide physical therapy treatment, the ratio of physical therapist to physical therapist assistants and the supervisory requirements, and the requirements for appropriate (ie, approved) continuing education courses and hours. The board or agency controlling the practice of physical therapy in a state should not be confused with the state chapter of the American Physical Therapy Association (APTA). The APTA is a national professional organization that promotes and protects the profession of physical therapy. Individual state chapters of the APTA serve that purpose on the state level. The APTA has a Code of Ethics and Guide for Professional Conduct, which all physical therapists should follow.[11,12] A violation of these professional guidelines is reported to, and handled by, that state's APTA chapter. The APTA may, in response, take action against the individual's APTA membership status. In contrast, a state physical therapy board exists

Chapter 5 / Employment Options

to protect the public and handles any violation of the state practice act and its regulations. The physical therapy board may, when appropriate, take action against the individual's license to practice physical therapy in that state.

There are also requirements on workplace safety as defined by the Occupational Safety and Health Association (OSHA), which has established guidelines on such behaviors as environmental safety, lifting guidelines, and the handling of blood and other body fluids, to name a few.[13] The requirements of external credentialing and accrediting agencies such as Medicare and the Commission on the Accreditation of Rehabilitation Facilities or CARF® require compliance with legal, regulatory, and accreditation standards.[14,15] A private practice owner or administrator must have a working knowledge of these laws and obligations, with established policies and procedures to support the employees and maintain compliance with employment laws and accreditation standards.

As an agent for the employer, the employee will commonly receive some type of evaluation or appraisal of work performance. This should be done on an ongoing basis to help the employee meet the objectives and standards of the business and to promote professional development in alignment with the business' needs and strategic objectives. Most employers will provide an annual performance review. This can come in many forms and can be used as a means to give merit raises in salary, identify areas for improvement, and reinforce the strengths of the employee. These reviews are typically based on the job description, adherence to policies and procedures, patient feedback, and compliance with external accreditation requirements. The system of performance review is a vital aspect not only in ensuring compliance but also in assisting the employee in developing the professional and personal skills that reflect the mission of the business. Performance reviews should be considered as ongoing support and nurturing of a vital and expensive investment of the business, the employee.

There are also additional external rules and regulations that influence the practice of physical therapy in specific settings that require their own understanding and compliance.

Setting Options

Acute Care Hospital

Medical personnel who are employed in an acute care hospital work with patients primarily to maintain the life of the acutely ill; maintain, restore, or minimize the loss of function; minimize the negative aspect of the hospital experience on patients; control pain, and manage the aspects of chronic diseases and their acute exacerbations. Hospitals typically employ full-time employees but will also have a pool of part-time and PRN employees to fulfill the needs of the patients as the hospital's census fluctuates throughout the year. This opportunity provides options for employment on a part-time or PRN basis, either on an individual basis or on a contractual basis with a practice/physical therapy office, to provide personnel as the need arises. This is often seen in the practice of traveling therapists or nurses who work for a company that assigns them to a specific hospital or clinic to provide their professional services for a specific period of time (Box 5.3).

In the acute care hospital, the patient is often assigned a particular physician, nurse, and physical therapist, as well as other health care professionals. Although the range of patient diagnoses, acuity levels, and reasons for admission vary depending on the services the hospital provides, there are some general guidelines that apply to the examination and delivery of services that apply to patients in the hospital setting (Box 5.4). Above all, the health care professional should be competent and confident to identify and intervene or assist with patients who are experiencing a medical compromised situation or event. Interprofessional communication is vital in this setting as the medical stability of the patients can rapidly change and the need for 24-hour care introduces a number of providers who care

BOX 5.3 • Traveling Therapist

Definition: A licensed physical therapist (PT) who is employed with a company that has contracts with several entities that require physical therapy staffing for a variety of reasons such as a short-term increase in demand, difficulty employing a full-time employee, or a short-term decrease in staffing arising from a leave of absence

Basic structure: The company assigns a recruiter to the PT to align the potential clinical sites to the skills the desires of the PT.

The company sends the PT to an identified site, typically on a 13-week assignment. (This is due to typical rental agreements for housing that require a 3-month lease at a minimum.)

The company receives a stipend for providing a temporary physical therapist and then pays the PT an hourly rate. The contract will state the minimum hours required to work and the number of weeks.

Typical salary and benefits: Generally, a higher pay rate than a regular full-time employee

Stipends may be provided for meals, incidentals, and housing. Other benefits may include health insurance, retirement fund contributions, malpractice insurance, relocation assistance, mileage reimbursement for work travel, if applicable. These will vary depending on the company.

Key points: Read the contract before you sign it, and ask questions for clarification. The contract may have a cancellation clause that will limit the anticipated time at the clinical site. Ask about reimbursement if that happens.

The PT is required to be licensed in the state of practice. Some states have compact agreements. These agreements create a way for PTs and PTAs to practice or work in multiple states. The PT Compact website lists current participating states and can be found on the APTA website.[1]

Clinical sites may require 1 year's experience before they will accept a traveling PT. Talk to the company's recruiter to see how common this is for their contracted sites.

The PT will be required to attend an orientation at the new site and learn how to use their electronic medical record and documentation requirements. This will occur at each site and will require additional learning by the PT.

For tax purposes, the PT should have a tax home. This is a permanent residence as defined by the Internal Revenue Service (IRS).[2] The PT should access the IRS website to ensure that they have a tax home.

There are several travel therapy companies that can be accessed via the internet. Be sure to find one that meets your needs. Example: WanderlustPT. Accessed July 14, 2023. https://wanderlustpts.com/

References:
1. APTA. Physical therapy licensure compact. Accessed July 13, 2023. https://www.apta.org/your-practice/licensure/licensure-compact
2. Internal Revenue Service. Business travel expense. Accessed July 14, 2023. https://www.irs.gov/taxtopics/tc511

---

for patients and make decisions on their management (Chapter 8). The physical therapist should take the time to become familiar with the unique requirements of the job, including the common physical therapy interventions (Box 5.5); increased diligence in monitoring the patient's response to treatment; the controls to decrease the risk of infection to both the provider and the patient (Box 5.6); and the policies and procedures established by the hospital to provide safe, effective, and compliant care.

Most hospitals are voluntarily accredited through an external organization such as *The Joint Commission on Accreditation of Healthcare Organizations* (JCAHO, referred to

BOX 5.4 • Common Examinations for an Acutely Ill Patient

Chart review
Medical status
Lab values (eg, ABGs, hematocrit and hemoglobin levels)
Isolation status
Medical restrictions
Appropriateness for physical therapy today

Patient
Vital signs: body temperature, blood pressure, heart rate, respiration rate, oxygen saturation, pain
Level of consciousness
Identification of lines and ports used in the medical management.
Bed mobility
Skin integrity/surgical site
Transfer skills
Balance
Functional mobility within the hospital setting
Gait pattern
Safety
Use of assistive devices
Ability to participate in self-care

Patient and Caregiver
General emotional status at time of visit
Ability to cope with current situation or recommendations
Knowledge and understanding of instructions
Ability to participate in a home program

as The Joint Commission).[16] A facility with a JCAHO accreditation has demonstrated that they have met the standards for patient care issued by the accrediting body that represents a body of their peers (eg, physicians, nurses, hospital administrators, other health care professionals). Facilities are accredited for a period of time, must regularly submit predetermined data to maintain their accreditation, and must be reaccredited after a specific period of time. Accreditation is an ongoing process with standards that generally address patient safety, quality of patient care, patient satisfaction, and performance measurement. It is expected that employees are familiar with the accreditation standards relevant to their position and may be asked questions regarding those standards during an unannounced site visit (ie, the hospital administration and employees will be notified in the morning that the site team is visiting the hospital that day).[16]

The goal of the services provided in the acute care hospital setting is to maintain the life of the patient and promote recovery and some level of independence, including mobility, given the current medical status of the patient. Once the patient is medically stable, based on the patient's needs and potential, the patient can be discharged to home, home care services, outpatient services, or an inpatient rehabilitation program.

Inpatient Rehabilitation

For a patient to be eligible for inpatient rehabilitation, there must be reason to believe that the patient has not met their full level of independence and has the potential to benefit

BOX 5.5 • Common Physical Therapy Interventions Used in the Acute Care Setting

Therapeutic exercise
Functional mobility
Aerobic capacity/endurance to activity
Balance and coordination training
Fall prevention
Body mechanics for bed mobility and transfers
Gait training/stair negotiation
Activities of Daily Living (ADL) training
Dressing
    Using the toilet
Device/equipment fit and training
    Use of crutches/walker
    Use of orthotics
Manual therapy techniques
    Range of motion
Joint mobilization
Pain management
Airway clearance techniques
Respiratory muscle training
Integumentary repair and protection
Provide discharge recommendations regarding therapy needs, patient and caregiver education,
    safety, and equipment needs.

Adapted with permission from Bobish T, Stanger M. Providing services in the clinical setting: neonatal intensive care unit and inpatient. In: Drnach M, ed. *The Clinical Practice of Pediatric Physical Therapy: From the NICU to Independent Living*. Wolters Kluwer Health/Lippincott Williams and Wilkins; 2008:115-140.

from rehabilitative services. The patient should also be able to tolerate several hours of therapy service a day and have the need for more than one type of rehabilitation service, such as physical therapy, occupational therapy, or speech therapy (Box 5.7). Inpatient rehabilitation provides an intensive comprehensive interdisciplinary approach to the restoration of function. An inpatient rehabilitation unit can be a free-standing facility or a specialized unit within an acute care hospital. The Centers for Medicare and Medicaid Services (CMS) criteria for admission to an inpatient rehabilitation hospital include a patient who is medically stable and able to tolerate a minimum of 3 hours of rehabilitation therapy a day for at least 5 days per week.[17]

The multidisciplinary inpatient rehabilitation team includes physicians, nurses trained in rehabilitation, dieticians, occupational therapists, physical therapists, speech pathologists, psychologists, social workers, and orthotists. Interprofessional communication is vital (Chapter 8). The patient's family and caregivers are an integral part of the team throughout the rehabilitation process. Multidisciplinary teams will function differently among rehabilitation facilities. Some teams may work as an interdisciplinary team or even a transdisciplinary team at times while in other facilities the team will remain a multidisciplinary team, with each discipline working separately on their own goals. In the ideal scenario, the team will work as an interdisciplinary team, with all members aware of and striving toward the same goals. Skills of working as a team member are important in this setting as

BOX 5.6 • Common Infections Seen in the Acute Care Setting

Three of the more common infections encountered in the acute care hospital are methicillin-resistant *Staphylococcus aureus* (MRSA), vancomycin-resistant *Enterococcus* (VRE), and *Clostridium difficile* (C. diff).

Patients with prolonged hospital stays and heavy antimicrobial therapy are at an increased risk for acquiring **methicillin-resistant *Staphylococcus aureus*** (MRSA). MRSA frequently colonizes in the nose, axilla, groin, and/or wound sites, including burns. The most common mode of transmission is by contact. Droplet/contact precautions are used for patients infected with MRSA.

Vancomycin-resistant *Enterococcus* (VRE) is a bacterium that colonizes in the gastrointestinal tract. Patients with prolonged hospital stays and antimicrobial therapy are at risk for acquiring VRE. The most common mode of transmission is by contact. Contact precautions are used for patients infected with VRE.

Clostridium difficile (C. diff) is a bacterium that colonizes in the large bowel or colon. It releases a toxin that causes diarrhea and abdominal pain. Patients who had abdominal surgery or are receiving antibiotics or chemotherapy are at an increased risk for acquiring C. diff. The most common mode of transmission is by contact. Contact precautions are used for patients infected with C. diff.

Reprinted with permission from Bobish T, Stanger M. Providing services in the clinical setting: neonatal intensive care unit and inpatient. In: Drnach M, ed. *The Clinical Practice of Pediatric Physical Therapy: From the NICU to Independent Living*. Wolters Kluwer Health/Lippincott Williams and Wilkins; 2008:115-140.

the coordination of care and the plans for discharge are significant factors. Weekly multi-disciplinary conferences, or care-coordination conferences, are held on most rehabilitation units to address the status of the patient, plans for discharge, teaching and equipment that is needed prior to discharge, and the status of caregivers' competency with carryover of care at home. This is a significant transition as the patient and the family lose the support and

BOX 5.7 • Common Admission and Discharge Criteria for Inpatient Rehabilitation

Admission:
The patient:
    is medically stable
    has not reached full potential for independence
    has potential to benefit from therapy services
    is able to participate in 3 hours of therapy a day
    is in need of more than one rehabilitative service
Discharge:
The patient:
    has reached his potential for independence or can achieve this on an outpatient basis
    no longer requires the comprehensive services of inpatient rehabilitation
    is able to be cared for at home
    can access the level of rehabilitation services on an outpatient basis

Reprinted with permission from Stanger M. Providing services in the clinical setting: rehabilitation and outpatient. In: Drnach M, ed. *The Clinical Practice of Pediatric Physical Therapy: From the NICU to Independent Living*. Wolters Kluwer Health/Lippincott Williams and Wilkins; 2008:141-172.

input of the intensive medical and rehabilitation services that are provided in the acute care and inpatient rehabilitation facilities. This can be a daunting time as families and caregivers are expected to assume more of the responsibility for the patient's care, especially if the patient has not recovered as the family or caregivers desired or anticipated (see Box 5.7).

In addition to federal laws and regulations that impact the delivery of health care, (eg, Health Insurance Protection and Accountability Act [HIPAA], OSHA, State Practice Act) most rehabilitation hospitals are accredited through an external organization such as the Commission *on Accreditation of Rehabilitation Facilities* (CARF).[15] The mission of CARF is to promote quality, value, and optimal outcomes of services through accreditation that centers on enhancing the lives of the persons served.[18] CARF accreditation signifies that the facility has demonstrated a commitment to continually enhance the quality of their services and to focus on the satisfaction of the patients served. Examples of values of quality of service are the inclusion of patients in the design of their treatment plans, services that are individualized to meet patients' unique needs, patients who are satisfied with the services they have received, and utilization of data from a continuous performance improvement system to manage the quality of services delivered to patients. As in the acute care hospital, the inpatient rehabilitation facility provides 24-hour supervision and care. The level of service is much higher than on an outpatient basis owing to the patient's medical status and their need for intensive rehabilitation invention.

Outpatient Rehabilitation/Outpatient Clinic

Criteria for admission to an outpatient program will vary among facilities but most require that, at a minimum, the patient is medically stable and has the potential to benefit from outpatient services. The services are typically delivered by one discipline, for a specific period of time (eg, 1 hour session), for a number of days per week, with periodic progress reports and reevaluations to determine the need for ongoing intervention. In this setting, the intensity of service delivery is much less, and more emphasis is placed on home exercise programs and caregiver education. Service provision in this setting also requires the patient to leave the home or be transported to the outpatient facility by a family member or caregiver, making the compliance with participation contingent on other factors, such as transportation and availability of a driver, if necessary. Individual facilities may also have specific admission criteria related to age (eg, pediatric), diagnosis (musculoskeletal injuries, cerebral vascular accidents), or skill set of the employees (sports medicine, pelvic health), and many will have policies that allow for discharge or discontinuation of the patient for frequent appointment no shows, cancellations, or a lack of demonstrated progress over a specified period of time (Box 5.8). This can be a challenging period (ie, episode of care) if the patient has not returned to their prior level of functioning by the end

BOX 5.8 • Discharge Criteria From Outpatient Facility/Clinic

The patient:
- has met the goals identified at the beginning of the episode of care
- has reached their potential for functional independence at this time
- is no longer benefiting from the interventions provided
- can access and safely utilize community resources/settings to address their health and wellness needs

Stanger M. Providing services in the clinical setting: rehabilitation and outpatient. In: Drnach M, ed. *The Clinical Practice of Pediatric Physical Therapy: From the NICU to Independent Living.* Wolters Kluwer Health/Lippincott Williams and Wilkins; 2008:141-172.

Chapter 5 / Employment Options

of the episode or if the patient has to adjust to, and accept, a new level of functioning owing to a chronic illness or acquired disability. Once again, communication is important (Chapter 8). Establishing patient-centered goals, realistic timelines, and ongoing patient and caregiver education on the effectiveness of the interventions, compliance with the plan of care, and the progress made or not made toward the identified goals are important in transitioning the responsibility for a patient's health and functioning from the health care provider to the patient.

Outpatient health care services differ from those provided in an inpatient rehabilitation setting in several key areas. Besides the availability of the patient, the other providers of services (eg, physician, other therapists) may not be readily available to consult or discuss the patient's progress, requiring more time to coordinate that discussion at a convenient time, typically by phone. Also, the provider must obtain patient consent to share information with each individual provider of care at other sites to ensure that the continuity of care, and the information provided about the patient, is efficient and timely. The patient's initial entry into outpatient services will vary among states depending on direct access regulations and state practice acts. Many states will require a prescription for outpatient physical therapy either at the onset of services or within a defined time period after the initiation of services. Third party payers will have different reimbursement structures and different visit allowances that impact the plan of care. These external factors can be a challenge and frustrate the delivery of care unless properly understood and managed. Maintaining a skill set or certification of outpatient therapists that provide specialty care, such as sports medicine or pelvic health, are also an additional factor in providing care in this setting (Box 5.9).

The progress that is often accomplished by a patient in the rehabilitation or outpatient setting can be very rewarding for all members involved and highlights the successful teamwork, care, and communication that contributed to the patient's optimal functional independence.

Home Health Agency/Home Care

When a patient is discharged from the acute care setting, they may not be appropriate for either inpatient rehabilitation or outpatient services. Home health care is a covered service under the Medicare Part A program and consists of part time, medically necessary, skilled care (nursing, physical therapy, occupational therapy, and speech-language therapy) that is ordered by a physician.[19] This setting offers an opportunity for the health care professional to work either full time or part time or as a PRN employee and typically has a lower daily visit expectation than other clinical settings. This is

---

BOX 5.9 • Examples of Clinics That Specialize in Particular Patient Diagnosis or Population (Typically Part of a Larger Health Care System But May Be a Private Practice)

Sports medicine
Pelvic health
Pediatric
Vestibular and balance
Pulmonary rehabilitation
Industrial medicine
Cardiac rehabilitation
Wound care

partly because of the traveling required to provide services in the patients' homes. There also documentation is required, especially if the patient is receiving home care services from a Medicare certified Home Health Agency (HHA)[20] (Box 5.10). The Outcome and Assessment Information Set (OASIS) is a group of standard data elements HHAs integrate into their comprehensive assessment to collect and report quality data to the CMS[21] (Box 5.11). A physical therapist is qualified to complete this comprehensive assessment, although a physical therapist assistant is not. Services that establish eligibility for the Medicare home health benefit include skilled nursing, physical therapy, and speech therapy but not occupational therapy, although an OT can complete the OASIS form. The amount of travel, documentation requirements, and lack of working directly with coworkers are some of the challenges of working in home care. But providing services in a patient's home can be both enjoyable and rewarding. Patients are generally happy to be home and enjoy their home environment. The provider gets to interact with others in the patient's family and the patient's circle of friends. But there are some unique features to this setting. Preventing infections, interacting with pets (which may be aggressive, protective, or just curious), limited available therapy equipment, maintenance of equipment that is in the home, encountering challenging family dynamics, and addressing environmental safety issues can be challenging and often require good communication, education, and working within the family dynamics and cultural practices that are more evident in this setting.

BOX 5.10 • Documentation Requirements

1. Documentation supporting the medical necessity of services should be legible, relevant, and sufficient to justify the services billed.
2. The plan of treatment is written and signed by the patient's physician in consultation with the therapists.
3. When documenting family member/caregiver training and education, the documentation should include the person(s) being trained and the effectiveness of the training and education.
4. The Outcome Assessment Information Set (OASIS) data should support the medical necessity of the services documented in the medical records.
5. The documentation should justify:
   - the individual is under the care of a physician or nonphysician practitioner
   - that the services require the skills of a therapist
   - that the services are of the appropriate type, frequency, intensity, and duration for the individual needs of the patient
6. For restorative/rehabilitative therapy, the documentation should establish:
   - variables that influence the patient's condition
   - services provided at the time of treatment
   - objective measurements that the patient is making progress toward goals
7. In maintenance programs, the documentation must reflect that skilled therapy is necessary to achieve the goals of the planned maintenance program.
8. Physician documentation must support the service coverage.
9. Under a restorative program, the therapist should adjust the exercise program when needed to meet the beneficiary's needs in response to a regular reevaluation.

Reference: Centers for Medicare and Medicaid Services. Medicare coverage database. Home health care physical therapy. Contractor information. Local coverage determination. Documentation requirements. Accessed July 18, 2023. https://www.cms.gov/medicare-coverage-database/view/lcd.aspx?LCDId=34564

Chapter 5 / Employment Options

BOX 5.11 • Elements of the Outcome and Assessment Information Set

Administrative information (eg, National Provider Identifier, patient ID number, patient's address, patient's Medicare number)
Hearing, speech, and vision (including health literacy)
Cognitive patterns
Mood
Behavior
Customary routine activities (eg, living situation, types of assistance)
Functional status (comprehensive assessment)
Bowel and bladder
Active diagnoses (including the International Classification of Disease code)
Health conditions (including pain and falls)
Swallowing/nutritional status
Skin conditions
Medications
Special treatments, procedures, and programs (eg, chemotherapy, respiratory therapy)
Participation in assessment and goal setting

Reference: Centers for Medicare and Medicaid Services. Outcome and assessment information set. OASIS-E manual. Published January 1, 2023. Accessed July 18, 2023. https://www.cms.gov/Medicare/Quality-Initiatives-Patient-Assessment-Instruments/HomeHealthQualityInits/HHQIOASISUserManual

Hospice

Hospice is a philosophy of care with a focus on providing palliative care to patients with a terminal medical diagnosis (Box 5.12). The word "palliate" comes from the Latin word, *palliure*, "to cloak." It is defined as making (the symptoms of a disease) less severe without removing the course. Goals of palliative care are directed toward physical comfort, emotional support, and quality of life. Although all hospices provide palliative care, not all palliative care reflects hospice care. It depends on the diagnosis, the choice of the patient, and how long the patient is expected to live (prognosis). Most hospice programs in the United States developed from grassroots organizations, mainly from home health care organizations. In 1982, the U.S. Congress included a provision to create a Medicare hospice benefit in the Tax Equity and Fiscal Responsibility Act of 1982 (P. L. 97-248).[22] This Medicare

BOX 5.12 • Common Diagnoses in Hospice Care

Alzheimer disease
Chronic obstructive pulmonary disease
Heart failure
Senile degeneration of the brain
Lung cancer
Parkinson disease

Reference: Dustman R. Top 20 principal hospice diagnoses for 2017. AAPC Knowledge Center. 2018. Accessed July 24, 2023. https://www.aapc.com/blog/42339-top-20-principal-hospice-diagnoses-for-2017/

hospice – a philosophy of care with a focus on providing palliative care to patients with a terminal medical diagnosis

BOX 5.13 • Physical Therapy Interventions and Some Examples of Their Application in Hospice

The physical therapist should be aware of the contraindications to the use of certain interventions and make an informed decision, along with the hospice team, including the patient and family, of the benefits versus the risk of an intervention's application. In some cases, it may be determined that the contraindication does not outweigh the palliative benefit of the intervention, given the terminal diagnosis.

Coordination/communication/documentation: Coordination of information and interventions. Remember, in a hospice program, time is of the essence.

Patient/client-related instruction: Body mechanics; transfers; positioning to optimize use of the upper extremities for eating or bathing; use of equipment. Reinforce pain management protocol. Instruct on nonpharmacological pain control measures (eg, heat, cold, TENS Unit, massage, relaxation, deep breathing techniques). Instruct home program to maintain strength, range of motion [ROM], balance, positioning to promote comfort. Teach safety measures/injury prevention.

Therapeutic exercise: To maintain function; promote a feeling of self-worth; pain management

Functional training: Self-care/home—strategies to bathe, dress, eat, groom, use the toilet; strategies to allow for participation in household chores or activities; being part of the family

Manual therapy (including mobilization/manipulation): For pain management

Prescription, application, and fabrication of equipment and devices: Identification, prescription, acquisition, and utilization of assistive technology

Airway clearance techniques: Chest physical therapy, assisted cough techniques, proper positioning to promote optimal air exchange, suctioning

Integumentary repair and protection: Education on risk reduction; skin inspection or wound management

Electrotherapeutic modalities: For pain management

Physical agents/mechanical modalities: For pain management or to promote relaxation

Reprinted with permission from Constantine C, Drnach M. Pediatric hospice. In: Drnach M, ed. *The Clinical Practice of Pediatric Physical Therapy: From the NICU to Independent Living.* Wolters Kluwer Health/Lippincott Williams and Wilkins; 2008:253-271.

benefit provides coverage for hospice care for terminally ill Medicare beneficiaries who elect to receive care from a participating hospice. The regulations established eligibility requirements and reimbursement standards and procedures, defined covered services, and delineated the conditions a hospice must meet in order to be approved for participation in the Medicare program. A Medicare certified hospice agency provides services such as nursing care, counseling, physician services, spiritual care, physical, occupational, and speech therapy, durable medical equipment, and short-term inpatient and respite care through a hospice plan of care. The physical therapy services provided in this plan are significantly different than those provided in other settings. The focus is on providing palliative care, education to the caregivers on transfers and use of medical equipment to ease the burden of care, and providing support to the family and patient as the patient lives out the rest of their life in the setting of choice (home or center). This fundamental shift in the focus of treatment can be challenging and often requires periodic educational training of the provider on the concepts of hospice and palliative care. The patient, as well as the family unit, are evaluated and reevaluated continually in hospice by a variety of professionals. This is an important aspect of care because it can identify needs as they arise and provides the family or patient with the opportunity to discuss emotional and difficult topics when they are ready. Physical therapy services may be requested to help the patient accomplish a

Chapter 5 / Employment Options

simple task such as to be able to attend a particular function (family event, school, social, etc) or participate in a family routine (see Box 5.4). These are achieved through the use of appropriate interventions, assistive technology, and caregiver education. Physical therapy services, as one part of the interdisciplinary hospice team, should strive to maintain patient independence through the dying process and to provide the patient and family with appropriate support, education, and assistance.

Physical therapy practice arrangements with hospices can vary from independent contracts providing PRN visits to full-time employment with a hospice agency. The lower and variable visit frequency can be financially challenging for the provider with per-visit arrangements. However, this may work well for health care professionals who wish to add additional hours to their current jobs or who are seeking part-time positions with more flexible hours.[23]

Hospice should be seen as a broader application of a combination of palliative care and interventions that promote functional skills delivered in a variety of settings from the hospital to the home (Box 5.13). Being at home and participating in the family is a highly positive and much desired goal.[24] Patients with terminal illnesses should be viewed as an inseparable part of the family unit, and the goal of hospice care should be to promote an optimal quality of life for both the patient and the family. The rewards and satisfaction of providing care in the hospice setting are powerful as people support and provide comfort to families and patients during this most significant stage of their lives.

Schools and the Individuals With Disabilities Education Act

Rehabilitation professionals, such as occupational therapists, physical therapists, and speech-language pathologist, also have the educational system as a market that utilizes these rehabilitation services in the education of children. The therapists can work as independent contractors or as full-time employees in this setting during the 9 months of the school year. The Individuals with Disabilities Education Act (IDEA, PL 108-446), the current reauthorization of the Education for All Handicapped Children Act of 1975 (PL 94-142), requires that eligible children receive rehabilitation services (referred to as Early Intervention Services under Part C and Related Services under Part B of IDEA) that optimize their ability to develop and learn.[25,26]

Early Intervention

The services provided through IDEA, Part C, Early Intervention, are unique in their focus on the family as well as the child, and those services are delivered in the most natural environment for the child, namely, the home or day care center. Service providers (which includes physical therapists) are often utilized to provide education and strategies to aid the family in their daily routines, coordinate services, and provide support to a family as they learn how to live and manage the day with their new infant. Early intervention services are based on early childhood development and the role of the family in that process. General principles for best practice include a family-centered approach to the delivery of services, where the parents are both recipients and providers themselves, a relationship between parents and providers in which they are both equally respected, and a team that shares the same goals and values while working collaboratively.[27] The providers and family construct

family-centered approach – a principle of care where the parents are both the recipients and providers of care and their input and that of the other professional providers is equally respected and considered in the development of a plan of care

BOX 5.14 • Elements of an Individualized Family Service Plan

A statement of the child's present level of functioning based on objective criteria

A statement of the family's resources, concerns, and priorities

A statement of the measurable results or outcomes expected, including preliteracy and language skills

A statement of the specific early intervention services based on peer-reviewed research, to the extent practicable, necessary to meet the unique needs of the child and family

A statement of the natural environment in which the early intervention services will be provided

Identification of the dates of service, including the intensity, frequency, and duration

Identification of the service coordinator from the profession most immediately relevant to the child's or family's needs

Identification of the steps to be taken to support the transition of the child to preschool or other appropriate services

Reference: Individuals With Disabilities Education Improvement Act of 2004. Public Law 108-446. (Sec 636 (d))

a living environment that benefits the family and child by influencing the child's development during the years that provide the most chance for remodeling the nervous system. A family-centered approach is reflected in the chosen services and interventions that are based on the concerns and priorities of the family and not primarily on the diagnosis or level of developmental delay of the child.

A child is determined to be eligible under the IDEA if the child is less than 36 months of age, has a diagnosis associated with developmental delay, presents with a developmental delay as determined by a licensed professional, or is at risk for a developmental delay if services are not provided (Sec. 632(5)(A)).[25] After eligibility has been established, an evaluation by the appropriate professionals is scheduled to future examine the capability of the child and needs of the family (Appendix 5A). Once complete, a meeting is held with the multidisciplinary team, including the family, to develop the Individualized Family Service Plan (IFSP). The *IFSP* is a plan written in family-friendly language (ie, a language that reflects the family's level of health literacy) that addresses the family's primary concerns, priorities, and resources, and identifies how the team can work together to improve the family's situation. The IFSP must include specific elements that form an individualized plan for the child and family and is the explicit contract for the provision of services (Box 5.14). Establishing outcomes for children in an early intervention program differs from the practice followed in other settings. The entire team, including the parents, using easily understood language, establishes the goals and outcomes. In addition, the outcomes are so written as to be attainable within a specific time period, typically within 6-months. The outcome should reflect the child's and parent's needs and be functional in nature. This may be as basic as "Mark will walk." The family must then state why they want Mark to walk. They may say, "We want Mark to walk so we don't have to carry him all over town." The outcome could then be: "Mark will be able to walk with his family on community outings." The team also documents what the child is doing currently in the process of achieving that goal, such as "Mark creeps all over his home as his main means of movement." The agreement of the measurement or activity that would indicate that the outcome has been reached is also identified. For example, the team could write, "Mark will walk in his home and community as his primary means of mobility."

Finally, the service coordinator talks with the family about transitioning out of the early intervention program. This transition plan is included in the IFSP in order to ensure a

transition plan – a formal plan that provides continuity between one program and another

Chapter 5 / Employment Options

seamless transition into the school system or other appropriate setting. The transition plan must officially appear in the IFSP before the child's third birthday, as specified by law, to allow the family time to decide and prepare for the transition from early intervention services to the appropriate environment (eg, home, preschool, day care).

Special Education

The IDEA Part B provides federal funds to states to assist them in providing a public education to children with disabilities within the state.[25] The practice of physical therapy in the public educational environment was clearly defined with the passage of Public Law 94-142: The Education for All Handicapped Children Act of 1975 (PL 94-142).[26] This law provided for a "free and appropriate public education" (FAPE) for all children with disabilities, beginning whenever the individual state provides public education to children who are not disabled. (Age 5 or 6 years depending on the state.) Contained in PL 94-142 are several provisions commonly encountered in the special education classroom today, including the individualized educational program (IEP), education in the least restrictive environment (LRE; to the extent appropriate, the education of students with disabilities with students who are not disabled, in a regular classroom), and the right to related services (services that assist a student with a disability to benefit from special education), which include, but are not limited to, audiology services, medical services for diagnostic purposes, occupational therapy, physical therapy, rehabilitation counseling, and speech-language pathology services. This federal requirement creates a market for the rehabilitation professional in the educational setting. Local school districts can decide to hire the professional as an employee or contract professionals as independent contractors to provide services as outlined in the students' IEPs as a related service to the student's education.

Related services are defined as those services necessary in special education for a student to benefit from special education. If a student does not need special education, they do not need a related service for special education. Understanding the role of a related service in special education is important in facilitating a collaborative approach toward achieving the IEP goals.[28] Many professionals are educated and trained to function independently within their profession rather than collaboratively with an educational team. Understanding the interrelatedness of the service providers, the educational relevance of the intervention, and the skills of each person involved with the student helps to foster a more collaborative and, hopefully, efficient system of service delivery (see Box 8.5 in Chapter 8).

Once a student has been determined to be eligible for special education, an IEP must be developed within 30 days (Sec. 300.323 (C) (1)).[25] Evaluations by the appropriate professionals are scheduled to future examine the capabilities and educational needs of the student, including the student's functional ability in the classroom and school environment (Appendix 5B). Once complete, a meeting is held with the multidisciplinary team, including the family, to develop the IEP. This is a legal document, developed by a team of professionals and parents to address the educational needs of the student. Adherence to the goals identified in the IEP and the agreed upon frequency of service delivery are required, unless formally changed by the team and appropriately signed. Professionals working in the school system are obliged to adhere to the established IEP, whether or not they took part in the construction of the plan.

IDEA does not require special education programs to maximize the educational opportunities of children with disabilities; it only requires that children receive some

related services – defined by the IDEA as those services necessary for the student to benefit from special education

educational benefit from the special educational program. That benefit should revolve around the students learning skills necessary to access opportunities that will allow them to participate in society after graduation. This distinction is important to understand when deciding on the frequency of services in the educational setting, which has a different focus from Early Intervention or other medical settings with which the family may be familiar.

A unique aspect of the educational setting is the billing and payment for services. As an exempt employee, a professional would be paid a salary for the services provided in a calendar or academic year. As an independent contractor, payment would be provided based on the terms of the contract. In 1988, the *Medicare Catastrophic Coverage Act* (PL 100-360) was signed into law, which allows states to obtain funds through public health insurance programs, namely, Medicaid, to pay for health-related services in special education as long as there is no cost to the family.[29] A family does not have to enroll in Medicaid in order to receive a related service.

Medicaid (Title XIX of the Social Security Act) is required to pay for the IDEA-related services that are medically necessary and already provided by the state's Medicaid Program, for Medicaid-eligible students. The services that are covered and listed on the IEP are subject to the state's Medicaid requirements for coverage, which may include the need for a physician prescription for the services, prior authorization, and appropriate and specific documentation of services rendered. Even if the state's practice act does not require a referral for the provision of services by a physical therapist, the state Medicaid Program may require a referral from a physician for payment to the school district. Proper documentation and submission of additional paperwork for those students eligible for Medicaid would be required. In addition, school districts are given the ability to bill third party payers for services, including physical therapy or other related services, mandated by a student's IEP, with the approval of the parents. In doing so, the state must ensure that there is no delay in the implementation of a student's IEP. Any insurance funding that requires copayments, decreases the lifetime benefit, or results in a loss or decrease in service benefit cannot be accessed without parent permission. Parents are not required to provide the school with their insurance information, and refusal by the parents cannot impair or jeopardize the student's right to an appropriate education.

Similar to IDEA Part C, Part B requires a transition plan included in the IEP in order to ensure a seamless transition from school to postschool activities. These postschool activities can include postsecondary education, vocational training, employment, continuing and adult education, adult services, independent living, or community participation in social programs.

These transition plans can begin at any time but must be identified in the student's IEP no later than the first IEP to be in effect when the student is 16 years old (Sec 614 (d)(1)(A)(VIII)).[25] Early discussions with the student and their parents to identify the student's interests and preferences after graduation are paramount to achieving the optimal outcome for the student. Identifying appropriate opportunities that are available for the student in the community, the degree of participation, the level of independence or assistance required, and the amount and type of employment or postgraduation activities are appropriate goals of a transition plan. Some of the transition services could include formal assessment of career skills or interests, job readiness or prevocational training, and specific job skills training. The therapist can assist in this process by clarifying the student's level of motor functioning and use of assistive technology to aid in activities of daily living, community participation, vocational training, workplace ergonomics, or postsecondary education, to name a few of the options.

Regular Education

Students not requiring specialized instruction (special education services) may still be eligible to receive rehabilitation or related services (services that assist a student with a disability to benefit from special education, including physical therapy services) in order to access the general curriculum and school activities under the *Rehabilitation Act of 1973* (PL 93-112).[30] This law prohibits the discrimination of an individual based on their disability in any program that receives federal funds. Generally applied to the issue of discrimination in the workplace and in the employment and training of adults with disabilities, this important piece of civil rights legislation also addressed the responsibility of the public schools to appropriately educate students with impairments in motor function and not cognition (eg, people with spinal cord injuries, amputation, visual impairments). It identified and established the need for rehabilitation services for the student with a disability in order to meet the student's educational needs as adequately as the needs of the student without a disability.[31] Often referred to by the section of the law that applies to the educational environment, Section 504, no formalized testing is required to determine the student's eligibility, but there are two main factors to identify and report: First, what is the impairment? Second, how does this impairment substantially limit the student's ability to participate in a major life activity (eg, walking, seeing, hearing, performing manual tasks)? If the student is determined to be eligible, the Section 504 Committee (similar to an IEP team) will create an accommodation plan, or a *Section 504 Plan*, for the student. There is no legal requirement for what should be included in the Section 504 Plan as in the case of an IFSP or an IEP, but it is an explicit contract. Basically, the plan should address the identified impairment or disability, how it impacts a major life activity, and how this impact relates to the student's education. The plan should also clearly spell out the necessary accommodations or modifications needed that would allow the student to access his educational program in the classroom or the LRE identified. The Section 504 Plan does not reduce the academic expectations of the student but provides the necessary modifications to enable the student with a disability or impairment to participate and have an equal chance to compete in the classroom.

Unlike an IFSP or IEP, the identification and recording of the frequency and duration of intervention in the Section 504 Plan is not mandatory under the Rehabilitation Act but may be a policy or procedure required by the state. Furthermore, the state's practice act will also dictate the need for a physician's referral and the supervisory guidelines for the utilization of a physical or occupational therapist assistant.

THE STUDENT WITHOUT A DISABILITY All students, with or without a disability, have the right to an appropriate public education, including the right to participate in physical education and extracurricular activities. The physical therapist can also contract with the school district to provide general screenings and examinations of the students' musculoskeletal and cardiopulmonary systems, nutritional screens, preparticipation screenings for sports, and education on prevention of injury, and sport-specific training.

Skilled Nursing Facilities

Long-term care programs provide a variety of services, from residential nursing homes, skilled nursing facilities (SNF), assisted living, or home care to people who are unable to live independently. All of these settings offer employment opportunities for the rehabilitation professional, from PRN to full time, or by contract with an independent practitioner, who provide interventions and plans that promote various levels of activity that have been shown to benefit the physical and psychological health of older adults.[32] Long-term care is not only for adults over the age of 65 years, but this population constitutes most of the consumers of these services.

An SNF is a nursing facility with the staff and equipment to provide skilled nursing care and, in most cases, skilled rehabilitative services and other related health services.[33] A typical resident is an older woman living alone on a fixed income, having experienced a health event that requires additional nursing and rehabilitation services after the acute hospital stay, who desires to return home. Rehabilitation services are provided to meet that goal or to promote optimal quality of life and functioning. It is important to note that most SNF are run for profit by a variety of ownership types.[34] The goal of maximizing profits has to be balanced with providing effective, appropriate, and safe care. The owners are responsible for carrying out the regulatory mandates regarding the mix and ratio of licensed and unlicensed personnel and adhering to the other regulations required by both the state (Medicaid certification) and federal (Medicare certification) governments and The Joint Commission, if participating in this peer-reviewed process. The health care provider is required to adhere to specific regulations that include the development of appropriate patient-centered rehabilitation plans of care, documentation, typically done electronically, recertification of the plan of care by a physician, done every 30 days, and the appropriate utilization of an assistant (eg, physical therapy assistant [PTA], certified occupational therapy assistant [COTA]), governed by the respective state practice act. The variety of providers and adherence to the processes that ensure compliance with regulations while promoting quality, cost-effective care require interprofessional communication and collaboration skills that support and make patient management efficient (Chapter 8). Understanding and working with insurances, including coverage limits, developing appropriate and objective plans for rehabilitation or maintenance programs, obtaining assessments of the home environment, and planning discharge from the SNF, requires good and efficient interprofessional communication, communication with the family and home caregivers, as well as interpersonal communication with the patient, to provide the optimal amount of patient-centered care for the best outcome.

Considering that most of the SNF are certified by Medicare, the regulations related to this certification, referred to as the conditions of participation, should be understood.[34] Medicare's intent to be financially prudent while providing quality care is reflected in the requirements to justify the delivery of service for payment of those services. These have included a retrospective reasonable cost basis (implemented at its inception in 1965), followed by a prospective payment system (implemented in 1997) that introduced categorizing the level of patient care anticipated into Resource Utilization Groups, or RUGs, based on the patient's level of severity or need, and then, in 2019, implemented the Patient Driven Payment Model (PDPM).[35] This current model attempts to improve payment accuracy by focusing on patient characteristics and goals, rather than volume of services.[36]

As the number of Americans over the age of 65 years continues to grow, and the advances in medical interventions continue to extend the life of the patient, the need for rehabilitation services for this population will continue to be in demand. Working in an SNF can be daunting as new regulations and processes are implemented to support cost-effective patient-centered care, but the rewards of assisting an elder patient at this stage in life is very rewarding and needed.

Higher Education/Faculty

There are a growing number of academic programs to prepare students to become doctors of physical therapy. This means there are more jobs for physical therapists who want to enter into the area of academics.[1] This can be accomplished on a full time, part time, or

Chapter 5 / Employment Options

adjunct (teaching a limited number of courses a year) basis, depending on the needs of the academic program, and the desires and credentials of the physical therapist. An employment contract will be prepared that outlines the job duties, typically referenced to a section of the Faculty Handbook that describes them in detail, the term of the contract, the salary, and benefits if provided (part-time faculty may receive some benefits; adjunct faculty typically do not). Academic faculty are typically expected to have a doctoral degree, commonly an EdD or PhD. Many academic programs have a mix of faculty who have earned a DPT and faculty who have earned an EdD or PhD. Other unique expectations in this area of employment established by the Commission on Accreditation in Physical Therapy Education (CAPTE) include the requirement to provide evidence on ongoing scholarly contributions through peer-reviewed venues, continuing education focused on the courses that are taught, and competency in teaching, which includes the development of lesson plans and assessments of student learning.[37] With the increase in distance education, faculty must also become competent in the use of the specific learning management system (LMS), such as Canvas™ or Blackboard™ and teaching strategies, tools, and communication platforms (eg, discussion boards, chat rooms, text messages, email, live video links), to support students' engagement and learning.

Section 504 of the Rehabilitation Act is applicable to the higher education environment. Students who are eligible for reasonable accommodations to their education program, typically in assessments and/or delivery of information, will have a 504 Plan or Accommodation Plan for faculty to follow. Similarly to the HIPAA, which protects a patient's private health information, the confidentiality of the student's educational record is also required to be protected under the Family Educational Rights and Privacy Act (FERPA).[38,39] This law prohibits educational institutions from disclosing personally identifiable information in education records without the written consent of the adult student or, if the student is a minor (under the age of 18 years), the student's parent.

Working in higher education as a faculty member can be a very rewarding experience, educating future practitioners as well as improving and keeping up to date on the current literature and practice patterns of the profession.

Summary

Physical therapists in the United States have several options in regard to practice settings and the level of employment, including working as a proprietor of a practice, working full time for an employer as an agent for the employer, becoming an independent contractor either on a full-time or part-time basis, working part time or PRN as a second job while maintaining full-time employment. These options provide the professional with a variety of ways to earn money to meet their financial goals while learning and applying a variety of skills that reflect professionalism and lifelong learning.

REFERENCES

1. Commission on Accreditation in Physical Therapy Education. Aggregate program data. 2022 physical therapist fact sheets. CAPTE. Accessed July 8, 2023. https://www.capteonline.org/globalassets/capte-docs/aggregate-data/2022-pt-aggregate-data.pdf
2. Internal Revenue Service. Independent contractor defined. Accessed July 13, 2023. https://www.irs.gov/businesses/small-businesses-self-employed/independent-contractor-defined
3. Internal Revenue Service. Self-employment tax. Accessed July 13, 2023. https://www.irs.gov/businesses/small-businesses-self-employed/self-employment-tax-social-security-and-medicare-taxes
4. Small Business Administration. Choose a business structure. Accessed July 13, 2023. https://www.sba.gov/business-guide/launch-your-business/choose-business-structure
5. US Department of Labor Statistics. Occupation outlook handbook. Work environment. Physical therapist. Published 2021. Accessed July 4, 2023. https://www.bls.gov/ooh/healthcare/physical-therapists.htm#tab-3

6. Thomson Reuters®. Fast facts about the employment at will doctrine. Published March 11, 2022. Accessed August 21, 2023. https://legal.thomsonreuters.com/en/insights/articles/at-will-employment-doctrine
7. Civil Rights Act of 1964 (PL 88-352). Title VII [42 USC § 2000e(2)]
8. US Department of Labor. Fair Labor Standards Act. Accessed August 21, 2023. Wages and the Fair Labor Standards Act | U.S. Department of Labor (dol.gov)
9. US Department of Justice, Civil Rights Division. Guide to disability rights law. Updated February 28, 2020. Accessed July 8, 2023. https://www.ada.gov/resources/disability-rights-guide/
10. US Department of Justice, Civil Rights Division. ADA update: a primer for small businesses. Updated February 28, 2020. Accessed July 8, 2023. https://www.ada.gov/resources/title-iii-primer/
11. American Physical Therapy Association. Code of ethics for the physical therapist. Updated August 12, 2020. Accessed July 8, 2023. https://www.apta.org/apta-and-you/leadership-and-governance/policies/code-of-ethics-for-the-physical-therapist
12. American Physical Therapy Association. Guide for professional conduct. *Phys Ther.* 2001;81(4):1073-1077. Accessed July 8, 2023. https://search.ebscohost.com/login.aspx?direct=true&db=s3h&AN=54633388&site=eds-live
13. United States Department of Labor. Occupational Health and Safety Administration. Laws and Regulations. Accessed April 2, 2024. https://www.osha.gov/laws-regs
14. US Centers for Medicare and Medicaid Services. Accessed July 9, 2023. www.cms.gov
15. Commission on Accreditation of Rehabilitation Facilities. Accessed July 9, 2023. www.carf.org
16. The Joint Commission. The Joint Commission FAQ. Accessed July 15, 2023. https://www.jointcommission.org/who-we-are/facts-about-the-joint-commission/joint-commission-faqs/
17. Centers for Medicare and Medicaid Services. Inpatient rehabilitation facilities. Accessed July 15, 2023. https://www.cms.gov/medicare/provider-enrollment-and-certification/certificationandcomplianc/inpatientrehab
18. CARF International. CARF's mission, vision, core values, and purpose. Accessed July 15, 2023. https://www.carf.org/About/Mission/
19. Centers for Medicare and Medicaid Services. Home health quality reporting program. Last modified May 24, 2023. Accessed July 18, 2023. https://www.cms.gov/medicare/quality-initiatives-patient-assessment-instruments/homehealthqualityinits
20. Centers for Medicare and Medicaid Services. Medicare coverage database. Home health care physical therapy. Contractor information. Local coverage determination. documentation requirements. Accessed July 18, 2023. https://www.cms.gov/medicare-coverage-database/view/lcd.aspx?LCDId=34564
21. Centers for Medicare and Medicaid Services. Outcome and assessment information set. OASIS-E manual. Published January 1, 2023. Accessed July 18, 2023. https://www.cms.gov/Medicare/Quality-Initiatives-Patient-Assessment-Instruments/HomeHealthQualityInits/HHQIOASISUserManual
22. Tax Equity and Fiscal Responsibility Act of 1982. PL. 97-248. Title I. Subtitle A. Part 1. Section 122. Hospice care.
23. American Physical Therapy Association. Developing a hospice physical therapy practice. Published July 2015. Accessed July 24, 2023. https://www.apta.org/your-practice/practice-models-and-settings/hospice-and-palliative-care/developing-a-hospice-physical-therapy-practice
24. Benini F, Ferrante M, Trapanotto M, Xacchello F. Palliative care in children: problems and considerations. *Riv Ital Pediatr.* 2004;30:205-209.
25. Individuals with Disabilities Education Improvement Act of 2004. Public Law 108-446.
26. The Education of All Handicapped Children Act of 1975. Public Law 94-142.
27. Carpenter B. Early intervention and identification: finding the family. *Child Soc.* 1997; 11:173-182.
28. Giangreco MF. Related service decision-making: a foundational component of effective education for student with disabilities. *Phys Occup Ther Pediatr.* 1995;15:47-68.
29. Medicare Catastrophic Coverage Act of 1988. Public Law 100-360.
30. The Rehabilitation Act of 1973. Public Law 93-112.
31. The Rehabilitation Act of 1973. Section 504. 29 USC § 794.
32. Agbangla NF, Séba MP, Bunlon F, Toulotte C, Fraser SA. Effects of physical activity on physical and mental health of older adults living in care settings: a systematic review of meta-analyses. *Int J Environ Res Public Health.* 2023;20(13):6226. doi:10.3390/ijerph20136226
33. Medicare. Skilled nursing facility (SNF) care. Accessed July 31, 2023. https://www.medicare.gov/coverage/skilled-nursing-facility-snf-care#:~:text=Skilled%20nursing%20facility%20%28SNF%29%20care.%20Medicare%20Part%20A,to%20use.%20You%20have%20a%20Qualifying%20hospital%20stay
34. Pete Welch W, Oliveira I, Blanco M, Sommers BD. Ownership of skilled nursing facilities: an analysis of newly-released federal data. Data Point. Assistant Secretary for Planning and Evaluation. Office of Health Policy. Published December 15, 2022. Accessed August 3, 2023. https://aspe.hhs.gov/sites/default/files/documents/fd593ae970848e30aa5496c00ba43d5c/aspe-data-brief-ownership-snfs.pdf#:~:text=Most%20

Chapter 5 / Employment Options

SNFs%20are%20for-profit%20%2871.7%25%29%2C%2022.5%25%20are%20non-profit%2C,as%20 corporations%20and%2016.2%25%20as%20limited%20liability%20companies

35. Prusynski R. Medicare payment policy in skilled nursing facilities: lessons from a history of mixed success. *J Am Geriatr Soc.* 2021;69(12):3358-3364. doi:10.1111/jgs.17490

36. Centers for Medicare & Medicaid Services (CMS), HHS. Medicare program; Prospective payment system and consolidated billing for skilled nursing facilities (SNF) final rule for FY 2019, SNF value-based purchasing program, and SNF quality reporting program. Final rule. *Fed Regist.* 2018;83(153):39162-39290.

37. Commission on Accreditation in Physical Therapy Education. Standard 4. Standards and required elements for accreditation of physical therapists education programs. Revised November 3, 2020. CAPTE. Accessed August 5, 2023. https://www.capteonline.org/faculty-and-program-resources/resource_documents/accreditation-handbook

38. Centers for Disease Control and Prevention. Health Insurance and Accountability Act of 1996 (HIPAA). Updated June 22, 2022. Accessed August 5, 2023. https://www.cdc.gov/phlp/publications/topic/hipaa.html

39. Centers for Disease Control and Prevention. Family Educational Rights and Privacy Act (FERPA). Updated June 27, 2022. Accessed August 5, 2023. https://www.cdc.gov/phlp/publications/topic/ferpa.html

APPENDIX 5A

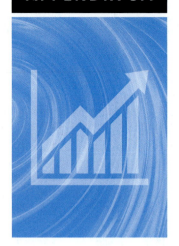

An Evaluation: Early Intervention Physical Therapy Evaluation

PHYSICAL THERAPY

General information:

Child's name: _____ _____ male _____ female

Exam date: _____

Parent's names: _____

Address: _____ Phone: _____

Date of referral: _____

Date of birth: _____ Chronological age: _____

Medical diagnosis: _____

Precautions: _____

Medications: _____

Pediatrician: _____

Other health care services/agencies: _____

_____

Medical and birth history: _____

_____

Other EI services: _____

Chapter 5 / Employment Options

Parent's concerns and priorities: _____

_____

_____

Systems review:

Child's current height: _____ Weight: _____

Communication: _____ verbal _____ non verbal _____ vocal _____ sign _____

device: _____

Vision: _____ Within Functional Limits (WFL): Impaired: _____

Hearing: _____ WFL: Impaired _____

Emotion/behavior during exam: _____ cooperative _____ uncooperative _____ passive

_____ other: _____

Motor control: _____ impaired _____ not impaired.

Motor learning: _____ impaired _____ not impaired

Sensation to touch: _____ impaired _____ not impaired

Oral motor skills: _____ impaired _____ not impaired

Additional comments: _____

_____

_____

Caregiver availability and capability:

_____ Lives with mom who is primary caregiver.

_____ Other: _____

_____ Also attends daycare center. Staff: _____

Tests and measurements:

Range of motion and muscle tone

_____ Range of motion and muscle tone are Within Normal Limits (WNL) throughout the

trunk and extremities

_____ Range of motion and muscle tone are WNL throughout the trunk and extremities

with the following exceptions: _____

Functional strength

_____ Able to touch the back of the head

_____ Able to touch the middle of the back

_____ Able to pronate/supinate the forearm

_____ Able to oppose fingers to thumb

_____ Able to rise from a chair

_____ Able to step up a six-inch step

Rises from the floor

_____ using half kneel

_____ via squat

_____ via modified plantargrade

_____ requiring: _____ assist

_____ Other: _____

Neuromotor development

Reflexes: Primitive reflexes _____ appear integrated _____ are present

Comments: _____

Reactions:

Righting _____

Protective extension _____

Equilibrium: _____ prone _____ supine _____ quadruped _____ sitting _____ kneeling

_____ standing

Balance: _____ not impaired _____ impaired

Sitting: _____

Standing: _____

Walking: _____

During ADLs: _____

Coordination: UE: _____ not impaired _____ impaired

LE: _____ not impaired _____ impaired

Chapter 5 / Employment Options

Mobility:

Transfers: _____ independent _____ dependent

Description with level of assistance needed: _____

Ambulation: _____ independent _____ assist _____ non-ambulatory

Gait pattern: _____

Assistive device: _____

Level of assistance needed: _____

Stair negotiation: _____

Child is independent in the developmental sequence _____

Self care (mark the level of assistance needed to complete the task)

_____ undressing _____ dressing _____ eating _____ toileting _____ bathing _____ other

Comments: _____

Assistive technology or adaptive equipment presently used:

_____

_____

_____

The following information was obtained by _____ report _____ observation

Accessibility of the natural environment:

_____

_____

Child's primary position during play/activities: _____

_____

Analysis of child's motor skills while playing: _____

_____

Analysis of child's participation in activities: _____

_____

List of family's leisure activities: _____

_____

116   Section 2 / The Decision

DEVELOPMENTAL SKILLS CHECKLIST

Developmental Checklist:

(Numbers in parentheses indicate the average age in months at which a child typically demonstrates this skill)

Gross motor

Prone suspension: head above body (2)
Bears weight through legs (4)
Props on elbows when prone (4)
Rolling: prone to supine (5); supine to prone (6)
Sits on floor (6)
Props on extended elbows when prone (6)
Assumes hand and knee (7)
Crawling (8)
Sits on floor for 10 minutes (8)
Transitions to sitting independently (9)
Pull to Stand (10)
Standing (10)
Stepping/walking (12)
Throws ball (13)
Squats (15)
Crawls up steps (15)
Walks independently for a few steps (15)
Begins to jump (18)
Climbs into adult chair (18)
Walking without holding onto anything (18)
Carries large toy two hands (19)
Walks backward (24)
Runs (24)
Stairs: step to step (24); alternates up (36)
Jumps with both feet off the ground (30)
Fine Motor
Grasp reflex (1)
Holds rattle for 10 seconds (2)
Reaches for object (3)
Hands to mouth (4)
Ulnar grasp (4); Palmar grasp (5); Radial grasp (6)
Picks up spoon (5)
Rakes and bangs (6)
Manipulates (7)
Plays with paper (7)
Holds two objects (8)
Developing precision grasps (8)
Hands used for separate functions (9)
Holds, bites, and chews cracker (9)
Uncovers toy (10)
Points (11)
Holds with one hand and manipulates with another (12)

Unwraps toy (14)
Holds three items (14)
Attempts to fold paper (24)
Turns pages of book separately (24)
Imitates vertical and horizontal line, and circle (27)
Holds crayon with thumb and index (30)
Copies a circle (36)
Cuts across paper with scissors (36)

Cognitive

Watches caregiver (1)
Smiles (2)
Looks at object for several seconds (2)
Follows object 180 (3)
Watches hand (4)
Localizes sound (4)
Laughs (5)
Discriminates strangers (6)
Resists removal of toy (6)
Mouths toy (6)
Bangs and shakes (7)
Understands the word no (8)
Responds to name (9)
Looks for object when dropped (9)
Looks for things when you hide them (12)
Looks when asks "Where is the ball?" (13)
Asks for objects by pointing (15)
Stacks objects (15)
Looks at pictures and turn pages (18)
Points to one named body part (18); 4 body parts (24)
Follows two-step directions (18); three-step directions (21)
Holds something in one hand while using the other (24)
Refers to self by name (24)
Understands size difference (27)
Knows full name (30)
Knows if they are a boy or girl (36)
Joins in song (36)

Language

Coos (2)
Produces single vowel sounds (2)
Turns head toward sound (4)
Squeals (5)
"ba," "ka," "na" (8)
shakes head no (9)
Ma Ma and Da Da (10)
Uses two words (12)
Looks at object when you name them (15)
Speaks in two-word sentences (21)

Asks for food when hungry (21)
Uses pronouns (24)
Uses plurals (36)
States first name when asked (36)
Asks "who," "what," "where," "why" questions (36)

Self-Help

Holds bottle (6)
Holds, bites, and chews (9)
Finger feeds (12)
Takes off hat or shoe (12)
Cooperates with dressing (12)
Pulls off socks (14)
Vocalizes or gestures wants (15)
Imitates housework (16)
Uses spoon (18)
Empties dish when done (18)
Uses toilet (18)
Puts toys away where they belong (21)
Attempts to put shoes on (22); Put on pants (24)
Takes off clothes (24); Undresses completely (36)
Uses spoon (24)
Will dry hands (30)
Dresses with supervision (33)
Unbuttons (36)

Emotional/Social

Calms down when spoken to or picked up (2)
Looks at your face (2)
Smiles when you talk or smile (2)
Crying decreases dramatically (3)
Stranger anxiety (6-8; then at 15)
Expresses protest (6)
Likes to look at self in mirror (6)
Shows several facial expressions (9)
Responds to verbal request (10)
Gives toy to adult on request (12)
Plays games with adults (12)
Wants to be near adults (14)
Shows affection (15)
Imitates grown-up activities (16)
Parallel play (18); Enjoys roll play (24); Associative play begins (33)
Helps to dress by putting or lifting foot or pushing arm through sleeve (18)
Notices when others are upset (24)
Shows what they can do by stating: look at me (30)
Follows simple routines when told (30)
Calms down within 10 minutes after someone leaves (36)

Chapter 5 / Employment Options

Impairments:

_____ impaired range of motion   _____ impaired respiratory function

_____ impaired motor learning   _____ impaired muscle strength

_____ impaired balance   _____ impaired motor control

_____ impaired coordination   _____ impaired mobility

_____ impaired endurance

Functional limitations:

_____

_____

_____

_____

Other services, equipment, or assistive device recommendations: _____ none

_____

_____

SUMMARY: _____

_____

_____

_____

_____

_____

_____

_____

_____

_____

_____   _____

Physical Therapist signature   Date

_____   _____

Parent's signature   Date

APPENDIX 5B

School-Based Evaluation, Documentation, and Outcome Forms

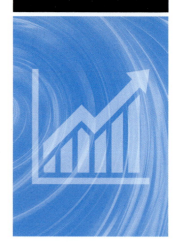

The clinical evaluation form provided is one example of the type of information gathered on students in special education. The form is self-explanatory. The following comments are presented to clarify the process:

Prescription for physical therapy: If needed, the physician's prescription for physical therapy should be obtained and filed in the student's educational record. Although there is no law stating how often the prescription needs to be renewed, best practice is to have a new prescription written annually.

Medical diagnosis: A student in special education may have one or more medical diagnoses that provide information on the possible impairments and prognosis for functional independence.

Medications: Medications play an important role in the general health of a student. They may also affect the interventions provided by the physical therapist. It is important that the physical therapist is aware of the medications that the student is taking and understands their possible effect on the student's performance.

Student's height and weight: An important objective measurement to obtain when considering equipment specifications, lifting requirement, and general growth of the student.

Range of motion: The range of motion chart contains two columns for comparison in measurements taken over time.

Muscle performance: Standard manual muscle testing may not be appropriate for students for a number of reasons. Since the testing is subjective, it is difficult to determine the results of a break test in a student who is very young or who has a cognitive impairment that could jeopardize the testing results. For these reasons, assessing the student's functional strength may provide more helpful information. Through observation, the physical therapist can determine how much functional strength or active range of motion a student has to perform daily classroom and personal care activities.

Educational concerns: Discussions with the teacher regarding the student's physical limitations and their educational goals is the reason for the evaluation. This is an important aspect of the evaluation and is instrumental in determining the need for a related service.

Goals: Note that there are no discipline-specific goals identified on this evaluation form. Goals for the student are created at the IEP meeting with input from all members.

Information for the Physical Therapist at School.

Student's name: _____

Parent's name: _____

Chapter 5 / Employment Options

My name is _____ and I am the physical therapist at your child's school. In order to ensure efficiency in the provision of service to your child, please complete the questions below and return this letter to the school.

The physical therapy examination for your child is scheduled on _____

If you have any questions, you can reach me by calling _____

Thank you.

1. What is your child's medical diagnosis? _____

2. Have they had any surgeries in the past? _____ Yes _____ No

   If yes, what was done and when?

   _____

3. Are you planning for any surgeries or purchase of special equipment in the next 9 months?

   _____ Yes _____ No *If yes, please explain.*

   _____

4. What equipment does your child use, or have, at home? How often is the equipment used? *(Please list.)*

   _____

6. Does your child receive therapy services at another facility, in addition to what they are receiving in the school? _____ Yes _____ No

   If yes, please describe: _____

   _____

Identification of services does not authorize contact. If contact with an agency or person is required, prior authorization will be requested.

Physical Therapy Evaluation Form

General Information:

Student's name: _____ Exam date: _____

School: _____ Classroom: _____

D.O.B.:_____ Age:_____ _____ male _____ female

Medical diagnosis: _____

Precautions: _____

Medications:_____ Prescription for PT.: _____ Yes _____ No

Service provision by: _____ IEP _____ Service Agreement.

Secondary insurance*: _____ N/A _____ MA _____ other:_____

Significant Medical History:

_____ See Parent/Guardian Report, attached

Other _____

_____

_____

_____

Previous physical therapy services: _____

Systems review:

Communication: _____ vocal _____ nonverbal _____ verbal _____ sign language

_____ device: _____

Vision: _____ WFL _____ Impaired

Hearing: _____ WFL _____ Impaired

Cognitive level by report: _____

Emotion/behavior during exam: _____ cooperative _____ uncooperative _____ passive

_____ other: _____

Student's height: _____ weight: _____

Is the student continent of bowel: _____ yes _____ no. of bladder: _____ yes _____ no.

Heart rate: _____ Respiratory rate/pattern: _____

Circulation: _____ impaired _____ not impaired _____

Edema: _____ present _____ present _____ describe: _____

Hand dominance: _____ right _____ left _____ not established

Motor function:

Motor control: _____ impaired _____ not impaired.

Motor learning: _____ impaired _____ not impaired

Sensation to touch: _____ impaired _____ not impaired

Oral motor skills: _____ impaired _____ not impaired

Chapter 5 / Employment Options

Additional comments:

Tests and Measures:

_____ Standardized Test: _____

Outcome: _____

_____ Additional tests or measures: _____

_____

Range of Motion:

_____ Range of motion and strength are WFL throughout the trunk and extremities

_____ Range of motion and strength are WFL throughout the trunk and extremities with the following exception: _____

_____ Range of motion and strength is present as follows

GONIOMETRIC MEASUREMENTS _____ PASSIVE _____ ACTIVE									
Dates	**ROM __/__**		**ROM __/__**			**ROM __/__**		**ROM __/__**	
UPPER EXT.	**L**	**R**	**L**	**R**	**LOWER EXT.**	**L**	**R**	**L**	**R**
Shld. Flex. 0-180					Hip Flex. 0-120				
Ext. 0-60					Ext. 0-30				
Abd. 0-180					Abd. 0-45				
Horz.Add. 0-135					Add. 0-30				
Int. Rot. 0-70					I.R. 0-45				
Ext. Rot. 0-90					E.R. 0-45				
Elbow Flex. 0-150					Knee Flex. 0-135				
Ext. 150-0					Ext. 135-0				
Wrist Flex. 0-80					Ankle Dorsi. 0-20				
Ext. 0-70					Plant. 0-50				
Rad.Dev. 0-20					Inver. 0-35				
Uln.Dev. 0-30					Ever. 0-15				
Forearm Pro. 0-80					Trunk				
Sup. 0-80					Neck				
Fingers					Toes				

Comment: _____

_____

_____

Muscle Performance

Muscle tone:

_____ is WNL throughout trunk and extremities with active and passive movements.

_____ is hypotonic in _____

_____ is hypertonic in _____

Functional Strength

_____ able to touch the back of their head

_____ able to touch the middle of their back

_____ able to pronate/supinate their forearm

_____ able to oppose their fingers to thumb

_____ able to rise from a chair

_____ able to step up a 7-inch step

Rises from the floor:

_____ using half kneel

_____ via squat

_____ via modified plantargrade

_____ requiring: _____ assist

_____ Other: _____

Student is independent in the developmental sequence to _____

Neuromotor Development

Reflexes: Primitive reflexes _____ appear integrated _____ are present _____
_____

DTRs are (0 +1 +2 +3 +4) in _____

Reactions:

Righting _____

Protective extension _____

Equilibrium: _____ prone _____ supine _____ quadruped _____ sitting

_____ kneeling _____ standing

Balance:

Sitting: _____

Standing: _____

Walking: _____

During ADLs: _____

Coordination:

UE: _____

LE: _____

Mobility:

Transfers: _____ independent _____ pivot _____ dependent

Description with level of assistance needed: _____

Wheelchair Mobility: _____ N/A _____ independent _____ assist _____ dependent

Description with level of assistance needed: _____

Ambulation: _____ independent _____ assisted _____ nonambulatory

Gait pattern: _____

device: _____

level of assistance needed: _____

stair negotiation: _____

Self-care in School (mark the level of assistance needed to complete the task)

_____ undressing _____ dressing _____ eating _____ toileting _____ grooming _____ other _____

Comments: _____

Orthotics: _____

Equipment: _____

The following information was obtained by _____ report _____ observation

Analysis of the school environment: _____

_____

_____

Student's position during educational activities: _____

_____

_____

Analysis of student's motor skills for education: _____

_____

_____

Analysis of student's participation in school activities: _____

Analysis of student's leisure activities: _____

_____

Educational concerns: _____

_____

_____

_____

Impairments:

____ impaired range of motion   ____ impaired respiratory function

____ impaired motor learning   ____ impaired muscle strength

____ impaired balance   ____ impaired motor control

____ impaired coordination   ____ impaired mobility

____ impaired endurance   _____

Functional limitations:

_____

_____

_____

_____

Summary/current level of functioning: _____

_____

_____

_____

_____

_____

_____

Chapter 5 / Employment Options **127**

Other services, equipment, or assistive device recommendations/considerations:

_____

_____

_____

_____

Signature, title, and date

This form should be kept in the student's file.

Physical Therapy Documentation Form

Student: _____   School year: _____

Frequency of services as noted on the IEP: _____

IEP GOAL	DATE	COMMENT
Monthly Summary:		

_____

Physical Therapist

County School District

Example of a Physical Therapy End of Year Report

Student: Alek Smith

Number of IEP goals: five

Number achieved: four

Goal achievement rate: 80%

PT service frequency on IEP: 60 minutes per week; direct.

Annual Summary:

During this school year, Alek has made significant progress in his prewalking skills, sitting skills, and moving skills. In October, we initiated bench sitting with the seat tilted forward. This activity was done to encourage a more upright posture of his trunk and to encourage him to move his trunk during seated activities. By December, he was able to move from bench sitting to stance with one-hand assist. In January, we initiated standing against the wall while holding onto a standard walker. By the end of the month, Alek had demonstrated the ability to maintain a grasp on the walker for 10 seconds, with both hands, independently! He received new braces in January, and we initiated walking forward with his walker by the end of the month. In February, Alek received a new wheelchair and made progress in his sitting posture and use of a standard walker during assisted walking exercises. By March, Alek demonstrated the ability to stand for 5 seconds independently and to walk with one hand held for 10 feet in the classroom. On March 12, he took one step on the right independently. By the end of April, Alek was able to walk 50 feet down the hall with one hand held, far enough to walk to the physical education class with his classroom peers. In May, Alek was demonstrating the ability to knee walk 3 to 5 feet, move from lying on his back into a full kneel independently, and move from a full kneel to stance with one hand assist. He can stand at the table in the art room for 5 to 10 minutes. His walking with one hand held has improved in speed, accuracy of foot placement, posture, and control.

During the school year, the classroom reports that Alek has demonstrated an increased use of his left hand. He is more socially interactive and has improved in his listening and following directions skills. Alek is making requests regarding his wants and needs more consistently, and he is compliant with physical activities during gym class.

Recommendations:

After consultation with Alek's teacher, the classroom staff, his parents, and other IEP team members, goals were developed and discussed at the IEP meeting. The IEP goals address Alek's functional skills in the classroom, as well as his mobility and walking skills. The need for direct physical therapy services was determined to be 30 minutes every other week, with indirect services provided to the teacher, parent, and classroom staff for 60 minutes once a month.

Physical Therapist

Chapter 5 / Employment Options

Example of an Annual Physical Therapy Program Report

School Year

Administrator:

During this school year, I provided physical therapy services to nine students at Central High School. Their end of the year reports are attached.

From the data collected, the overall goal attainment rate for this group of students was 78%. This reflects all of the goals identified on their IEPs that were addressed with physical therapy as a related service. If you eliminate the one outlier from the group, who had a 50% goal attainment rate for this year, the group rate increases to 83%.

It has been great working with you again. You have a great program. Keep up the good work.

Professionally:

_____

Physical Therapist

CHAPTER 6

Entrepreneurship

DAVID EDWARDS

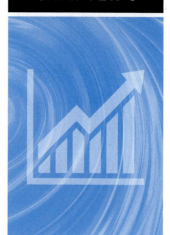

Learning Objectives

The reader will

1. Define and understand the key characteristics attributed to entrepreneurs.
2. Make use of the available internet resources to start a small business.
3. Understand the unique features of the practice of physical therapy in the digital age.
4. Outline the components of a business plan.
5. Summarize the steps needed to begin a practice, from establishing an organizational structure to the strategies for employee retention.
6. Utilize the information in this book to develop a general plan to become a physical therapist entrepreneur.

Many physical therapists (PTs) who want to start their own practice may find that they have not been adequately prepared by their basic education or experience to structure and manage the complexities of planning and operating their own business. The intent of this chapter is to contribute to the reader's understanding of the benefits, inherent challenges, and risks of ownership and provide experience-based guidance for becoming a small business owner for those PTs pursuing this entrepreneurial career path.

Basic Entrepreneurial Skills and Attributes

"An entrepreneur is one who creates a new business in the face of risk and uncertainty for the purpose of achieving profit and growth by identifying significant opportunities and assembling the necessary resources to capitalize on them."[1] Although being an entrepreneur can include a very diverse set of personal attributes and skills, this chapter presents a summary of the most common findings in an entrepreneur's profile.

Action Minded

In making the decision to start a physical therapy practice, being action minded is at the top of the list of attributes a practitioner should possess. Taking action is important not only in the day-to-day operations of running a business once it is started but also, crucially, in the early phases of actually starting the business.

Chapter 6 / Entrepreneurship

As doctoral educated practitioners, PTs are typically very inquisitive, analytical, and thoughtful people. After all, they just invested close to 7 years of learning exactly how to examine every aspect of a patient case down to the very last detail. Careful and extensive planning are part of their everyday thinking. Unfortunately, this extensive level of detailed planning and wanting everything to be just right can, in fact, be a roadblock to starting a business. Learning and extensive planning are necessary, but often, people spend too much time intellectualizing rather than just taking action.[2] When starting a business, a practitioner may not have all of the exact details perfectly in place, but the important thing is to take action and take the first step to actually start the business. A statement frequently heard in the business world is "80% is good enough"[3,4] This is a belief that in business not everything will be perfect, or flawlessly planned. Some things may not be perfectly planned, and unexpected situations will arise. The location of the practice may not be the one preferred, or the equipment desired may be too expensive at this stage of development. But this does not mean that the practitioner should not take actions to start the business. Perfection can be the enemy of starting or advancing a business.

Careful forecasting and extensive problem solving will always be the mainstay of starting and running a business, but a practitioner/entrepreneur should not let a focus on perfection stop progress on actually starting a business or making strategic decisions once the business is started.

Leadership Skills

In starting a business, the practitioner should expect to be in a leadership role. A practice owner will have to lead a group of both clinical and nonclinical employees, collaborating with outside vendors, patients/clients, third-party payers, and other people involved in the business of health care. Leadership skills are of utmost importance in hiring and retaining talent, introducing new services, and ensuring efficiency within the business.[5]

Although there are many leadership styles that are beyond the scope of this chapter, it would be wise to reflect on the type of leadership style one would like to employ as a practice owner. Central to any leadership style is that the owner creates an environment where employees feel a sense of collaboration and inclusiveness with day-to-day operations and business decisions. Possessing the skills to motivate others, providing mediation when needed, and having strong communication skills are essential to running a business and are traits of strong leadership.

Strong leadership skills, and confidence in being a leader, are valuable assets, especially when collaborating with a group of outside vendors or contractors. Having the ability to stand in front of a group of people and help them to succeed in a goal is expected of a leader. This is often how new business partnerships are formed or current partnerships flourish.

Any new practitioner should get comfortable with the idea of leading a group of people. The exact leadership style can be decided based on one's personality style, but demonstrating strong communication skills, having a clear vision for the practice, possessing motivation skills, and collaboration skills are central to being a successful entrepreneur.

Resilience/Tenacity

Entrepreneurial resilience is defined as the processes an entrepreneur utilizes to develop and deploy capabilities in order to adapt and respond to adversity encountered in the

entrepreneur – a person who creates a new business in the face of risk and uncertainty for the purpose of achieving a profit

entrepreneurial resilience – the ability to adapt and respond to adverse business situations

entrepreneurial role.[6] When starting a business, it is inevitable that there will be obstacles and hurdles to overcome. Very rarely, if ever, does one start a business and not have some things deviate from the plan. Having the ability to bounce back from these negative events or circumstances, learn from them, and then move on is a vital trait for any entrepreneur. Many would even call this resiliency trait a skill or capability.[6] "Resiliency" is also often seen as a trait, whereas "resilience" is seen as a process.[7]

It has been noted that obstacles that would typically defeat an individual do not dissuade entrepreneurs from continuing on and progressing their business.[1] Resilient individuals have a tendency to see adversity as a challenge and see themselves as having the skills to overcome these obstacles.[7,8] Because they are more likely to take proactive measures to solve business problems, they tend to have higher business survival rates.[7,8] Having a resiliency mindset through the process of starting and running the business is of vital importance. It has been proposed that while resiliency may be a personality trait, it can be improved with experience over time.[9] So encountering business obstacles and overcoming them could ultimately strengthen this trait or skill.

Remember, negative events will occur, but the entrepreneur has the ability to accept this as part of the process and knows that the ability to solve the problem and then learn from it is crucial and necessary. No entrepreneurial endeavor comes without obstacles, and it is an expectation that an entrepreneur will have the ability to navigate them when they arise.

Willingness to Work Hard

Entrepreneurs work hard to build their companies, and there are no shortcuts around a dedicated workload.[1] Hard work is an expectation with any career endeavor, but when someone decides to start a business, they should be prepared to work above and beyond that of a typical employee. It is a well-held belief that entrepreneurs typically capitalize on opportunity through sheer hard work. Entrepreneurs are often willing to operate at a workload, especially when the business is new, that other people are unwilling to do.[1] It is not uncommon when starting a physical therapy practice to dedicate after-hours time to business development, financial planning, facility upkeep, and other tasks that nonbusiness owners typically do not perform. A new physical therapy practice owner may, for example, decide to take a patient on a Saturday morning or meet with a potential referral source for dinner on a weeknight at 8:00 pm because this is what will drive the business forward. Hard work is just an expectation of starting and running a physical therapy practice.

Comfortable Being Uncomfortable

Entrepreneurs frequently have a high tolerance for ambiguity, changing business situations, and evolving environments in which they operate.[1] A physical therapy practice owner may be treating a patient with an acute anterior cruciate ligament tear at 2:00 pm and be in a business meeting to develop a partnership with a local school at 3:00 pm. An entrepreneur will frequently be placed in situations where rapid change in environment and business practices will occur. They will also have to be comfortable being uncomfortable. A business owner will wear many hats, and some of these hats will be comfortable, whereas others will not. A successful entrepreneur will engage in these uncomfortable/unsteady situations, learn from them, and then evolve to move the business forward.

Basic Finance Skills

Failure to understand basic finance skills is a common mistake among those wanting to start a business.[1,10] Nearly 40% of small business owners report being financially illiterate,

Chapter 6 / Entrepreneurship

yet 81% of business owners manage their own finances.[11] Basic financial and money management skills are vital to running a business successfully.

Oftentimes, the best approach is to seek out a good accountant to help explain the details of things like maintaining a profit loss sheet, tax payment expectations, and hidden costs associated with running a business such as payroll tax and workers compensation fees (see Chapter 1). Entrepreneurs manage endeavors on how to bring in new revenue and consider the cost or expense it is going to take to actually run the practice. Key pieces to understanding a business's finances are the Balance Sheet and the Income Statement[1] (see Chapter 2). The most fundamental statement of the financial health of a physical therapy practice is the Income Statement, also called a Profit-and-Loss Statement. This statement compares expenses against revenue over a certain period of time to show the business' net income or earnings.

The Profit-and-Loss Statement is typically done in monthly, quarterly, and yearly format. It provides a moving picture of a business profitability over a period of time[1] (see Chapter 9). The net income is, essentially, the earnings the business owner has after collecting the payment for contracts and services and then subtracting the operating expenses required to run the business such as employee payroll, rent, and supplies. Again, it is commonplace for new business owners to calculate their earnings based only on the revenue they bring in, without taking into account the expenses it will take to run the business. Keeping a low overhead or business expense line is often a good practice early in a business' startup. As a new physical therapy practice, one likely does not *need* the $6,000 machine and can likely get by with lower cost equipment and clinical tools, which reflects well on the earnings at the end of the quarter. As the practice grows, and income is generated, larger equipment and supply purchases can be considered. Deciding to lease or buy a clinic space is also an important decision. Keeping the lease payment in a manageable range is vital to ensuring that the practice's expenses do not exceed the revenue potential. If an owner leases a clinic space that costs $10,000/month but plans to see only 40 patients per week, this will create a challenging net profit scenario. Remember, the higher the expenses are, the higher the revenue collections must be to make a profit at the end of the month.

Entrepreneurs consider how they will make money. In a physical therapy practice, this is done typically through the provision of physical therapy services to patients and clients. An important key to this practice, especially when starting a practice, is to know how much the practice will actually get paid for providing the services. For example, if the practice decides to contract with an insurance company and discovers that for an hour's visit, they will only be reimbursed $25 for that service, this information must be considered in terms of revenues and expenses to operate the clinic for that hour. How much expense is associated with that hour of service, and will the revenues obtained cover those costs and add to the profit margin? The practice owner would need a rationale for contracting with the insurance company and the benefit it brings to the practice. The practice owner can decide to operate in a private pay model, and charge $100 per visit, if the market would bear such a price, eliminating a third-party payer altogether (see Chapters 1 and 9). It may be determined that a more reasonable rate of $125 per visit would be appropriate based on the practice's cost and the demographics of the local market. Again, often physical therapy practice owners know how to treat their patients and how to complete the service but really need to focus on how much they will be paid for the service to ensure the financial health of the practice.

Forecasting a Profit-and-Loss Statement with expected expenses and planned revenues based on a market analysis is vital to any physical therapy practice. This will help a new practice owner to better understand the financial aspects of the practice and identify targets or benchmarks needed to guide the practice toward its goal of providing effective services and achieving long-term financial success. Ongoing evaluation of the financial targets and key performance indicators (see Chapter 9) are important guides to navigate the practice through the turbulent environment of health care in the United States.

Communication Skills

Basic communication skills, although it seems like a given, are of utmost importance to an entrepreneur (see Chapter 8). During the startup phase of a business, having productive interactions with members of the community, referral sources, and potential contract partners is vital. A PT may possess exceptional clinic skills and have the ability to help many patients at a startup physical therapy practice, but if they cannot exude confidence when communicating with potential patients/clients and members of the community, maintaining adequate visit numbers may be challenging.

Communication with employees is also vital to ensuring efficient, safe, and effective service delivery and adherence to the clinic's processes. Open, clear, and direct communication as far as productivity expectations, promoting a strong clinic culture, and adhering to the clinic's values are important. In addition, communicating effectively to patients is important in promoting optimal outcomes, which will, in turn, improve business, through new customers and word of mouth referrals (see Chapter 9).

Having the ability to communicate the practice's mission and values is also important for marketing and branding initiatives.

Branding/Marketing

In the health care field, branding and marketing are often afterthoughts when planning and running a business. Creating and maintaining an identity for the business is important in building community and patient relationships. Branding can be defined as "communicating a company's unique selling proposition to its target customers in a consistent and integrated manner."[12] Creating a brand that is clear and easily identifiable to the customer is one of the easiest ways to differentiate a business from others. Companies that establish a definite brand typically benefit from increased customer loyalty, have the ability to hold higher prices, have greater visibility and increased name recognition.[12] Establishing a definite brand does require a clear vision of the business, with key attributes of the company communicated to the customer consistently and in an integrated manner.

Marketing often works hand in hand with the businesses branding model. Marketing is how a practice owner promotes and sells the services or products of the business (see Chapter 7). Although a full description of the different strategies for marketing are beyond the scope of this chapter, some basics are necessary to know. Marketing a new or existing physical therapy practice does not have to be expensive. There are many venues for marketing, including social media, hosting seminars or workshops, or sponsoring a community event as examples. When starting a physical therapy practice, it is important to identify a need in the target market that will influence the marketing efforts to this specific market (ie, niche). For example, if a new physical therapy startup practice focuses on running-related injuries, it will be important to ensure that marketing efforts reach the local running groups, local gyms, or racing events. Options for marketing to this niche market can include social media posts, email marketing, hosting workshops/seminars (eg, preventing running injuries), sponsoring local community events (eg, 5K Fun Run), volunteering to assist in a community event (eg, PT tent for runners at the end of the race), creating and running a blog, offering loyal customer programs, and hosting community events at the clinic (eg, flexibility screenings). Many online marketing options (eg, Facebook, Google Ads)

---

branding – communicating the business' unique selling proposition in a consistent and integrated manner

marketing – how a practice owner promotes and sells the services or products of the business

Chapter 6 / Entrepreneurship

will allow you to select geographic location and even target customer attributes such as interests or social media group affiliations. Also, one of the best strategies for marketing is to provide an exceptional patient experience so that the patients become the biggest fans and turn into *brand ambassadors*.[12] These patients often end up telling their friends and family about how great the experience was, creating new customers. Ensuring that the marketing efforts are in line with the branding/mission and that the marketing actually reaches the target customers is vitally important.

Small Business Administration

Post World War II, the federal Office of Small Business was created because business failures were believed to result from a lack of knowledge or expertise in the management or running of a business.[13] Brochures and trainings for business owners were provided to help aid in successful business management and operations for small business entrepreneurs. In 1953, the Small Business Act was passed by Congress, creating the Small Business Administration (SBA). The SBA is an organization that helps people start, grow, and build their business.[13] This was an additional resource to promote the success of small businesses in the United States because the federal government vowed to ensure a fair proportion of government contracts and sales of surplus property to small businesses.

The SBA today has grown significantly. SBA programs now include financial and federal contract procurement assistance, management assistance, and specialized services for women-owned businesses, minority-owned businesses, and armed-forces–veteran-owned businesses.[13] The SBA also provides loan assistance during natural disasters and pandemics (eg, COVID-19 of 2020).

The SBA has resources in each state that provide assistance to those interested in starting a business. In-person counseling is an option in many states to ensure that the appropriate steps are taken and followed when starting a business. These state SBA offices often offer in-person counseling and business planning help along with other electronic options.

The SBA offers online training and access to business-related materials, including how to complete market research and analysis, writing a business plan, calculating startup costs, funding your business, picking a business location, choosing a business name, registering your business, getting federal and state Tax ID numbers, applying for permits, opening a business bank account, attaining business insurance, managing finances, hiring and managing employees, paying taxes, staying legally compliant, marketing and sales, preparing for emergencies, and so on.[14] The SBA also offers a "10 Steps to Start Your Business" guide that can be accessed on their website[14] (Box 6.1).

BOX 6.1 • The Small Business Administration Road Map

1. Conducting market research
2. Writing a business plan
3. Funding your business
4. Picking a business location
5. Choosing a business structure
6. Choosing a business name
7. Registering your business
8. Getting federal and state tax ID numbers
9. Applying for licenses and permits
10. Opening a business bank account.[14]

136   Section 2 / The Decision

The SBA is a valuable resource for any new or existing business owner. For the physical therapy practice owner, the SBA is a valuable and logical resource for information, guidance, and support when starting up a practice.

Practice in the Digital Age

Web Page Basics

Today, the average American will spend 7 hours per day consuming online content.[15] Modern customers expect to be able to get information about a business in an online format. There are currently many company options such as Wix™, SquareSpace™, and GoDaddy™, for a business owner to self-create a company website, or a business owner may also choose to hire an outside company or consultant for this aspect of the business. Having a visually appealing and highly effective website is crucial to being discoverable as a business and in attracting new customers. Small businesses are investing more time into developing and updating their websites, optimizing their sites to achieve top search engine rankings, making their sites mobile friendly, and encouraging customers to post reviews.[1] A potential customer expects to be easily able to find the business website and to have access to fast and meaningful information. Most small businesses also encourage communication through the website through tactics such as "message now" or "schedule now" links.

To maximize a company's website performance, it is crucial that the site is easy to navigate, contains meaningful content that is easy to find and understand, is visually appealing, provides a snapshot of the businesses brand and offers an easy contact option (phone, email, message) or schedule option for the customer.

A common mistake in business website design is to make it too busy and not simple. A website with too many click options, too many click channels, or busy wording is often

---

BOX 6.2 • Tips by Cornwall and Scarborough for Setting Up an Effective Website[1]

- Avoid clutter, especially on the site's home page.
- Use less text on the home page, landing page (ie, where the customer lands after accessing a link to the webpage from an email or other website), and initial product or service page.
- Avoid huge graphic headers.
- Make the site easy to navigate.
- Minimize the number of clicks required for a customer to get to any particular page in the site.
- Incorporate meaningful content in the site useful to visitors that is current, well organized, and easy to read.
- Include a Frequently Asked Questions (FAQs) section.
- Avoid fancy typefaces and small fonts that make reading difficult. Limit the font and color choices to two or three to avoid an unprofessional appearance.
- Avoid using small fonts on busy backgrounds; no one will read them.
- Choose colors carefully, keeping color palettes simple and limited.
- Use the website to collect information from visitors, but avoid providing too much information for the visitor to consume (eg, lengthy registration process).
- Make sure the page is visually appealing.
- Remember that simpler is almost always better.

Source: Scarborough NM, Cornwall JR. *Essentials of Entrepreneurship and Small Business Management.* 9th ed. Pearson; 2019.

Chapter 6 / Entrepreneurship

> ## BOX 6.3 • Key Strategies That Can Be Used Within a Social Media Marketing Platform[20]
>
> - Use a Call-to-Action button—Through video or visual, explain to a viewer why they need an offered service, and attach a schedule or *call now* button to take action.
> - Social proof—Display positive patient testimonials, customer ratings, or success stories that present the strengths and value of the business.
> - Video content—Low production or no cost production, recording educational videos or simply clinic update videos, is a great way to capture viewers' attention. Videos are often far more engaging than a still photo or text.
> - Periodically evaluate the need for a new platform or different content style—Consider utilizing different social media platforms for different ad styles/schemes on a yearly basis. Review the success, or lack of success, on a particular platform or with a particular content style.
> - Get others' perspectives—Consider consulting with other successful social media professionals or marketing experts. Also consider consulting with other business owners who have a great social media presence.
>
> *Source:* Decatou P. The 5 offensive formations for a championship social media strategy. Impact. 2018. Accessed September 11, 2022. https://www.ppsimpact.org/the-5-offensive-formations-of-a-championship-social-media-strategy/?print=print

off-putting to the customer. Simplicity and ease of navigating the site is usually preferred (Box 6.2). A website should include a simple design, be easy to navigate, have consistent color schemes, and contain clear "Call to Action" (an invitation to perform a desired action such as *Schedule Now*) on each page.[1] In a recent survey, 64% of online shoppers said that they seek a site that offers simplicity and a streamlined shopping experience.[16]

It is also recommended that the business owner frequently visit the website to ensure links are working and all information remains current. If errors are discovered or link issues occur, it is vital to rapidly correct them.

Electronic Communication

Communication with patients/customers typically takes place in one of three modes. These modes are phone, email, and text.[17] Modern communications typically bypass the traditional route of phone calls and have made a significant move to electronic communication. More than ever, people prefer or expect quick and reliable communication by means of email or text message.

Electronic communication through secure patient messaging systems is a way to encourage efficient patient communication and typically improves patient satisfaction. Email messaging is one means to ensure timely communication, but many practices are now using text messaging or secure messaging systems that are often built into the patient's documentation system. Utilizing secure patient messaging allows the patient to ask important clinical or therapy-related questions quickly and efficiently and encourages a collaborative and active role in recovery. Ease of communication and speed at which this can be done is greatly improved with these messaging formats.

Attracting and scheduling customers is also typically much more efficient through email or text messaging systems. With phone-based communication, a game of phone tag is often the case when a new patient is trying to schedule or a current patient is simply trying to reschedule an appointment. With messaging systems, the patient can simply send a text/secure message or email to make this request or change. This is often appreciated by the patient and greatly improves time efficiency in scheduling practices.

Privacy is a concern with message-based medical communication, so a Health Insurance Portability and Accountability Act (HIPAA)–secure messaging platform or text messaging system should be used. Many systems, such as PtEverywhere™, offer secure messaging within a patient app. Text message systems through companies such as Google Voice™ also offer HIPAA-compliant text messaging with a business associate agreement that ensures privacy. When protected health information is shared, the business owner should request a business associate agreement that ensures privacy compliance whenever contracting with a company to use their text, email, fax, or messaging systems. It is prudent to have the patients/clients sign a messaging acceptance and acknowledgment form to ensure that they understand that process of messaging and the potential risk of privacy breaches (eg, A message is sent and a relative is holding their phone at that time.) It is also best practice to include a statement that messaging through text or email can be inherently less private than phone communication. It is recommended that all patients receive and sign an acknowledgment form with consent to their preferred communication styles, including phone, email, or text message. They can then use the secure messaging platform to communicate protected health information, including results of clinical tests and measures, rather than through basic text messaging. Practitioners should also use discretion as to what they decide to discuss in a messaging platform versus in person or on the phone.

As with other aspects of a business, messaging systems or automated appointment reminder systems come with a cost. As the business grows, the benefit to having these systems in place greatly outweighs the cost.[17] Quick and convenient communication between provider and patient does keep the patient happy and often reflects a sense of caring.[17] The ease of communication with the provider and timely responses are often a major factor in patient retention. The use of automated systems decreases the need for an administrative staff sitting at a desk, waiting for patients to call to schedule or reschedule appointments. Messaging-based systems can also reduce costs by allowing clinicians to be involved with simple tasks such as moving patient appointments or answering simple questions through messaging systems. Administrative support hours could be reduced, thus reducing one aspect of a business' overhead cost.

Social Media Marketing

Regardless of a personal opinion about social media, it is hard to argue that social media marketing is now vital to growing a business.[18] Social media marketing can be a cost-effective way to present a brand, communicate easily with new customers, and stay in touch with past customers who may end up as return customers. Many business owners view social media as a gateway to building awareness for the company's brand, bringing people to the company's website, and generating leads for more business.[1] Now, more than ever, people are using smartphones and devices to view social media on a daily, if not hourly, basis. Seventy-six percent of internet users participate in at least one social networking site, which is more than double that in 2008.[19] It is now an expectation that a business has a social media presence (see Chapter 7).

There are many platforms for social media advertising, such as Facebook™, X (formerly Twitter)™, LinkedIn™, and Instagram™. Facebook™ is typically viewed as having an older audience, and a business would benefit from posting between 1:00 pm and 4:00 pm, 2 to 3 times per week, when people from this demographic typically access the media.[18] Facebook™ allows for a wide range of posts, including photo, text, and video. A clinic may want to focus on the clinic's brand, the personality of a clinician, interesting educational topics that are available, or news from the clinic's offered services.[18] X (formerly Twitter)™ is typically seen as having a younger audience, and the recommendation is to post there 3 to 5 times per week between 1:00 pm and 3:00 pm.[18] A large focus on interesting hashtags

Chapter 6 / Entrepreneurship

(used to identify content on a specific topic) and the number of retweets/replies/comments is the typical focus of X (formerly Twitter)™. Instagram™ can also be utilized, but it primarily uses brief visual (photo/video) posts, so items such as brief patient testimonials or interesting photos would be appropriate on this site.

Most of the social medial services also offer targeted ads where a geographic area and select patient demographic can be chosen. These are often paid ads but are very cost effective and allow for a very targeted approach, thus reducing marketing cost.

There are several strategies that can be used with a social media platform[20] (Box 6.3). A practice can ask patients to *Check In* when they are at the practice to further increase viewership and advertisement. *Schedule Now* buttons are also efficient and effective when integrated into a social media platform, allowing the interested customer/patient to simply click a button to schedule.

Basics of Virtual Visits

With the COVID-19 pandemic, the practice of telehealth and virtual visits was put center stage for a period of time. Virtual visits are encounters between a provider and a patient using electronic communication and video interaction when both the provider and the patient are in different physical locations. Patients may choose to stay home for different health reasons or may simply prefer this mode of delivery for its convenience and time-saving attributes.

Before beginning virtual visits, a PT must check the state's practice act to ensure virtual visits are allowed within the state and investigate the specifics of such a service delivery in the state's bylaws.[21] For example, in many states, the patient must be located in the state in which the PT is licensed. So, if the PT is licensed in Ohio, the patient must be sitting in a location that is in the State of Ohio.

A provider must also investigate the payers of services, especially third-party payers, to ensure that they reimburse for virtual visits.[20] Some third-party payers may reimburse for these services at the established rate, a lower rate, or not at all. The financial aspect of a virtual visit is as important as the infrastructure and privacy assurances that are put into place in order to provide this type of visit. As with in-person visits, a practitioner needs to obtain a HIPAA-compliant virtual visit service that includes a business associate agreement.[20] This is not a standard across the video service market, so this must be identified and required by the video service prior to forming an agreement to protect the health information of the patient. Many new physical therapy documentation systems such as PtEverywhere™ offer a HIPAA-compliant virtual visit platform. Other outside business such as Doxy™ also offer a good option for health care providers. It is also prudent to contact the physical therapy practice's malpractice insurance carrier to verify coverage of virtual visits.

Most virtual visits systems are going to require a secure and stable internet connection; a working microphone and camera; and an uncluttered, quiet environment to carry out the visit.

The provider and the patient should be in a location where other people cannot overhear the discussion. Communicating these requirements to the patient prior to the visit is important for a safe, efficient, and private virtual visit. If a patient cannot ensure that all of these requirements can be met, then a virtual visit may not be the best option for providing care. For example, if a patient does not have a stable internet connection, the visit may

virtual visit – a visual and auditory encounter that utilizes electronic means to connect people at different physical sites (eg, telehealth) be constantly interrupted by connection issues, impairing communication, which can be detrimental to the patient. The same could happen if the patient does not have a private and quiet place to participate in the virtual visit. Also, the provider should practice using this type of delivery system through test runs prior to involving patients and feel confident in this type of interaction. The provider should come to the virtual visit prepared with any therapy tools or educational material that may be needed for the visit. In the practice of physical therapy, many of the objective tests and measures will need to be altered because the patient cannot be physically touched in these encounters (eg, manual muscle testing, goniometric measurements). Instead, observation of movement, biomechanical analysis of movement, functional movement screens, repeated movement examinations, functional strength examinations, and other more virtual visit–friendly objective measures can be used.

It is also important for the provider to know the emergency plan if something should happen to the patient during the virtual visit. The patient's alternate and emergency contact phone numbers and the patient's local emergency medical response phone number should be readily available to the provider if and when needed.

Documentation for virtual visits is the same as for an in-person visit, with a few additions. Documentation of the virtual visit should include the reason for the virtual visit versus an in-person visit, the location of both parties, the date, and the start and stop times of the visit. If anyone besides the provider and the patient are present during the virtual visit, this should also be documented.

How to Begin

Components of a Business Plan

Before a practitioner can start a business, a road map in the form of a business plan should be developed. A business plan is a document that identifies the business' objectives, operating structure, general strategies to achieve the identified objectives, and financial goals. Research has shown that businesses that engage in formal business planning prior to launching a business outperform those that do not.[1] It has also been shown that potential new business owners who write a formal business plan are nearly two-and-a-half times as likely to actually start the business.[22] Scarborough and Cornwall define a business plan as, "a written summary of an entrepreneur's proposed business venture, [its] operational and financial details, [its] marketing opportunities and strategy, and [its] managers' skills and abilities."[1] The business plan can help a new business see the potential for success once everything is written down on paper, and it also provides information for a potential investor or business partners, if desired. The business plan should present the purpose of the company, the goals, where the business wants to be in the market, and how it intends to get there.[1] This requires the entrepreneur to dedicate the necessary time to market research, financial planning, and business forecasting. The primary function of a business plan is to support the viability of the business after the development of a mission statement, operating structure (including services to be offered), budgets, and financial forecasts in order to convince potential lenders, potential employees, and investors/partners of the viability of the business.

When starting a business, the entrepreneur will have to secure funds to finance the business. This can be done by the entrepreneur with personal funds or by securing financing in the form of a loan in order to purchase equipment, pay the rent/mortgage, and pay for

business plan – a written document that outlines the business' objectives and the actions to be taken to achieve those objectives in a stated period of time

Chapter 6 / Entrepreneurship

staff expenses and other startup costs. To obtain financing, typically, a sound business plan is needed that shows there is a market for the practice, that it fulfills a need or can compete with local competitors, and that it will provide value to the potential customer. A business plan used to obtain financing through a lending agency should make the lender confident that the business endeavor can generate funds to pay back the loan and to show that the business is feasible, is needed, and can be financially successful.

It is recommended that a business plan be 10 to 20 pages in length.[1] The first step in developing a business plan is to create the mission statement, which states the purpose for the business and what it intends to become in the market. The business plan should succinctly state what the business does, how it does it, and for whom (target market). The plan should include a cover page with the business logo. In addition, the five key elements that should be included in a physical therapy business plan include an executive summary, the business objectives/goals, a marketing plan, general statements of the day-to-day operations, and financial information[23] (Box 6.4). The executive summary should address the target patient/client population or niche at whom the services provided by the business are targeted and how the services are different or better than the competitors. It should address the growth projection of the business/practice, the overall financial and funding plans, any necessary physical/service equipment and space requirements, and the initial marketing effort to attract patients. The business objectives/goals should describe what the business will bring to the community and how it can help the target population (eg, it will help high school athletes safely return to play after injury), the long-term goal for business growth (eg, what is the vision for the clinic, both in patient/client numbers and financially, in the near future?), and a plan for business/staff expansion, such as eventual staff numbers and geographic reach. The marketing plan should detail how the business intends to communicate its services (social media, radio, etc), the marketing budget, the message and branding that will be delivered, identification of the target market, and the business' strengths/advantages over other clinics in the area. The day-to-day operations should be presented with items such as proposed staff, workflow, materials/supplies needed for clinic operation (fax, documentation systems, etc), and the organizational structure detailing who is responsible for what parts of the business practices (see Chapter 5). The business plan should have a financial plan with proposed balance sheet, income statement, and break-even analysis for the lender, investor, or partner to review (see Chapters 1 and 2).

It is also advisable to seek help from resources such as the Small Business Development Center (SBDC)[24] or the Service Corps of Retired Executives (SCORE)[25] in writing a business plan. These agencies offer helpful guides and, in some cases, personal assistance in drafting the plan.

Staff Selection

When recruiting and selecting staff, there are several factors to consider, especially since staff recruitment, training, and retention are significant investments made by a business. The first step is to establish what type of services are going to be offered; the expertise of the staff needed; the physical space that will be required to deliver the services; and the administrative support that would be required to efficiently deliver, bill, and collect for the services rendered. A projection of how many patients/clients will be seen in a month will provide a working number of how many PTs, physical therapist assistants (PTAs), aides, and administrative staff will be needed to deliver the services. This type of information is commonly included in a business plan and used to make a successful argument on the amount of startup capital/money needed. Keep in mind that the total cost needed (eg, rent, utilities, equipment, supply purchases, liability insurance) must be covered by the anticipated revenues in order for the business to be profitable.

BOX 6.4 • Key Elements of a Business Plan

i. Executive Summary
   a. Describe the business, location, legal status
   b. Mission Statement
   c. Stage of development and growth projections
   d. Services offered and equipment needs
   e. Target market(s)/patient population
   f. Marketing strategy to attract customers
   g. Competitor(s)
   h. Operational location(s) and space needs
   i. Management and organization
   j. Financial information
   k. Long-term goals
   l. Funds sought, uses, and estimated return on investment

ii. Business Description, Objectives, and Goals
   a. Mission (state what does the practice do best, to whom, and where)
   b. Industry analysis (describe industry, current trends and opportunities, economic cycles, supply and demand data)
   c. Long-term goals (vision, what will happen to the business in the future?)

iii. Marketing
   a. Market analysis and target market(s) (demographics, describe ideal customers)
   b. Competitor analysis (who and where, market distribution, position of competitors, barriers to entry and opportunities for growth)
   c. Marketing plan, goals, and strategy (how will services be made known? What is unique to the proposed business?)
   d. Marketing budget
   e. Branding

iv. Synopsis of operations and location(s)
   a. How will the business be run? capacity, productivity, quality control, map, photos, construction plans for location(s)
   b. Organizational structure (lines of authority, board, advisors, principles, management experience, consultants, key employees, management style)

v. Financial Information
   a. Personal capital being applied (personal financial information—how much capital does the owner have, how much money is needed, when, for what purposes?)
   b. Equipment list (priorities, vendors, and costs)
   c. Break-even analysis
   d. Balance sheets (personal and business if it already exists)
   e. Cash-flow analysis (estimate of first year month by month and annually for years 1-3)
   f. For existing business, current audited tax returns, and other significant financial data

vi. Supporting Documents
   a. Resume(s) of principle(s), managers, key personnel
   b. Letters of intent
   c. Letters of recommendation
   d. Current contract(s)
   e. Job description(s)
   f. Special awards, achievements, relevant recognition
   g. Equipment photos

Chapter 6 / Entrepreneurship 143

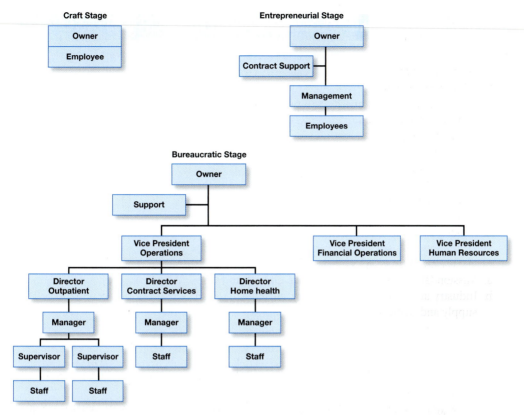

Figure 6.1 The organizational chart should represent the actual structure, not a desired culture or set of relationships. (Adapted from Nosse L. Internal environment: physical therapy. In: Nosse LJ, Friberg DG, eds. *Management and Supervisory Principles for Physical Therapists*. 3rd ed. Wolters Kluwer Health/Lippincott Williams and Wilkins; 2010:105-127.)

The next step is creating an organizational or operating structure to deliver and coordinate the services that are delivered to meet the common goal or mission. The **organizational chart** is a graphic representation of an organizational operating structure. Using boxes, lines, and occasionally other geometric shapes, an organizational chart becomes a graphic representation of the parts of the business/organization. Typically, solid lines represent direct reporting relationships. Direct reporting relationships indicate both accountability and responsibility. Organizational structures are most often pyramidal, representing the hierarchy of the management structure. In a pyramidal structure, the most senior management position would be placed at the pinnacle of the triangle. Subordinate positions and departments would follow in the order of organizational position from high to low. Traditionally, the organizational chart describes the authority and responsibilities of positions within the organization. In small businesses, the structure is typically reflected in a craft, entrepreneurial, or bureaucratic style (Figure 6.1). The organizational chart should represent the actual structure, not a desired culture or set of relationships.

The third step is the development of policies and procedures on the provision of services (including the documentation of services, billing, and the collection of fees) and the adherence to established laws of the operations of a business (eg, Equal Employment Opportunity Commission, The Occupational Safety and Health Administration), which is vital to ensure that all employees understand their role in fulfilling the mission and purpose of the

organizational chart – a graphic representation of an organizational operating structure

BOX 6.5 • Example of a Job Description's Duties and Responsibilities for a Physical Therapist Position and Possible Structured Interview Questions to Ask During an Interview

Duties and Responsibilities

1. Will perform examinations on patients/clients seeking physical therapy services.
   Interview question: Tell me about how you generally conduct an examination of a patient; what is the process you go through and what information do you find vital to the process?
2. Will keep the patient informed of their progress regarding the established plan of care.
   Interview question: Describe to me how you educate your patients/clients on their progress. How do you address the issue of noncompliance with recommendations made or lack of progress toward the established goals? What do you do if the patient/client achieves the goals on the plan of care sooner than was initially anticipated?
3. Will oversee the plan of care, supervise, and collaborate effectively with the assigned PTA.
   Interview question: Are you familiar with the supervisory requirements of PTA in this state? What do you think are the key components of effective collaboration between a PT and a PTA?
4. Will produce, submit, and maintain appropriate clinical documentation in compliance with the clinic's and external accrediting agencies' requirements.
   Interview question: What are your strengths and weakness in clinical documentation? What do you find most challenging in clinical documentation?
5. Will maintain appropriate licensure and other certifications as deemed necessary for the job.
   Interview question: Tell me how you decide on which continuing education program to attend? How do you keep track of the Continuing Education Unit requirements for licensure?

PT, physical therapists; PTA, physical therapist assistant.

---

business. Remember the business/practice is owned by an entrepreneur or group of people that have a vested interest in providing services to a particular market. Those individuals who are employed to assist in that endeavor require a framework in which to operate that is consistent with the values and expectations of the owner(s). Written policies and procedures provide that framework as does a job description.

A job description is a written description of the responsibilities of the position and commonly lists the general duties, decision-making authority, work standards, minimum job requirements, responsibility for the work of others (eg, PTAs, aides, students), and the methods of coordinating/collaborating with other members of the organization. It lists the duties required of the position in order to achieve the goals of the business. It is also used in developing a structured interview for potential employees, focusing the questions on the needed duties to be performed (Box 6.5).

The next step in the process is deciding on where and how to advertise for the position. What demographics is the practice looking to hire? For example, if the practice will operate a sports clinic, it may decide that the PTs should be certified clinical specialists in sports in order to better serve the intended patient population. If the practice blends physical therapy and fitness, it may seek out professionals with more advanced certifications or knowledge base not only in physical therapy, but also in the area of overall fitness. What is the target market for patients? Will the staff selected in some way reflect the demographics of the patients served? Regardless of the medium a practice owner decides to use to advertise for staff, they

job description – a written description of the responsibilities of a position, commonly listing the general duties, decision-making authority, work standards, minimum job requirements, responsibility for the work of others, and the methods of coordinating/collaborating with other members of the organization

Chapter 6 / Entrepreneurship **145**

should consider the market/population that accesses that medium or source. What are the demographics for people who use social media, read the printed newspaper or magazine, view posted announcements in the grocery store or library, or live or drive in the area where a public announcement (eg, billboard) is posted? Is the practice looking for staff who are bilingual? Are the advertising efforts available to people who are bilingual? Overall, the practice should make sure the advertising campaign is aligned with the business' mission and brand.

Once the recruitment process is complete, the hired staff will require training to ensure that the new employee understands the policies and procedures of the practice and the expectations of the job description, the productivity expectations, billing, and accreditation standards that must be followed. Often, a new employee will be put on a *probationary status,* indicating that for a period of time, typically measured in months, additional time will be allocated for understanding the procedures and delivery systems of the practice. During this period, productivity standards are typically decreased to allow for the training and assimilation of the new employee into the practice. It is important for the owner, or supervising therapist, to intentionally set time aside to review the work of the new employee and provide feedback, education, and guidance toward the expected behavior.

It is clear that the process of staff selection and orientation is a costly expense for a business. It is important that the practice owner support and nurture their investment with efforts to assure continued compliance with work expectations along with fostering employee satisfaction with the work and work environment of the clinic. Providing clear directions and structure, listening to employee concerns, facilitating a work culture of teamwork and shared responsibility, providing for flexibility in the schedule whenever possible, and celebrating the success of the employees and business can help in the retention and satisfaction of this valuable resource, the health care employee.

Profit Centers

A profit center is a branch or division of a company that directly adds to the company's bottom line profitability.[26] These separate segments of the business can often be treated as a separate entity with their own Profit-and-Loss Statement. Sometimes, profit centers are separated as different departments and operate under the umbrella of the main business/company. For example, a physical therapy practice may also decide to offer personal training for fitness within the same facility. Although this may not be the primary business, it is a way to generate profit. A business many have multiple profit centers operating within the business. Oftentimes, it is up to the business owner to keep these centers separate and then decide, through profit loss comparison, which ones are the most profitable, align best with the mission, reflect the brand, and are worth the continued investment. For example, a physical therapy practice may offer merchandise sales, fitness/personal training, and massage services in addition to physical therapy services. These could each have their own profit loss statement, and at the end of the quarter or the year, the business owner could determine which of these are generating the most profit and showing the best alignment with the practices' mission and financial goals. Profit centers are a benefit if they are bringing in more revenue, but they can also act as an advertising or marketing effort to get more customers in the door. For example, a person receiving personal training services provided through a physical therapy practice may be more likely to use the physical therapy services if the need arose.

Vendor Relationships

Maintaining a collaborative vendor relationship is important to ensure that a practice has the required supplies and materials to operate. A vendor is really anyone who is supplying

profit center – a component or department of a business that brings in revenues in excess of its costs, adding to the profitability of the business

the practice with the goods, materials, supplies, or equipment that is needed to operate the practice. This could range from a vendor company that provides dry needles; a company that provides electronic medical records services and support; an office supply company that provides the practice with paper and printing materials; or the equipment company that maintains/provides the physical therapy equipment, durable medical equipment (DME), or modalities.

Oftentimes, there can be a cost savings if a practice signs an agreement with specific vendors to routinely order supplies or purchase them in bulk from a vendor. These buyer–supplier agreements are commonplace and are created with a clear set of expectations, including costs. Having a good relationship with vendors is especially important in instances of last-minute need for assistance or for specific supplies. When starting a business, it is a good practice to create a list of supplies or materials that are needed and then identify a specific vendor that the practice will utilize to obtain these items. There will likely be more than a few options, so this would be a good time to research items such as pricing or ease of communication or even check with other business owners on their experience with that specific vendor. A business owner does not, for example, want to purchase a piece of equipment, only to find that there is no local vendor/servicer to complete yearly maintenance of that piece of equipment. Having clear expectations for the speed at which items can be obtained or the speed at which assistance can be provided is vital to a good relationship with vendors and an asset to the practice.

Creating and Keeping a Great Team

Creating a team with a good business culture is one of the major keys to longevity in any physical therapy practice. A business owner cannot do everything alone and will need administrative and clinical personnel to make the practice a success. The first step is the hiring process. Now, more than ever, new physical therapy graduates can be more selective about their place of employment. Administrative personnel will also be selective about the environment in which they choose to work. New graduates report that flexibility and work-life balance are the two most important aspects of a job.[27] Therefore, it is vital for a practice to have clear and intentional recruitment, selection, and retention programs. Having discussions with applicants and employees on topics such as work-life balance, exceptions to expectations while at work, the culture of the business, and the skills and responsibilities of other staff are vital in fostering and maintaining a work environment that is supportive and nurturing.

Nearly 50% of PTs reported in 2020 that they felt more burned out than ever, with only 19% reporting that they did not feel burned out.[28] Although the pandemic could have been a significant factor, it is widely accepted that employee dissatisfaction and burnout in the physical therapy profession is a problem. Many PTs and administrators who work in physical therapy centers are reporting that they are disgruntled, lack job satisfaction, and are eager to leave at the end of the day. Obviously, if employees are not happy, or do not find fulfillment and job satisfaction, this will create problems for the practice both in terms of culture but also in the financial aspect of the business. A lack of autonomy, lack of advancement, and lack of appreciation are cited as three of the most common reasons for employee dissatisfaction.[28] As a business owner, it is vital to provide employees with some level of autonomy. It can be said that a practice owner is better off presenting to the employees the outcomes or what needs to be done, rather than operations or directions on how things have to be done.[28] Giving employees options and flexibility for achieving tasks will often create happier employees. As a physical therapy practice owner, giving the staff PTs autonomy in the way they practice rather than limiting them to one specific treatment approach is one example of supporting autonomy. Offering opportunity for advancement

Chapter 6 / Entrepreneurship **147**

or professional growth is also vital. Clearly asking employees, "which areas do you want to grow" is a simple question but provides a clear path for advancement. Maybe a PT wants to develop manual skills and attain a dry needling certification. An easy response to foster growth would be to offer to pay for the dry needling certification. If an employee would like to develop management skills, providing them with the opportunity to manage certain aspects of the practice and mentoring them in the process could also foster job satisfaction and a culture of support. Appreciation seems like a commonsense trait that any supervisor would express, but, unfortunately, sometimes it does not happen. Simply telling an employee that their hard work is noticed and commenting when they go above and beyond is a simple practice to make a significant impact. If the practice is doing well, meeting target goals, it is great to let the employees know that they contribute to this success. Another way of showing appreciation is through stepwise increases in pay. If an employee is performing well, and the practice is, in turn, performing well, it only seems right and fair to show appreciation by rewarding that employee monetarily.

At times, difficult conversations are necessary with an employee. Perhaps they are not performing up to the standards expected, or the patients are not satisfied with the care they received. Having timely, open, and honest conversations and providing clear goals to improve performance is vital. An employee cannot improve if they are not aware of the underperformance. Having quarterly or yearly reviews is a common way of completing performance evaluations or having dedicated time set aside to discuss the goals of the employee and the goals of the practice. Frequency and timeliness of feedback allows the supervisor to address negative or potentially negative issues early and take corrective actions sooner (see Chapter 10).

Having a collective understanding of the goals of the business and of the culture is imperative. Again, the interview process is the correct time to make every attempt possible at identifying if the applicant will be a good fit in the practice. For example, a component of the business culture may be that in the process of getting athletes to return to play appropriately and safely, there is an environment of fun and encouragement. This may require the practice to see injured athletes on the same day of injury or to see those athletes when they are not scheduled to be in clinic. If an employee decides that they do not want to participate in same day appointments or see occasional unexpected visits to the clinic and act negatively or with a lack of enthusiasm when asked to do so, they may not be a good fit for the practice. Conversely, the practice owner must promote a good work-life balance for the employees, so if that employee has an activity with their child or simply has another out-of-work event, the practice owner should allow for reasonable accommodations (ie, flexibility) to the work schedule. Promoting and maintaining a good work culture is an ongoing collaboration between the practice owner and the employee and will often create a long-term commitment in the employee.

Subcontracting

Subcontracting is the practice of assigning, or outsourcing, part of the obligations and tasks under a contract to another party.[29] Typically, a business will subcontract with another company when that company has an established product/service that would benefit the business. Oftentimes, the business owner also determines that it may be cheaper to simply outsource and hire the subcontractor to carry out the task. For example, if a physical therapy practice owner decides that they would like to offer massage services at the practice, it may be more cost effective to subcontract to a massage therapist who already has

> subcontracting – the practice of assigning, or outsourcing, part of a contractual obligation to another party

an established and flourishing massage practice. This massage therapist may also be well established in the community, so it may make more sense to hire through a subcontract than trying to grow and establish a new business segment. Another example would be hiring a personal trainer, who already has an established business, to perform the fitness screens for a new contract with a local employer. Both contracts (the local employer and the personal trainer) would be between the business and the PT practice, but the work would be out-sourced to and provided by the subcontractor. Subcontracting can take many forms, and it is important to remember that if the subcontractor is operating under the PT practice umbrella, the liability for the subcontractor's actions may still be the responsibility of the PT practice.

A Few Tips From the Author

Grit Matters

Starting and running a business will be hard and will require grit and perseverance to succeed. Nothing that is extremely easy is typically worth much, and this is true of running a business/private practice. The practice owner can expect to encounter their fair share of obstacles. This attitude will save the owner time and support their mental health when obstacles or unforeseen events occur. Things will be hard; figure out the problem, solve the problem, and keep moving forward.

Getting the Right Help

Asking for help from someone of trust is recommended. When seeking advice, it is important to consult someone who is experienced and who has a reputation for giving good advice. There are many online business gurus that will provide business advice but that may not have the practice's best interest in mind or an understanding of the demographics of the local market. It is advisable when starting a private practice to find a business mentor who actually has experience running a physical therapy practice or, at the very least, who has experience starting and running a successful business. If a mentor is not readily identifiable, there are several other resources that can help provide the necessary guidance and background information needed to start a private practice (Box 6.6). In general, a PT should begin by assessing personal strengths and weakness, set reasonable expectations, identify when and what assistance is needed, and set out a plan for developing and implementing decisive actions toward the established goals.

BOX 6.6 • Getting the Right Help

- Discussing private practice with owners of private practices and consultants
- Reading professional journals and books from many fields, including materials from the American Physical Therapy Association (APTA)
- Consulting community business organizations such as the Chamber of Commerce and the Better Business Bureau
- Attending meetings of national associations, including the APTA and other local, state, and national organizations
- Seeking advice from governmental sources like the Small Business Administration (http://www.sba.gov) and Service Corps of Retired Executives (http://www.score.org)
- Acquiring further education through continuing education courses or for-credit courses offered by educational institutions
- Exploring internet business resources

Honesty With Staff and Customers

Honesty and ethics in business is very important. Transparency will almost always be appreciated. If there is a mistake with a patient/customer, it is best to apologize and be honest. People understand, as long as they are treated with respect and honesty. If an employee isn't performing up to standards or needs to improve in an area of patient/client management, take the employee aside and professionally state the concerns along with a plan to address them. Be willing to listen, educate, and provide direction and support to make sure the employee understands the expectation and what the owner will do to help them meet that goal. Conversely, if the supervisor/owner makes an error of judgment or in delivery of information, apologize. The owner's behavior and work ethic should reflect the expectations of all the employees of the practice.

Private Pay or Insurance-Based Reimbursement?

With the current decline in insurance-based reimbursements for services and the expectation of efficient administrative tasks, such as timely documentation and obtaining authorizations, many physical therapy practice owners are deciding to move to a private pay model. This means that the patient pays "out of pocket" for their services, typically at the time of the visit. Many practices will provide the patient with a super bill to allow the patient to turn in receipts in order to claim reimbursement from their insurance company for the services provided as an out of network claim. This eliminates the need for the practice to collect reimbursement directly from the insurance company, which can often be a lengthy and time-consuming process.

The private pay model allows for more autonomy as the practice is not under the direction of a patient's insurance policy. For example, many insurance companies do not cover dry needling services. When operating in a traditional in-network model, the PT may not be able to complete that technique without billing a separate charge because the insurance will not cover the intervention. In a private pay model, as long as the PT operates within the scope of practice within his or her state, the PT has more freedom to provide interventions that they feel are most appropriate for a patient's plan of care. In addition, many insurance companies do not cover fitness or wellness services that are within the scope of a PT's practice. In a private pay model, these services can be billed and the cost recovered.

Insurance-based models do have some positive attributes. Most consumers see this model as the typical route for physical therapy, and most people have a health insurance plan that will cover physical therapy services. Capturing new patients/clients is easier with this model because it is the norm and, depending on the plan, may sometimes be less expensive for the patient/client.

Monitor Spending

When making decisions on the type and number of pieces of equipment and supplies needed for the practice, keep spending low. In an orthopedic/sports practice, for example, it is possible to spend less than 8,000 dollars to start the practice and still be able to provide outstanding treatment. Remember that physical therapy is provided by a person, a PT. Equipment only adds options. Typically, a practice with a focus on orthopedic/sports would purchase free weights, a treadmill, resistance bands, a treatment table, an exercise mat, a power rack, and an instrument assisted soft tissue tool to start. It may seem great to have force decks and underwater treadmills, but a practice does not *need* them to start. The option of subleasing a space in a local gym, fitness studio, or health care facility that has equipment already can lower the startup costs for a new practice owner.

Also remember, patients/clients care more about their overall experience with the practice. If the equipment is clean and organized and works, they will likely be happy. If the clinic space itself is clean and smells fresh, they will likely be happy. If the administrative staff treats them well and greets them with a smile, they will likely be happy. If the PT is attentive and genuinely cares that the patients get better, they will likely be happy. Expensive equipment will not impact these factors. In summary, don't go into debt for things that are not needed!

Direct Access and Practitioner of Choice

PTs are the practitioner of choice for movement disorders/impairments and should have direct access (the ability of the consumer to self-refer to a service, such as physical therapy, without the approval of a gatekeeper, such as a physician) to people seeking their care. Act like it! Do not rely solely on physician referrals, which has been a prime marketing strategy for years. (eg, Physician X, I am very good at fixing knees so when your patient's knee hurts and they need PT, please recommend me as an option.) A practice should market to referral sources and develop working relationships with them, but don't make that the only means of recruiting new patients/clients. Another strategy would be to have a balance of direct-to-consumer marketing (eg, Hey Mr Football Player, your knee hurts and I am good at making knees feel better, call my clinic and come see me), online marketing to target markets, community-wide marketing, health insurance network marketing, and marketing to other health care practitioners. Make sure the practice engages with the community (see Chapter 11) and is seen as a trustworthy and valuable member of the community. The marketing efforts must be honest, and the practice must deliver to the patient, client, referral source, or community on what it promises.

An aspect of professional autonomy requires that PTs identify and refer a patient to another health care provider if the patient is not appropriate for physical therapy (eg, perhaps they need a radiograph). This is a valuable aspect of establishing a working relationship with other specialists and service providers in the community.

First Impressions Matter

When someone walks into a business and meets the staff for the first time, it takes less than 10 seconds to make a first impression.[30] If the potential patient/client walks into the clinic and (1) the clinic smells clean, (2) is neat and organized, (3) was easily accessible, and (4) the person receives a friendly greeting and is offered assistance, the potential patient/client will likely form a good first impression of the practice. If the first experience does not meet the expectations of the potential patient/client or if a negative event occurs (eg, rude behavior by the staff, difficulty with parking or access to the clinic, or excessive clutter in the front office), the potential patient/client is likely to have a bad first impression that can be difficult to correct. So make sure that the equipment is organized and clean and that the clinic, including the floors, windows and bathrooms, are clean. Show appreciation that the person chose this practice to seek services instead of going to another clinic. Live up to the expectations.

After the first impression, the practice must ensure that the patient continues to receive a positive experience throughout their plan of care and that the value of what is being delivered is evident. Engage with the patient, giving them your full attention. Provide

> direct access – the ability of the consumer to self-refer to a service (eg, physical therapy) without the approval or referral from a gatekeeper (eg, physician)

Chapter 6 / Entrepreneurship

education on home exercises, work modifications, or sport-specific skill development and the progress being made from the services delivered. The benefits of physical therapy are numerous, but it is as important to value the person in front of you, which is reflected in the PT's behavior, attitude, and interactions.

Summary

This chapter provides an overview of the skills and attributes desired in an entrepreneur who wants to develop a physical therapy private practice. There are many positive aspects to becoming a private practice owner as well as certain skills and attributes that are commonly seen in practice owners. In addition to the knowledge and skills of a health care provider, the entrepreneur possesses skills in leadership, managing change, willingness to work hard, effective communication, basic financial management, and marketing the business. Small businesses are the backbone of the American economy. Entities are available to assist a PT in starting a business such as the Small Business Association, the SBDC, the American Physical Therapy Association, or the SCORE. If a PT desires to have the freedom and understands the commitment to owning a small business/private practice, support for their endeavors is available to assist in the adventure.

REFERENCES

1. Scarborough N, Cornwall J. *Essentials of Entrepreneurship and Small Business Management*. Pearson; 2019.
2. Franklin R. The importance of taking action as an entrepreneur. Forbes. Published October 27, 2021. Accessed January 27, 2022. https://www.forbes.com/sites/forbesbusinesscouncil/2021/10/27/the-importance-of-taking-action-as-an-entrepreneur/?sh=2725106964ba
3. Pozin I. 80% is good enough: grow your business by delegating. Forbes. Published December 17, 2012. Accessed March 27, 2022. https://www.forbes.com/sites/ilyapozin/2012/12/17/80-is-good-enough-grow-your-business-by-delegating/?sh=e825847218ca
4. LeBauer A. *The CashPT Blueprint*. Lulu Publishing; 2019.
5. Advanced Business Portal. Why is leadership good in entrepreneurship? Accessed March 22, 2022. https://www.icsid.org/uncategorized/why-is-leadership-good-in-entrepreneurship/#1
6. Williams TA, Gruber DA, Sutcliffe KM, Shepherd DA, Zhao EY. Organizational response to adversity: fusing crisis management and resilience research. *Acad Manag Ann*. 2017;11(2):733-769. doi:10.5465/annals.2015.0134
7. Garret R, Zettel L. Entrepreneurial resilience. *Business Manag*. 2021. doi:10.1093/acrefore/9780190224851.013.314
8. Chadwick IC, Raver JL. Psychological resilience and its downstream effects for business survival in nascent entrepreneurship. *Entrep Theory Pract*. 2018;44(2):233-255. doi:10.1177%2F1042258718801597
9. American Psychological Association. Building your resilience. Published February 1, 2020. Accessed March 29, 2022. https://www.apa.org/topics/resilience
10. Cote C. Must have entrepreneurial skills for aspiring business owners. Harvard Business School online. August 25, 2020. Accessed April 3, 2022. https://online.hbs.edu/blog/post/entrepreneurial-skills
11. Quickbooks Survey: More Than 40 Percent of Small Business Owners Identify as Financially Illiterate. *Intuit*. November 13, 2014. Accessed April 2, 2024. https://www.businesswire.com/news/home/20141113005240/en/QuickBooks-Survey-More-Than-40-Percent-of-Small-Business-Owners-Identify-as-Financially-Illiterate
12. Collie M. Marketing your practice? Then ensure your provide an exceptional patient experience. Impact. Published 2018. Accessed May 2, 2022. https://www.ppsimpact.org/marketing-your-practice/
13. U.S. Small Business Administration. Organization. U.S. Small Business Administration. Published 2022. Accessed June 6, 2022. https://www.sba.gov/about-sba/organization
14. U.S. Small Business Administration. Business guide. U.S. Small Business Administration. Published 2022. Accessed April 8, 2023. http://www.sba.gov/business-guide
15. Brandon J. New survey says we are spending 7 hours per day consuming digital media. Forbes. Published 2022. Accessed August 22, 2022. https://www.forbes.com/sites/johnbbrandon/2020/11/17/new-survey-says-were-spending-7-hours-per-day-consuming-online-media/?sh=cc1b3436b466
16. Retail Wire. New study reveals consumers are uninspired by online shopping. April 3, 2014. www.Retailwire.com/discussion/new-study-reveals-consumers-are-uninspired-by-online-shopping/

17. Rckless D. How technology can help create a patient for life. Impact. Published 2018. Accessed September 12, 2022. https://www.ppsimpact.org
18. Strauch A. Using social media to drive new patients. Impact. Published 2019. Accessed September 9, 2022. https://www.ppsimpact.org/using-social-media-to-drive-new-patients/
19. Pew Research Center. Social media usage: 2005-2015. Published 2015. Accessed April 15, 2023. https://www.pewresearch.org/internet/2015/10/08/social-networking-usage-2005-2015/
20. Decatou, P. The 5 offensive formations for a championship social media strategy. Impact. Published 2018. Accessed September 11, 2022. https://www.ppsimpact.org/the-5-offensive-formations-of-a-championship-social-media-strategy/?print=print
21. American Physical Therapy Association. Implementing telehealth into your practice. Published 2020. Accessed September 9, 2022. https://www.apta.org/your-practice/practice-models-and-settings/telehealth-practice/implementing
22. Lia J, Gartner W. Are planners doers? Pre-venture planning and the start-up behaviors of entrepreneurs. SBA Advocacy. Published 2009. Accessed April 15, 2023. https://permanent.access.gpo.gov/LPS109715/LPS109715/archive.sba.gov/advo/research/rs339.pdf
23. McKee K. 5 elements of a successful physical therapy business plan. WebPT. Published 2020. Accessed September 12, 2022. https://www.webpt.com/blog/5-elements-of-a-successful-physical-therapy-business-plan//
24. Small Business Administration. Small Business Development Center. Accessed April 15, 2023. https://www.sba.gov/local-assistance/resource-partners/small-business-development-centers-sbdc
25. Service Corps of Retired Executives. Published 2023. Accessed April 8, 2023. http://www.score.org
26. Segal T. "Profit Center". Investopedia. Published 2020. Accessed October 20, 2022. https://www.investopedia.com/terms/p/profitcentre.asp
27. WebPT. The state of rehab therapy. Published June 1, 2021. Accessed October 20, 2022. https://www.webpt.com/downloads/state-of-rehab-therapy-2021/
28. Gourlay J, Plisky P. The three biggest contributors to employee disengagement and what to do about it. Impact. Published March 3, 2022. Accessed October 20, 2022. https://www.ppsimpact.org/the-three-biggest-contributors-to-employee-disengagement-and-what-to-do-about-it/?print=print
29. Khartit K. Subcontracting. Investopedia. Published 2020. Accessed October 20, 2022. https://www.investopedia.com/terms/s/subcontracting.asp
30. Gorman C. Seven seconds to make a first impression. Forbes. Accessed November 30, 2022. https://www.forbes.com/sites/carolkinseygoman/2011/02/13/seven-seconds-to-make-a-first-impression/?sh=69667af12722

CHAPTER 7

Marketing

MARK DRNACH

Learning Objectives

The reader will

1. Identify the components of a SWOT analysis and an action plan used in the marketing process.
2. Recognize basic marketing principles and their application to a health care service.
3. Identify the components of a basic marketing mix and the additional components that apply to the service sector.
4. Understand the basics of digital marketing.
5. Apply the principles of marketing to a personal marketing plan.

Marketing

Marketing can be defined as the activities and processes for creating, communicating, delivering, and exchanging goods or services that have value to the customer, client, partner, or society at large.[1] It encompasses a broader set of activities than the distribution of goods and services and the collection of revenues from those exchanges. It is more than selling. Selling is a specific process that deals with the negotiation and exchange of something the *seller has to offer* to a potential customer, whereas marketing deals with the exchange of something the *customer desires* and the seller produces.[2] The difference requires the private practice owner to understand how to acquire information about the customer, identify, develop, and deliver the desired product in a cost-effective manner and effectively communicate the value of those services to the customer, client, partner, payer, or society at large. In health care, the goods or product could be identified as the outcome of "improved health." That is what patients desire. The service that is provided is the program or skills that are used by the practitioner to achieve that outcome. The goal of marketing is to capture the business of a percentage of the people in a given geographic location and to deliver a specific volume of product to sustain and grow the practice. Marketing decisions are intimately related to business decisions, and just as knowing the basics of business is necessary for financial success, knowing the basics of marketing is necessary for meeting the needs of the customer and being successful, financially. This chapter will present the basic principles of marketing and how they apply to a private practice, specifically, a physical therapy practice. It will also apply those marketing principles to individuals who may find at graduation, or when desiring to work for another employer, the need to market themselves.

153

SWOT Analysis

Successful marketing starts with the identification of the customers and the needs of those customers, along with an analysis of the strengths and abilities of the practice, and aligning those with the needs of the customers.[3] This process of identifying the strengths and weaknesses of a practice and the opportunities and threats in the external environment is known as a SWOT analysis. First conceptualized by Robert Stewart in the 1960s, the SWOT analysis is one of the earliest participatory planning frameworks used by businesses for strategic planning purposes.[4] The process involves stakeholders who individually identify the current strengths and weaknesses of a business or practice along with their understanding or view of the opportunities and threats in the external environment that can impact the business' future. This information is then shared with the managers and owners, executives of the business, who use this data, along with their own, to conceptualize the current strategic position of the business and the opportunities available in the external environment for consideration, as well as the threats they may encounter (Table 7.1). This process uses the brain power and judgment of the business' employees, and other stakeholders, to create a culture of participation. The information gained is used in the development of strategic goals for the future. These goals are supported by an action plan that sets clear expectations for addressing and reporting on the status of the goal's achievement. An action plan at a minimum should include a goal, an objective measure to know when the goal is met, the target date for meeting the goal, the person or job title responsible for addressing the goal, and a progress reporting timeline (Table 7.2).

The SWOT analysis is the first step in a marketing process that involves the assessment of a practice's internal environment (ie, strengths and weakness) and the external environment (ie, opportunities and threats) that make it possible to develop an effective marketing strategy.

Table 7.1 SWOT Analysis Template			
Name of the Business: **Date:** **Contributors:** **Internal Environment**		**External Environment**	
Strengths	*Weaknesses*	*Opportunities*	*Threats*

marketing – the activities and processes for creating, communicating, delivering, and exchanging goods or services that have value to the customer

selling – a specific process that deals with the negotiation and exchange of something the seller has to offer to a potential customer

SWOT analysis – a participatory planning framework used for strategic planning purposes. The acronym stands for strengths, weaknesses, opportunities, threats

action plan – a detailed description of the expectations for addressing and reporting on the status of a strategic goal's achievement

Chapter 7 / Marketing   155

Table 7.2 Action Plan Template				
Name of the Business: **Today's Date:** **Dates of the Plan from Start to Finish:** **Author of the Plan:** **Date Plan Approved by Management:**				
Goal	*Outcome*	*Target Date*	*Responsible Person*	*Interim Report Due Date*

Basics of Marketing

Historically, the need to market a health care business was not a priority when the demand exceeded the supply. One just had to open a shop (a private practice or hospital department), and the patients would come. But with the growing US population, more access to payment structures for health care services, and an informed and demanding consumer with options for health and wellness services, there is a requirement for practice owners and hospital departments to have a basic knowledge of business practices and engage with other stakeholders to survive and thrive in the current health care environment. Business knowledge, including basic marketing principles, was not part of a professional health care education curriculum. The current health care environment in the United States, which is greatly influenced by cost, makes this information necessary to deliver services that are not only evidence based or supported by best practice but are also cost effective and meet the needs of the consumers, the patients.[5]

In order to understand the consumer of the service, a provider can begin by understanding the demographics of the people in a certain geographic location. Demographics are the characteristics of a select group of individuals. These characteristics can include the average and range of ages, education levels, marital status, gender, occupations, or household incomes. Awareness of the demographics in a select geographic region will provide the practitioner with an understanding of the availability and possible needs of the people in a given area. This is useful information when considering various programs to offer, such as exercise classes for pregnant women or a fall prevention program for the older adults. Before developing a program, it would be helpful and strategic for the practice owner to know the demographics of the local area. Are younger people of child-bearing age moving into or out of the area? This information will provide an indication of the possible demand. What is the education level of the people in the local area? This information will be helpful when creating marketing and educational material for the participants or promoting health literacy in the community. The average household income would be helpful in deciding if the program should have a cash-only payment structure or utilize health insurance for the revenue stream. These are only a few questions that are appropriate to ask during the initial stages of program development. Demographic information provides the practitioner with an understanding of the potential customers and therefore allows for the development of programs that will be able to meet their needs and lead to a successful and sustainable business. Demographic information can be obtained through various federal and state government agencies and is available on the internet.

> demographics – specific characteristics of a select group of individuals in a certain geographic region

BOX 7.1 • Demographic Information Sources

US Census Bureau—Information on population estimates by age, gender, health insurance coverage status, and economic information. Available at https://data.census.gov/

Bureau of Labor Statistics—Information on unemployment rate, average hourly earnings, disability information, and educational attainment. Available at https://www.bls.gov/

Centers for Disease Control and Prevention (CDC) National Center for Health Statistics—Information on vital statistics (births, deaths), prenatal care utilization, and workers' health and mortality. Available at https://www.cdc.gov/

Local Department on Economic Development—Information on the cost of living, home ownership rate, local industries. Search for Economic Development Board for a specific state.

US Department of Commerce. Bureau of Economic Analysis. Information on personal income and consumption expenditures by state. Available at https://www.bea.gov/news/glance

Websites accessed on November 27, 2023.

It may take some time to understand the local community, but acquiring this basic information will support the future development of programs and the creation of an effective marketing strategy (Box 7.1). Determining how much information is needed is a function of the practice's management and/or leadership. The risk of making a poor decision resulting from lack of additional information must be balanced against the cost (including time and effort) that it will take to obtain more information. A point is achieved when the practice owner decides that the volume and type of information obtained are sufficient to address an acceptable level of risk and that the demographic information supports the initiative to further develop a specific program or service. (eg, yes, there is a growing number of young adults moving into the area. Or, yes, there is a significant number of people over the age of 80 years in the area.) This is a personal choice. Once a set of demographic data is obtained, it is important to track that information over time to identify any trends that may lead to a different choice in the future. (eg, expanding a pediatric program for infants when there is a declining adult population moving into the area may not be prudent.) It is also important to clarify the specific market where the services will be delivered and the product will be exchanged.

A market is a place, either physical or virtual (ie, online), where people with something to sell and buyers with a specific need or want gather to exchange goods or services for money. The potential buyers in a given location will seek out a service in a specific area (eg, hospital, outpatient clinic, web page) to fulfill a need or want. In health care, this potential buyer and decision maker could be a patient or client, a referral source, a parent, another professional, or an insurance administrator. The market for patients can be defined by their demographic characteristics, and then a select subgroup of them, with specific characteristics or needs (eg, pain), can be identified for a specific type of service (eg, health care). This process is called market segmentation, or dividing a market into groups with common characteristics. In health care, they have common symptoms or needs. The goal of market segmentation is to identify specific subgroups within the market that share similar traits, making it easier for a business to tailor marketing efforts to meet their specific needs.[6] The potential customers in the subgroup can then be categorized in a variety of ways, namely,

market – a place, either physical or virtual, where people with something to sell and buyers with a specific need or want gather to exchange goods or services for money

market segmentation – the process of dividing a market into groups with common characteristics

Table 7.3 Market Segmentation and Target Market

Market Segment	Target Market	Possible Services
Adult workers employed in the manufacturing industry. Have a high school education and health insurance. Earn an average income. Support a family.	Middle-aged workers who have a history of reoccurring back pain. Use medications for pain relief. Continue to work but periodically have to take days off owing to back pain.	Multidisciplinary team of physician, pharmacist, and PT PT available after work hours and on weekends Written home programs provided Assessment of job duties and workplace ergonomics Health insurance to pay for rehabilitation. Self-pay for maintenance program with follow-up visits 2 times per month **Information available** through social media, workplace posting, or mail
Parents of a child with a disability. Have a high school or college education. Earn an income above the federal poverty level. Use public and private transportation.	Parents of school-aged children who are 14 years of age or older. Enrolled in public education. Have an IEP. Use assistive technology.	Multidisciplinary team of physiatrist, social worker, equipment supplier, and PT Care's focus is on function and Activities of Daily Living (ADLs), caregiver skills Support identification of skills and plan to participate in community soon after high school. Social worker to help with guardianship paperwork once student reaches the age of 18 years Flexible schedules to accommodate family's schedule and transportation needs Electronic reminders of appointments **Information available** through packets sent home by the school, postings at school-sponsored events, presentations at parent meetings or groups
Older adults over the age of 80 years who live alone. Have a high school or college education. Use public transportation. Yearly income exceeds the state average. Have Medicare Insurance Parts A, B, and D.	Older adults with co-morbid diagnosis that makes them a fall risk or who have a fear of falling. Important to maintain their independence and functioning. Are on medications for a variety of reasons. May use a standard cane or walker. Travel periodically to visit family or friends.	Multidisciplinary team of physician, social worker, pharmacist, OT, and PT Group exercise programs with a focus on maintaining balance and independence. Programs offered during the daylight hours owing to possible transportation restrictions. Home care and environmental assessments for safety and proper ergonomics. Provides a subscription service for PT so former patients can call for basic information or follow-up visits on an as needed basis **Information available** through religious publications, physician offices, postings at pharmacies, or mail

by age, income level, gender, occupation, health status, etc. For example, people who work in manual labor occupations and are experiencing, or who have a history of, low back pain can be targeted for a specific set of services designed by the seller. This is called a target market—a select group of people with a specific need (ie, relief from chronic low back pain) and an interest in a specific service (ie, physical therapy). By identifying the target market, the provider can then package specific programs and communicate them to the target market through appropriate communication channels (Table 7.3). This optimizes resource utilization by focusing on people with specific needs who would most likely become customers.

target market – a select group of buyers with a specific need and an interest in a specific service

Knowing the size of the market (eg, the number of people over the age of 80 years in a given market) and the number of people with specific characteristics who could be served by the practice, the practice owner can determine the market share, or percentage of a market that purchases or has the potential to purchase a product from a business. For example, if in a given market, there are 5,000 people over the age of 80 years (information from the US Census Bureau) and the practice is providing services to 1,000 people annually in that market of people who are over 80 years of age, then the practice has 20% of the market share. A goal of a practice may be to obtain a certain percentage of the market share in order to have a sustainable practice. This can be influenced by the intentional positioning of the practice in the market. Market positioning is the decision of the practice on how it presents itself in a specific market. It is the way a practice is perceived by the customers in relation to other health care businesses. What makes the practice unique or valuable to the customer? There are several options that a practice can consider when it comes to market positioning: Does the practice want to be perceived as a *leader* in providing the most advanced, evidence-based, treatment techniques? An *innovator* providing services to patients and the community in a unique and socially responsible manner? Or a *consumer-centric* practice, providing services that are desired or needed by the customers?[2] Does the practice want to be perceived as providing *reliable services* that are effective and efficiently delivered? A practice that is *socially responsible*, offering programs that support the *community and that is engaged in community projects? Or have a branding position that promotes* customer loyalty?[7] In the competitive environment of private practice, where similar positions and approaches are directed at the same target market, a new practice may feel challenged to enter the market owing to the established positions of others who are considered leaders or innovators in a specific area of care. In this market, it is helpful to explore possible alternatives to the same target market.[8] (eg, Provide two-way texting or video options to support the home program. Have a mobile clinic that goes to the patient's home instead of the patient coming to the clinic. Partner with a durable medical equipment provider to expedite the acquisition of specialized equipment.) The new practice can also consider addressing the needs of a niche market, a specific target market that can be identified for a specific service that is distinctly differentiated from the competitors but that meets a specific need of a specific group. Some examples include a pelvic floor care program for women, a group exercise program for seniors, sports-specific training and rehabilitation for the high school athletes, therapeutic horseback riding for children with cerebral palsy, or physical therapy for people with Parkinson disease. Niche marketing can be effective for small practices that cannot afford the diversity of services, and the marketing expenses, associated with services provided to a larger market. It may also be helpful for a practice or sole proprietor that simply chooses not to serve a larger market but to focus on one type of patient for one area of care. Choosing the right segment of the market is key to achieving the sales volume and revenues that can make this strategy financially successful.[2]

The percentage of the target market (or niche market) that purchases the product of the practice at least once in a given time period provides information on market penetration.

market share – a percentage of a market that purchases or has the potential to purchase a service or good from a business

market positioning – the decision of the practice on how to present itself to the market

niche market – a specific target market that can be identified for a specific service that is distinctly differentiated from the competitors but meets a specific need of a specific group

market penetration – the percentage of the target market that purchases the product or services of the practice at least once in a given time period. It is a measure of the extent that the practice captured the target market

Chapter 7 / Marketing

This is a measure of the extent that the practice captured the target market during a period of time. Expanding in a market can be accomplished in a variety of ways, by forming partnerships, lowering prices, targeting new markets, or introducing new services. One goal of market penetration is to have patients come to the practice repeatedly for a variety of the services offered, instead of going to a competitor. In order to achieve this goal, the practice should have a good brand. A brand is the expressed promise of value.[9] It is an intangible asset that is intended to create distinctive images and associations in the minds of stakeholders, thereby generating an economic benefit for the practice.[1] It is not simply a logo or advertisement, but a feeling of trust and respect. It should set the practice apart from its competitors, add value, and enhance the experience of the patient.[10] It should answer the questions of who you are, what you exclusively do, and what this product or service does. Fill in the blank:

Our practice is the only ____ that ____.[10]
Examples: Our practice is the only outpatient clinic that produces value-based outcomes.
Our practice is the only locally owned business that provides comprehensive rehabilitation programs for seniors.
Our practice is the only physical therapy clinic that provides virtual visits and flexible scheduling.

The brand should align the needs and wants of the customer with the ability of the provider. It should drive marketing and be reinforced in the communications with all stakeholders. The brand should focus on what the practice does best and reinforce the value of the products and services that are delivered by the practice (Chapter 6) (Box 7.2).

The marketing process begins with the identification of the demographics of a population, segmenting that population based on specific characteristics, and, from that subset, targets a specific group with certain characteristics, symptoms, and needs that can be met by the practice. The practice has to decide on the image it wants to adopt, and the position it wants to take, to address this target market. It should clearly articulate its brand and repeat it aggressively to stakeholders. The practice should monitor its market penetration and market share in order to make strategic decisions about the future and the sustainability of the services or programs offered. These decisions will clarify the market planning process and focus the business decisions to efficiently use available resources to achieve its business and financial goals.

BOX 7.2 • Key Elements of Effective Branding

1. Invest in marketing communication to improve potential customer awareness and understanding of the product's value.
2. Create and sustain good internal communication so the employees are aware of the customers' needs and wants, market trends, company initiatives, and customers' needs and wants.
3. Contribute to the local community to improve the practice's reputation.
4. Improve service quality to improve market position.

Gray BJ. Benchmarking services branding practices. *J Mark Manag.* 2006;22(7-8):717-758.

---

brand – the expressed promise of value

Marketing Mix

Neil Bordon, a professor in the area of Marketing at Harvard University, is credited with coining the term marketing mix.[11] This term is widely used to describe the variables that a business uses to satisfy the wants or needs of a market. Originally, the four P's of marketing—product, price, place, and promotion—have been expanded to include other aspects associated with providing a service. These additions include packaging; physical evidence of effectiveness; processes that instill a sense of confidence; and the selection, training, and skills of the personnel in the business.[12]

Product

A product is the goods or services that are provided by a business. In health care, marketing should be driven by what the customer wants or needs so that the practice can build a sustainable relationship with the customers.[5] This is typically the end product of the services provided: fulfilling the need or want of the customer. How does the practice offer a service that best achieves that outcome? What product or service is necessary? How many products could be offered? Government policies, social trends (eg, the use of wearable biometric recording devices), information technology development (eg, tracking health information and reporting on health status is acceptable and desired by some), legal issues (eg, state practice acts), and business trends (eg, virtual visits) can all impact the behavior and decisions of the customer and provider. These factors should be taken into consideration when developing a product to ensure the product is marketable and profitable. Considering the perspective of the customer is vital in this process.

Price

The cost of producing the product is a significant factor in the price and an important component in the decision-making process of both the consumer and the producer. An understanding of the cost associated with the service or product must be identified and understood by the provider in order to set a price that is acceptable to the customer and is conducive to the financial viability of the practice (Chapter 1). Once the cost is known, the provider can then decide on the minimum price needed to cover the costs plus any profit margin that is desired. The price should not be so high as to exclude people from purchasing the service nor so low as to jeopardize the financial sustainability of the product or practice. There are pricing strategies, such as the *market or going rate*, the *break-even or cost method*, or the *mark-up method*, that can be adopted to position the product in the market. Tracking the trends in demand as it relates to the price is an important financial indicator to monitor (Chapter 1).

Place

The place is the physical location and aspects of the service delivery where the product is delivered. This environment should match the expectations of the customers. If the practice is providing pediatric services, then the physical environment should have child-friendly furniture, family bathrooms, and a play area for children while they wait. If providing sports-specific services for adolescents, the physical environment should be different from

marketing mix – a term used to describe the variables of product, price, place, and promotion that a business uses to satisfy the wants or needs of a market

the pediatric practice. It may have private seating areas to wait, video screens that provide relevant information to this population, and free Wi-Fi. In addition, the concept of place includes the hours of operation; the physical accessibility to the location and services; the location of the practice within the community; parking availability; and proximity to the referral source, other health care partners, or health care services. The place can also be virtual. If the practice has a website, it should be easy to navigate and have accessibility options for the text to be read out loud or have the ability to change the font size for easier reading. The website must be kept up-to-date to facilitate engagement with the patients who should find the content relevant and easy to access and understand. The virtual place should be responsive to the user's requests to support and sustain the relationship between the patient and the practice. Websites are also a vehicle to recruit other professionals into partnerships with the practice. Out-of-date information may have a negative impact on the practice's image or brand, so keeping the site current, functioning, and free of grammatical and typographic errors is important.

Promotion

Promotion is a strategy used to communicate with potential customers the product or service that a practice has to offer. It is the process by which the customers (or target market) become aware of the product. There are several methods that a practice can employ to communicate to a target market: advertising in publications, podcasts, or on websites; written advertisements posted at community venues and events; through a referral source or direct mailing campaigns; and by word of mouth, either in person or electronically, which can be efficient and cost effective. Electronic media allows the practitioner to set up a communication channel with existing patients to permanently communicate with them, providing updates or general health and wellness information to retain them as loyal customers. Promotion efforts should attempt to persuade the customer to prefer the practice's product over the competitors and to use the practice's services repeatedly. It should have the intent of producing customer loyalty. But, remember, although promotion *informs* the customers about a product, it is the personal, or expert, source of information that *legitimizes* the value of the product or service.[5]

Packaging

How the product is packaged or viewed by the customers is as important as the science that went into its development. The promotional materials, the attitude of the employees toward the customers, and the physical setting in which the product is delivered are all important components of the package. In general, patients show higher satisfaction when health care providers pay attention to their individual needs and treat them with kindness and when patients feel that they participate in their own care.[13] Studies also found that physical features, such as room temperature and cleanliness, are associated with the perception of quality.[14] With the trend toward value-based and patient-centered care models in health care reimbursement structures, patient satisfaction and value-based outcomes should be a marketing objective for every health care practice.

Physical Evidence of Effectiveness

Many patients do not understand the intricate details of the education or expertise of the health care provider treating them. They know who the physical therapist is by the designator PT or MD or DO. Having a license to practice in a state is another indicator of the health care provider's educational background and ability to provide health care services in the state. These are the basic requirements to provide care that is expected, by the patient, to be effective in addressing their concerns or needs. There are other sources of physical evidence to help them judge if they are about to receive a higher quality product and if it will be effective in meeting their needs. Such sources include items such as testimonials from patients or other community members associated with the practice and the displaying of state licenses, board certifications, community or professional association awards, accreditations, or publications by the health care providers. Through these means, a sense of quality and effectiveness of the care provided is communicated. Having partnerships with other health care professionals and providing value-based care and outcomes shows collaboration and the desire to meet the needs of the patient in an efficient and, hopefully, effective manner. The publication of annual reports, including the benefits obtained by a target market, is a way of communicating the effectiveness of the services provided. Quality is also communicated through the physical appearance of the clinical setting and staff, the cleanliness of the clinic, the age and condition of the furniture and equipment, and how staff speak to one another.[2] Every potential and actual customer has expectations of the practice. Meeting these through various forms of physical evidence can give them confidence that they will be treated appropriately.

Processes

The experience when buying a product is becoming more important as the customer becomes more educated on what they need and on what to expect from the provider. Poor adherence to processes can lead to a poor customer experience, which impacts the likelihood of a return visit and possibly communicating a negative opinion of the practice to people in the community. It is important to consistently reflect a patient-centered, customer-oriented approach in the service delivery and interactions with the public. All employees should have knowledge of the policies and procedures of the practice, especially as they pertain to the interactions with the customers. Do the processes instill confidence in the customer? Are the processes for the payment, scheduling of appointments, and cancellation of appointments clear and fair? Is written information, a hard copy or electronic, free of typographic or grammatical errors and appropriate for the customers' level of health literacy (Chapter 12)? Do the processes treat people, both customers and employees, with respect and support their needs? Do they provide the employees with clear guidance and expectations on professional development, adherence to external and internal standards, and development of new programs or production of value-based outcomes (Box 7.3)? As with the marketing aspect of place, people should be treated with respect and observe a clinical environment that is consistently professional, clean, and orderly.

BOX 7.3 • Five Steps to Prepare for Value-Based Care and Payment

1. Standardize documentation to ensure uniformity of data collection.
4. Adhere to appropriate clinical practice guidelines and clinical protocols to standardize care.
5. Identify and use a set of appropriate outcome measures that are relevant to the practice.
6. Adopt and use technology to prepare the practice for data collection at the population level.
7. Create and follow procedures to collect, analyze, report, and communicate outcome data at a minimum on an annual basis.

Gainer K, Smith H. The shift toward value-based payment. American Physical Therapy Magazine. Published October 1, 2017. Accessed November 22, 2023. https://www.apta.org/apta-magazine/2017/10/01/compliance-matters -the-shift-toward-value-based-payment

Chapter 7 / Marketing

Personnel

All employees in a practice can impact the customer's perception of quality. Image matters. That image is cultivated by how employees are recruited, selected, trained, and supported in their professional growth and development. Annual training and performance reviews assist the employee in maintaining and demonstrating the skills that will move the practice forward. It is a time to reflect and reinforce the expected behaviors that support the brand of the practice. Personnel with specific training (eg, information technology) or certification in a specialty area (eg, treatment of pelvic floor dysfunction) are a necessary component of a practice that delivers those types of services. The recruitment and retention of these employees with specific skills is vital to the brand and the service that is delivered. All staff members should act professionally: be kind and courteous; greet patients and coworkers; offer assistance; ask for clarification and understanding. The interactions with patients, coworkers, and partners should reflect professionalism and an understanding of the current literature and/or clinical practice guidelines that optimize the patient's outcome and promote a sense of caring and understanding of the patient's condition and concerns (Chapter 8).

The practice owner should nurture a culture that supports and promotes the marketing mix of the services and products offered. The concept of the marketing mix highlights the importance of the various factors that are used in a marketing strategy. How a practice defines these components helps to determine a marketing plan for business success. It is important that the employees of the practice understand the product they are delivering and how the services provided help the patient to gain that product, namely, better health.

Digital Marketing

Digital marketing uses electronic media to connect with potential buyers in a market. This can include marketing through search engines, websites, mobile devices, or social media platforms. Given that people in the United States spend hours a day on an electronic device, this form of advertising can reach a large number of potential customers and can be cost effective when advertising to a target market. Digital marketing is one of the most powerful and popular ways of marketing today. For optimal results, a practice owner should know the characteristic of the target market and which electronic media outlet would work best to communicate with those individuals.

A wide range of digital marketing strategies are available, but social media marketing, search engine optimization, pay-per-click advertising, mobile marketing, and email marketing are among the more common ones used.

Social media marketing (SMM) uses platforms such as Facebook, YouTube, WhatsApp, Instagram, and LinkedIn, which have a worldwide audience and millions of users who daily search for information and share ideas with other people online. Having a social media presence and/or advertising on these sites has the potential to reach a significant number of people far removed from the clinic's site. The practice owner should be realistic, given the restrictions of third-party payers and state practice acts, and may focus advertising on a specific target market, filtered by demographic information such as age and distance from the clinic's site. This is a more cost-effective and targeted approach to digital marketing. But digital marketing is more complex than simply posting a comment online.

digital marketing – a marketing approach that uses electronic media to connect with potential buyers in a market

social media marketing – marketing that uses platforms such as Facebook, which have users who search for information and share ideas with other people online

The practice has to create a consistent message, post and manage the content regularly, and routinely gather and evaluate the performance of the posts. SMM can have a significant impact on the practice's reputation and brand, making it necessary to allocate sufficient funds and time to its management.[15,16]

Search Engine Optimization (SEO) is a process of structuring a website, so search engines, such as Google or Yahoo, rank it higher on its results page. This is based on several factors such as key words or phrases that are frequently used on the site, links to other websites, and an easy-to-use navigation page. Google provides a free SEO Starter Guide to assist a person on how to set up and promote online content.[17] Part of this process recommends updating the content frequently, making sure the content is mobile device friendly, and the content is of good quality. Posting patient reviews is also helpful and of interest to the consumer when deciding on which practice or clinic to visit.

Pay-Per-Click (PPC) advertising is a model of digital marketing in which advertisers pay a fee each time one of their ads is clicked. Essentially, it's a way of buying visits to the site, rather than attempting to obtain those visits through SEO. Targeted search engine advertising is one of the most popular forms of a PPC strategy.[18] By limiting the advertisements to a target market and tracking the conversions from clicking on the ad to making a call or visit to the clinic, the practice can evaluate the benefit of this advertising on growing market share and market penetration. There are relatively inexpensive multiple call tracking systems available online that can assist in tracking conversions and providing summary reports.

Mobile marketing is done through a mobile device, such as a cell phone, which has a Subscriber Identify Module (SIM) that allows for the identification of the device and, ultimately, the owner or user. In order to get a message out to a potential customer, a practice has to advertise where the customer will see the advertisement; and the customer is using his or her phone. Mobile marketing is cost effective and makes it easy to reach a target market. It is also a quick form of communication that increases the risk of sending information containing errors. It is also important to obtain the patient's permission or acknowledgment that this type of message will be sent and that the message sent will be useful to the receiver.[19] Failure to do so can lead to patient irritation and a negative opinion of the practice.

Email marketing is a strategy of sending emails to past patients or interested potential customers to capture their attention and foster or sustain a relationship. As with text messages, the information has to be succinct and of interest to the receiver. Creating a clear message in the subject line will alert the receiver of the general intent of the message. Failure to use email marketing judiciously can result in the marketing efforts being diverted to the trash or spam folder.

Digital marketing is a form of promotion that provides the customers or target market with persuasive information, delivered electronically, about the product or services a practice has to offer. But, remember, promotion informs the customers about a product. It is the actual personal interactions and the benefits received by the patient from the services that legitimizes the value of the product.[5]

search engine optimization – a process of structuring a website so search engines, such as Google, rank it higher on its results page

pay-per-click – a model of digital marketing in which advertisers pay a fee each time one of their ads is clicked by a user

mobile marketing – marketing done through a mobile device, such as a cell phone, that allows for the identification of the device and ultimately the owner or user

email marketing – a strategy of sending emails to past patients or interested potential customers to capture their attention and foster or sustain a relationship

Chapter 7 / Marketing

Marketing Yourself

The purpose of marketing is to communicate to a target consumer relevant information in a manner that will persuade the consumer to decide to purchase the product. This section of the chapter will present a framework that an individual, either a new graduate or a physical therapist (PT) considering a new job, can use to market the product they have to offer, the service of physical therapy. (The term PT will be used in the following sections, but PT student is also implied.)

The first step in this process is to organize information about the *course of one's* life, in Latin, curriculum vitae (CV). This document should provide the reader with an overview of the professional aspects of a person's education, professional career, and life experiences that closely reflect who that person is today. It is a report on the education, work experiences, community involvement, and achievements one has accomplished. In contrast to a résumé, which is French for *summary*, the CV can be a lengthy document depending on the accomplishments and years of employment. (Note: A resume is typically 1-2 pages and covers a shorter time period, typically, the past 2-5 years.) There are several formats that can be used to present the information in a CV, and each person should structure a CV that reflects a personal style but should be organized and professional in appearance (ie, single spaced with double space between groups, same font size throughout, no more than two different font style changes, no typographic or grammatical errors, avoid excessive use of bullets) (Box 7.4). There are some basic items that should be included in a professional CV. This information includes the PT's contact information and a preferred method of communication (eg, email, text, phone call). It should list the educational degrees earned, starting with the most current degree awarded. A PT can be licensed to practice within a state or hold multiple licenses. A list of the state(s) and the status of the license (active, inactive) and the license number would be appropriate, as well as any certifications that the PT holds, such as cardiopulmonary resuscitation (CPR), advanced first aid, or board certification. The CV can also be a helpful document in professional development and monitoring of the specific guidelines and timelines for licensure renewal or recertifications. Having this information in the CV not only communicates that information to a potential employer but also serves as a reminder to the PT as to when license renewal is due or a certification expires. A potential employer will also want to know about the PT's previous work experience, both full-time and part-time employment. This information should include a brief listing of the responsibilities of the job or job duties, which duties would be listed in the job description and identified from the PT's personal experience while working at the job. This is one area of information that can be tailored to meet the needs of the audience who is reading the CV. For example, if a PT is working in a hospital outpatient clinic and has both patient treatment and department administrative duties but is applying for a management position in a free-standing outpatient clinic, the PT may elaborate on the administrative aspects of the hospital job and condense the information on the treatment responsibilities. Conversely, if the PT is applying for a staff position at a free-standing outpatient clinic, the PT may elaborate on the treatment responsibilities and condense the administrative aspects of the hospital job. Both versions would contain truthful and accurate information but emphasize different aspects of the job duties depending on the wants or needs of the target audience (or target market of one, the potential employer). Information on publications; presentations in peer-reviewed venues; and other professional activities such as grant writing, membership in professional societies, and consultative and advisory positions held communicate a level of effectiveness and quality. Acknowledgment from peer groups or other agencies who view the PT as a valuable source of information to include in their publications, presentations, or advisory boards is perceived as a reflection of

BOX 7.4 • Sample Outline of a Curriculum Vitae

Curriculum Vitae
Name:
Address:
Phone:
Email:
Preferred method of communication:

Education
Institution:
Location:
Degree/Date:

Licensure Information/Registration Number
State   Licensure number PT-(active)

Certifications
Type:
Certifier:
Dates of certification:

Full-Time Employment
Title/Position:
Institution:
Location:
Duration:
Responsible for

Part-Time Employment
Title/Position:
Institution:
Location:
Duration:

Publications
Books
Book chapters
Peer-reviewed publications
Professional presentations
Abstracts/Poster presentations
Invited publications/Articles

Grants
Authorship/Participation:
Amount of funding requested:
Nature of project:
Date and source:

BOX 7.4 • Sample Outline of a Curriculum Vitae (*continued*)

Membership and Positions Held in Scientific-Professional-Honorary Societies

Consultative and Advisory Position
Title:
Agency:
Duration:

Community Service
Title:
Agency:
Duration:

Continuing Education
Name of sponsor:
City/State:
Date of course:
Course title:
Instructors:
Credits:
Brief description and relationship to professional development:

quality. Many PT practices also value community engagement and know the importance of this activity on their brand. Listing the participation, past or present, in the community, especially as it relates to health or the social determinants of health (Chapter 11), can also be tailored to reflect the potential employer's brand.

Keeping track of the continuing education and the continuing education units (CEUs) that have been acquired during a specific time period (eg, 1 or 2 years) is necessary for several reasons. First, it is necessary in order to maintain a PT license to practice in a state. Having a list will help the PT manage the acquisition of CEUs in a timely and intentional manner and avoid having to look for *any* online continuing education offerings in the last month before license renewal. Second, it is evidence of a professional development plan. When documented in an organized fashion, a PT can review the past continuing education topics and seek additional topic areas that complement the knowledge already gained or identify gaps in current knowledge to explore. As with job duties and community service, continuing education listings can be tailored to meet the needs of the potential employer, expanding on the description of the course as it relates to the needs or wants of the employer. And, finally, it can be used to justify the currency of knowledge on specific topics that are taught in a physical therapy program (Chapter 5). If a PT wants to teach in higher education, either as an adjunct or as a full-time faculty member, and the Doctor of Physical Therapy program is in need of a faculty member to teach the topic of therapeutic exercise, the PT could show evidence of continuing education and current competency to teach in that area (see Box 7.4). In view of the number of continuing education courses a PT is required to attend for licensure, this section of the CV can be made into a separate document that is available on request, and only the most recent continuing education (eg, taken in the past 2 years), or the most relevant to the potential job, can be listed in the CV.

A Personal SWOT Analysis

A SWOT analysis should be a part of any business' strategic marketing planning process. This analysis can also be done on an individual level (see Table 7.1). It is important for a PT to periodically take inventory of their professional life, and an organized CV serves as a document that facilitates that reflection and also as a collection of past patients' feedback or testimonials and the PT's history of performance appraisals (Chapter 5). Identifying strengths can be an internal reflection with personal justification but should be supported by external validation reflected in the accomplishments listed in the CV or another source document (eg, letters from past patients, satisfaction surveys, outcome reports). From the strengths, weaknesses may become evident from the same source documents or internal reflection on the need to develop skills that are important in future practice. Weaknesses should be viewed as areas for growth and professional development and be treated as such by creating an action plan to address the identified weakness (see Table 7.2). A key difference is that the responsible person in this action plan is you. Identifying areas for professional and personal growth is part of a professional development program and a key aspect of being a professional.[20]

Strengths and weaknesses relate to the PT personally, the internal environment. The external environment is what is happening in the larger area of physical therapy and health care. Environmental scanning is an efficient way to capture and monitor what is happening in the external environment of health care (Chapter 1). The American Hospital Association publishes an annual environmental scan report that provides concise information on what is happening in the external environment of health care in the United States.[21] From this report, the PT can gain information on the trends in health care and the identified needs or opportunities in the market. Information on the local external environment can be obtained from resources that provide demographic information for both national and local areas (see Box 7.1). The sources of information on the external environment can be evaluated as to whether the information identifies a threat to the practice of physical therapy or an opportunity to practice physical therapy in a particular market. Participation in the state's chapter of the American Physical Therapy Association (APTA), local chamber of commerce, and word of mouth from people in the community are other sources of information on the opportunities and threats in the external environment of health care. From this information, the PT can begin to see how their personal strengths can be used to take advantage of the opportunities in the market, while also taking actions to address any weaknesses and monitor any possible threats to a successful career.

Personal Marketing Mix

As expected, a personal marketing mix includes personal factors in the decisions on what and how to market a PT (ie, you) to a target market. These include the desire or *passion* of the PT, how the PT wants to *practice* physical therapy, including the clinical setting, the geographic area or *place* where the PT wants to live and practice, and the amount of income or *payment* that can potentially be earned (Box 7.5).

BOX 7.5 • Steps in a Personal Marketing Mix

Step 1. Identify your passion.
Step 2. Explore the options available to practice.
Step 3. Decide on the place to practice and how to practice in that place.
Step 4. Determine the payment level needed to meet a desired level of income

Passion

An individual who goes into the field of health care does so for many reasons but commonly out of a desire, or passion, to provide a service to others, which is the motivator for the investment of time and effort needed for the acquisition of knowledge and a license to practice. This passion is the driver that motivates a PT to develop professional skills (a service) in a specific area that will benefit a specific type of patient (a target market) that will result in their optimal health (the *product*). This passion can become a reality when the PT actively reflects on their personal strengths and makes an honest evaluation of that aspect of an internal SWOT analysis. A PT may think they have the desire to help those without the financial resources to adequately access rehabilitation services, but may never have participated in a pro bono clinic or other services that help those individuals. A PT may think they have a desire to work with pediatric patients but may never have interacted, professionally, with that population. There is a difference between desire and interest. A desire is something the PT honestly wishes to do and has the internal motivation to do so because it provides a sense of self-actualization and fulfillment (Chapter 1). Their past behavior reflects this passion and desire. An interest is something the PT thinks they should do. Both would support the development of a viable product, but a passion would be a stronger motivator. It is important to identify the underlying passion that validates the opportunity costs associated with the PT's decisions and more clearly defines the *product*, the population of interest, and the personal brand that the PT will market. The PT should also be intimately familiar with how the product or service reflects their ability to produce a positive outcome from the services provided (ie, *physical evidence of effectiveness*). The passion should be supported by the PT's knowledge of the evidence in the literature of its effectiveness, the application of the relevant clinical practice guidelines, and the management aspects of service delivery (ie, *process*) to promote confidence in the potential employer and/or target population. (How exactly will the product be delivered, and why will it be delivered in that manner?) These attributes should clarify the differences between the PT and the competitors in the target market.

Practice

There are many settings and patient populations, or markets, where a PT can practice, from an independent contractor to an employee (Chapter 5). If working with children is what a PT desires to do, they can work in the neonatal intensive care unit of acute care hospital, the early intervention program under Individuals with Disabilities Education Act (IDEA), Part C, the school setting, private practice, or an outpatient setting that provides services to children. The populations and target markets are generally well identified by the nature of the practice setting. But the actual demographic characteristics of the population, their specific features, can vary depending on the geographic location. (eg, many of the people in the area do not speak English as their first language) Do the people in this market possess the appropriate characteristics this service would provide (eg, are they the appropriate age, have an appropriate level of functioning, have an inherent need)? What type of income do they earn or health insurance do they possess (Chapter 4)? What is the educational level of the people? What languages are spoken in the community? Understanding more about the population allows the PT to align their specific skills and passion toward meeting the needs of the population (see Box 7.1).

If the PT wants to practice as an employee of an established business, then they market themself to a target employer. Information about the potential employer and the services provided can be found on an employer's web page, job posting, advertisements, or public

passion – an internal drive that motivates a person toward a life's goal

records. A public record is a document filed with the state or federal government agency in the course of doing business that is viewable by the public (eg, financial reports, court actions). Information can also be obtained directly from the potential employer or by word of mouth from people associated with the business, such as vendors, or other health professionals. All this information can provide the PT with a better picture of the employer's practice and expose any areas of strengths, weaknesses, or concerns. A good marketing strategy is to understand the potential employer well enough to go into an interview and discuss how the skills and abilities of the PT can meet the needs of the practice, help to strengthen its brand, support its mission, and add value to the outcomes produced. This is an intentional process and can take some time and effort to gather valid information, evaluate the data, and create questions that bring clarity to the decision-making process. But it is a marketing strategy that allows the PT to differentiate themself from the other competitors for the job.

Place

Where does the PT plan to participate with this target population/market? The desired location is often a result of several factors that go into that decision, such as availability of family or friends who live in the area, familiarity with the location, a desire to live in a certain environment (eg, urban, or rural), and the opportunity to work in the desired area of practice. People have many reasons for wanting to live in and work in a particular area and in a particular area of practice. These reasons can then be compared to the opportunities possible in the identified market. Options can include volunteering; acting as a consultant; or being an independent contractor, a private practitioner, or an employee of a company that is already providing services in the area. Employment can be full-time, part-time, or as needed (PRN) (Chapter 5). How to practice PT in this place or location depends on both the availability and the desire of the PT and the needs of the people in the area (ie, target market). Clarifying these needs for both the PT and the target market allows the PT to create a *package* of services or skills, supported by their CV, that *promotes* the value of the services in meeting the needs of the target market. It should convince the target market of the PT's ability to provide the product of better health not only through the delivery of physical therapy services but also through the delivery of exceptional service. Creating value in the services can be shown through the PT's use of professional resources (eg, clinical practice guidelines), participation in professional and community organizations, the comfort and competence with technical skills and social media, demonstration of effective communication skills, and a working knowledge of the business aspect of health care. People and employers are looking for exceptional providers of health care. This aspect of marketing can help the PT to be successful in obtaining a place to practice.

Payment

A fundamental factor in the business of physical therapy is being paid for the services provided and earning enough money to sustain the level of participation and lifestyle desired. Payment comes in the form of cash provided either directly by the patient or by a third-party payer of the services, the health insurance company. A common question is, how much money do you need? The answer to that question can become clearer by the following process:

1. Determine your financial need by completing a personal budget of current expenses. (Chapter 12).

public record – a document filed with the state or federal government agency in the course of doing business that is viewable by the public

Chapter 7 / Marketing

2. Access the Bureau of Labor Statistics Occupational Outlook Handbook for salary information in the state or region for a PT.[22]
3. Use an estimated salary based on the median for the area, and add it into the revenue section of your budget.
4. Subtract the expenses from revenues. The difference should be a positive number. If it is not, then adjust the salary/revenue number until it covers all the expenses, or examine the expenses to see if any can be reduced.
5. Rework this process until a revenue number is achieved that will cover the anticipated expenses. This is the salary/revenue that is needed. (The salary *wanted* is a different number.)
6. Review your CV, and identify those areas that support the potential employer's mission or brand or that add value to the services already offered. These factors can be used to promote your skills and experience and educate the potential employer on why you are the best applicant for the job. Be thoughtful. Most job duties require the employee to adhere to certain standards and laws and interact with other members in the organization and may include inventory management, cash management, or customer relations. All businesses have a certain brand, be it explicit or implied. Employees must support that brand. They are expected to behave in a manner that promotes customer satisfaction and implement strategies to promote customer loyalty. Having good communications skills is often emphasized. All these are key attributes of most jobs duties that are also reflected in the practice of physical therapy. They can also be used as justification for the added value, and fair payment, for the skills that exceed the basic requirements of the job. (eg, A PT who has an undergraduate degree in communications may possess an added value to a business.)

Another significant factor in determining how much money is needed to live in a certain area is the cost of living. The cost of living is the average amount of money needed to purchase the basic necessities of life, such as food, clothing, and shelter, in a specific geographic region and therefore provides information on how expensive it is to live in one area or city compared to another. There are cost of living calculators available online. This comparison puts into perspective the amount of discretionary income that would be available to the PT if the salary were the same (eg, $90,000) in two different cities. Earning a salary of $90,000 in Wheeling, West Virginia, provides more discretionary income after expenses than a $90,000 salary in Honolulu, Hawaii. It is not only how much money a PT can earn in a given area but how much money it costs to live there that should be considered in the decision-making process.

Understanding the amount of money needed to meet the PT's current needs, what the market is willing to pay, and the value placed on additional skills the PT possesses puts the PT in a better position to practice as they desire in a market and be satisfied with the income earned.

Summary

Historically, marketing has been the responsibility of a group of people within a company, the marketing department. Today, all employees are involved in marketing. This is more evident in the service industry, where the product that is being sold isn't so tangible. The patients' perception of the quality of the service provided and the value of the results of those service, or the product, is influenced by many factors of the practice, especially the provider of the service. It is important for health care providers to understand the impact

cost of living – the average amount of money needed to purchase the basic necessities

of their behavior, verbal and nonverbal communication, and physical appearance, in supporting a practice's brand and their responsibility in developing and sustaining patient loyalty. Marketing can also be done on an individual level. The value of physical therapy in optimizing movement and improving the health of society should be clearly communicated to the public, through both the businesses that provide physical therapy and the physical therapists themselves.[23] In the move toward payment for value-based care and value-based outcomes, the value of physical therapy is worth marketing.

REFERENCES

1. American Marketing Association. Definitions of marketing. Published 2017. Accessed November 25, 2023. https://www.ama.org/the-definition-of-marketing-what-is-marketing/
2. Friberg D. Marketing basics. In: Nosse L, Friberg D, eds. *Managerial and Supervisory Principles for Physical Therapists*. 3rd ed. Lippincott Williams and Wilkins; 2009.
3. U.S. Small Business Administration. Market research and competitive analysis. Updated November 8, 2023. Accessed November 25, 2023. https://www.sba.gov/business-guide/plan-your-business/market-research-competitive-analysis
4. Puyt R, Lie F, Wilderom C. The origins of SWOT analysis. *Long Range Planning*. 2023;56(3):102304. doi:102304.10.1016/j.lrp.2023.102304
5. Purcarea VL. The impact of marketing strategies in healthcare systems. *J Med Life*. 2019 Apr-Jun;12(2):93–96. doi:10.25122/jml-2019-1003. PMID: 31406509.
6. Langford S. Market segment vs. market target: what's the real difference? Product Market Alliance. Published October 2, 2023. Accessed November 27, 2023. https://www.productmarketingalliance.com/market-segment-vs-target-market/
7. Coffie S. Positioning strategies for branding services in an emerging economy. *J Strateg Mark*. 2018;28:321-335.
8. Elrod JK, Fortenberry JL. Target marketing in the health services industry: the value of journeying off the beaten path. *BMC Health Serv Res*. 2018;18(suppl 3):923. doi:10.1186/s12913-018-3678-5
9. Nair MN, Ahmad FS. Will branding engage perpetual bonding in healthcare? *Int J Bus Soc*. 2023;24(1):343-361.
10. Baghouri S. Healthcare branding: the definitive guide. UNNUS. Published 2023. Accessed November 29, 2023. https://unnus.com/medical/healthcare-branding/
11. Borden NH. The concept of the marketing mix. *J Advert Res*. 1964;4(2):2-7.
12. Booms B, Bitner MJ. Marketing strategies and organizational structures for serve firms. In: Donnelly JH, George WR, eds. *Marketing and Services*. American Marketing Association; 1981:47-51.
13. Al-Jabri FYM, Turunen H, Kvist T. Patients' perceptions of healthcare quality at hospitals measured by the revised humane caring scale. *J Patient Exp*. 2021;8:23743735211065265. doi:10.1177/23743735211065265
14. Xu J, Park S, Xu J, Hamadi H, Zhao M, Otani K. Factors impacting patients' willingness to recommend: a structural equation modeling approach. *J Patient Exp*. 2022;9:23743735221077538. doi:10.1177/23743735221077538
15. Cho Y, Sutton CL. Reputable internet retailers' service quality and social media use. *Int J Electron Commer Stud*. 2021;12(1):43-64. doi:10.7903/IJECS.1877
16. Basit A, Lum Wai Yee A, Sethumadhavan S, Rajamanoharan I. The influence of social media marketing on consumer buying decision through brand image in the fashion apparel brands. *Int J Contemp Archit*. 2021;8:564-576.
17. Google. Search engine optimization (SEO) starter guide. Updated December 1, 2023. Accessed December 2, 2023. https://developers.google.com/search/docs/fundamentals/seo-starter-guide
18. Bender H. Digital marketing. Impact. Private Practice Section of the American Physical Therapy Association. Published November 2018. Accessed December 2, 2023. https://www.ppsimpact.org/digital-marketing/
19. da Silva ASL, Rabelo Neto A, Luna RA, de Oliveira Cavalcante GT, de Moura AR. Mobile marketing: an approach on advertising by SMS. *Revista De Administração Da UFSM*. 2019;11(4):1012-1029. doi:10.5902/1983465918134
20. American Physical Therapy Association. Ethics and professionalism. Accessed December 3, 2023. https://www.apta.org/your-practice/ethics-and-professionalism
21. American Hospital Association. Environmental scan. Published 2023. Accessed December 3, 2023. https://www.aha.org/environmentalscan
22. US Bureau of Labor Statistics. Occupational outlook handbook. Published September 6, 2023. Accessed December 4, 2023. https://www.bls.gov/ooh/
23. American Physical Therapy Association. Guiding principle to achieve the vision. Updated September 25, 2019. Accessed December 5, 2023. https://www.apta.org/siteassets/pdfs/policies/guiding-principles-to-achieve-vision.pdf

CHAPTER 8

Communication in Health Care

MARK DRNACH

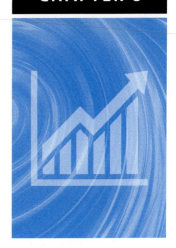

Learning Objectives

The reader will

1. Understand the key aspects of verbal, nonverbal, and written communication in health care.
2. Value the unique factors of interprofessional communication with other providers, including the payer of services.
3. Demonstrate a basic understanding of coding and how to use the Medicare Physician Fee Schedule Calculator.
4. Appreciate the costs associated with Medicare's Resource Based Relative Value Scale for setting reimbursement for a Current Procedural Terminology (CPT) code.
5. Understand the basic process of communicating with a payer of health care services.

Health care has evolved over the past century into a multibillion-dollar business. The need to communicate effectively and remain financially solvent has put pressure on both for-profit and not-for-profit organizations, whether it's a single provider or a group of providers working together as a single business unit. Constant pressure to produce positive outcomes, achieve a level of patient satisfaction, and maintain a positive bottom line (making a profit) has expanded the role and responsibilities of the health care provider. The provider can no longer only focus on communicating with patients regarding their treatment, but must also have the ability to effectively communicate with others to achieve patient/program outcomes, satisfaction with services offered, and meet financial targets that make a practice sustainable. Even in the realm of not-for-profit or charitable health care organizations, pressure to manage or reduce expenses, and the focus on long-term financial viability, is constant. Health care providers, including physical therapists, whether they are working in a for-profit or not-for-profit organization, have to communicate with many interested parties in order to obtain the desired outcomes and justify the payments for the services rendered. These parties typically include patients, many of whom have access to more health care information via the internet; third-party insurance companies who seek justification for payment of services rendered; outside accrediting agencies who advocate for the patient and want assurances of compliance with industry standards; as well as federal and state governmental agencies.

This chapter will cover basic communication skills that are used in the delivery of services to patients and to third-party payers, including the use of standard codes for payment.

174 Section 2 / The Decision

Understanding basic communication skills and the language of coding will allow the provider to communicate more effectively to patients and payers and promote more efficient and effective delivery and payment for services rendered.

Basic Elements of Communication

Communication in health care today is done through a variety of ways: in person, through electronic media, and through writing. It is an important aspect of health care as specialization and access to providers grows and more patients are seen by multiple providers and in multiple clinical settings. Clear, succinct, and timely communication is vital to assure continuity of patient care and to optimize the benefits to the patients. Poor communication can have a negative impact on the outcomes of service delivery, including disrupting the continuity of care, jeopardizing patient safety, and promoting patient dissatisfaction with the care provided, and is thus an inefficient use of a valuable resource in health care, namely, the provider's time.[1]

Communication is always a two-way process, and the person delivering the information, verbally or in writing, should remember that the information sent may not be the same as the information that is received. Each participant both sends and receives information within their own context of the interaction. Within the act of communicating, there is an exchange not only of information but also of emotions and perceptions that are influenced by experience, expectations, cultural factors, and beliefs. In a broader sense, communication is the development of a mutual understanding that is dependent on the sharing of information and arriving at an agreed-upon meaning.[2] That mutual understanding begins with the level of health literacy of both parties. Health literacy is the degree to which individuals have the ability to find, understand, and use information and services to inform their health-related decisions and actions.[3] Ways for health care providers to assess patients' health literacy is to ask them to describe how they will follow the instructions or medications that were prescribed, what they understand about their current health condition, or what services are available in their community to assist them with their health care needs. One role of all health care providers is to educate their patients on their current health condition and management. That should include an assessment of the basic understanding of their health literacy. The ultimate goal of communication is collaboration to produce mutual understanding.

Although the pervasiveness of electronic communication and the use of electronic medical records (EMRs) is evident in health care today, it should not be assumed that these factors alone improve communication between providers or between providers and patients.[4]

Verbal Communication

In verbal communications, voice characteristics are used to add meaning to the information being conveyed. Voice characteristics include such aspects as articulation, intensity, pitch, speed, and emphasis placed on chosen words. The voice conveys the speaker's emotions by a combination of these speech characteristics. To pick up these subtle changes in face-to-face communications requires active listening skills. Remember that the message

> communication – a process of exchange, either verbally or nonverbally, that leads to the development of a mutual understanding that is dependent on the sharing of information and arriving at an agreed-upon meaning
>
> health literacy – the degree to which individuals have the ability to find, understand, and use information and services to inform their health-related decisions and actions

Chapter 8 / Communication in Health Care **175**

sent is not necessarily the message received. The fidelity of the reception and interpretation of a verbal message is dependent on how well the receiver is listening and attending to the speaker's verbal and nonverbal signals. Active listening is a skill demonstrated through nonverbal actions and behaviors of the receiver and can support communication to validate the verbal exchange and understanding between both parties. A health care provider should recognize that in interpersonal communication encounters, it is important to listen more than to speak. A health care provider can use active listening as a response to a patient to validate understanding in the conversation and to build provider-patient rapport. This is critical when participants are mutually intent on discovering something from or about each other.[5-7] Active listening is a core behavior of physical therapists, a necessary component of the patient management model of care, and an essential component of patient-centered care.[8,9] Engaging in active listening requires the health care provider to resist engaging in the righting reflex, which is a natural reaction to speak up and impose solutions before understanding the patient's full story.[10]

Patient-centered care is promoted by an understanding of the patient's perspective of the illness or medical condition, showing empathy and concern throughout the encounter, and facilitating the development of agreed-upon goals for the plan of care.[11] This can be fostered by asking patients open-ended questions during the encounter, not interrupting the patient as they provide information in the manner in which they feel comfortable and necessary, and for providers to demonstrate active listening behaviors (Box 8.1). It is not only what is said but how it is said that is important. Using people-first language shows respect and acknowledgment that the person is not the disease or condition; the person is of primary importance, the condition is secondary.[12] People-first language is a style of communication that places the person first when communicating verbally or in written form (Table 8.1). Never identify people solely by their diagnosis or disability. They may not view their disability as an affliction, or themselves as victims. Even using terms such as "normal" or "healthy" implies that people with disabilities are not normal or healthy, which is not always true. It is important to understand and respect how patients view their conditions and not place labels on them or additional barriers to their identity. It is often said that people in society can disable people, by their attitudes and actions, more than the person is disabled.

The provider should also acknowledge that it is sometimes difficult to maintain a professional demeanor when working with people throughout the workday. Having a personal reminder of the role and responsibility of a health care provider, such as taking a deep breath before entering a room, pausing before responding to a comment made, or taking a few moments, eyes closed, to mentally rest and reset, can be helpful and necessary in maintaining a professional demeanor and displaying effective verbal and nonverbal communication throughout the workday.

Health care providers may also encounter patients for whom English is not their first language or who do not speak or understand the English language. Although there are many phrase books for medical terminology and electronic applications that will interpret words spoken into another language, the use of a medical interpreter is vital to ensure that accurate information is both conveyed and understood. The use of medical interpreters can result in fewer errors in communication, improved patient satisfaction, and lower malpractice risk and is also associated with shorter hospital stays and reduced remission rates.[13]

righting reflex – a natural reaction to speak up and impose solutions before understanding the patient's full story. Can be a barrier to active listening

people-first language – a style of communicating that recognizes the person before the descriptors of that person

BOX 8.1 • Basic Communication

Verbal

Show respect. Use people-first language. Do not show judgment of the patient's emotions.

Observe the patient's ability to comprehend, and adjust your language to allow for a better understanding.

Ask open-ended questions. What can I do for you today? Tell me more about that experience. What do you think caused this issue?

Validate the patient's feelings/emotions. Yes, that is difficult. Yes, pain can be very limiting. I understand why you are upset.

Be clear. Let me summarize what I know so far. OK, so here is what we are going to do. Do you have any other concerns today?

Nonverbal

Maintain eye contact. Look at the person speaking. Limit documentation while the person is speaking to objective data that are important. Avoid looking at the time or away while the person is talking.

Maintain an appropriate facial expression. Show interest or surprise by raising your eyebrows. Nod or smile to show understanding or agreement. Maintain a neutral expression is situations that may be embarrassing to the patient, such as a loss of bowel or bladder control. Show comfort with respectful silence.

Assume an open body posture. Orient your body with the patient's in sitting or standing.

Lean slightly forward to show interest in certain aspects of the patient's communication. Do not cross your arms or talk with your hand on your face.

Active Listening

Listen to understand, not to respond.

Do not interrupt when others are speaking.

Periodically *nod* or provide verbal agreement of understanding what was said so far in the conversation.

Maintain appropriate eye contact, facial expression, and body posture during the conversation.

Table 8.1 People-First Language

Situation	Appropriate Term	Inappropriate Term
Disability	Person with a disability	Handicapped, crippled, differently abled, challenged
Person with a disability	Person who has multiple sclerosis (MS)	Suffers from MS, afflicted with MS, a MS patient
Person who incurred a disability	Person who sustained a spinal cord injury (SCI)	Victim of an SCI
Person with a mobility disability	Person who uses a wheelchair or walks with the assistance of crutches	Wheelchair bound, confined to a wheelchair, crippled, invalid, lame
Person with a mental illness	Person with a mental illness	Lunatic, psycho, crazy, mental
Person recovering from a health condition	Person recovering from a stroke	Stroke victim, brain damaged, a stroke patient
Person without a disability	Person who can walk, see, hear	Normal person, healthy person

DHS Office for Civil Rights and Civil Liberties. A guide to interacting with people who have disabilities. US Department of Homeland Security. Accessed May 2, 2023. https://www.dhs.gov/sites/default/files/publications/guide-interacting-with-people-who-have-disabilties_09-26-13.pdf

Nonverbal Communication

Nonverbal communication, or the messages conveyed through body language or nonverbal responses while someone is speaking, are comprised of movements and gestures that are made during a conversation (Box 8.1). Nonverbal communication includes the eye contact made with the speaker, head nodding by the listener, which can convey agreement or understanding, and the facial expressions made by the listener that communicate the listeners' feelings to what is being spoken. Every nonverbal reaction gives an intentional or unintentional message that impacts the response and, if noted by the speaker, impacts the understanding of how the message is being received. There is an inherent imbalance in power between the person with health knowledge and the person seeking that knowledge. The health care provider must be sensitive to that imbalance and assure the patient that the provider is actively listening and cares about the information being provided. When speaking, using appropriate facial expressions, positive gestures, such as nodding the head, and limiting unpurposive movements, such as hand gestures, can have a positive impact on patient satisfaction and the patient's perception of the encounter.[14,15] In addition, appropriate nonverbal communication helps to promote active listening by the patient and conveys a sense of empathy and compassion by the provider or speaker.[16]

In clinical practice, the provider should demonstrate the attributes of effective communication, which include appropriate eye contact, an open body posture of the speaker, speaking concisely, providing an explanation of the provider's thoughts, and providing a summary of the next steps as a result of the information gathered.[16]

Written Communication

Written clinical documentation is a professional responsibility and a legal requirement. It is more than just a record of services provided and outcomes achieved to provide justification for services rendered: documentation is critical to ensuring that individuals receive appropriate, comprehensive, efficient, patient-centered, and high-quality health care services throughout the episode of care.[17] Written communication encompasses both grammatical skills and the art of effectively and succinctly communicating in written form. The speaker, although in writing, is challenged with capturing and sharing information stated in a way that optimizes the reader's understanding of the content conveyed without the immediate verbal and nonverbal feedback that is available with verbal communication. Written communication/documentation is created to convey information that is assumed to be understood by the reader, that can be used to collectively show the progress, or lack of progress, with the interventions provided, to capture data to show the goal attainment rate that can be used in forecasting future visits, and to show justification for the provision of care or the need for input from/referral to other professionals. Clinical documentation is the record of care, the data used in clinical decision-making, and the evidence of the effectiveness of interventions provided that shows the pathway to patient outcomes. It is not just an administrative task but a vital aspect of the management of patients and clients.

Documentation requirements will vary depending on the setting in which physical therapy service is provided. Hospital-based and ambulatory services are required to capture information in compliance with external accrediting agencies such as the Joint Commission (formerly known as the Joint Commission on Accreditation of Healthcare Organizations) and/or the federal government programs of Medicare and Medicaid. Early Intervention

nonverbal communication – messages conveyed through body language while someone is speaking, comprised of movements and gestures that are made during a conversation

Services and school-based services are required to include documentation in accordance with the Individuals with Disabilities Education Act (IDEA), Parts C and B, respectively. Home Care services that are paid by Medicare are required to capture certain information pertaining to the Outcome and Assessment Information Set (OASIS) form. It is necessary for the physical therapist to become familiar with the documentation requirements for the setting in which they are practicing in order to be compliant with the law, external accrediting agency, patients/clients, and payers of services.[18] Knowledge and understanding of this information should be part of the new employee orientation process and, at a minimum, be reviewed annually (or when the information of pending requirements is released) with all the staff to keep them current on the documentation requirements for the external accrediting agencies, the practice's data collection needs, and the information required by the payers of services. Box 8.2 lists some of the basic elements of clinical documentation.

Written documentation is a vital resource of data that shows the progress of the patient/client in their plan of care and how the patient/client responds to the interventions provided. Using objective data, the physical therapist can determine the effectiveness of an intervention provided, whether this is to increase functional movements, improve muscle strength, decrease pain, or increase endurance. The data can also justify the use of an intervention. If the data do not show a change in the impairment under consideration, a different intervention should be chosen to attempt to facilitate the desired result. Objective data can also be used to forecast the anticipated time to reach a goal, or the overall goal attainment rate (Box 8.3). This type of information is key to a successful argument for the justification of services provided and for reimbursement.

The use of objective data, succinct sentences, and an organized format can help make written documentation less time consuming for the practitioner. The use of standard formats for documentation in the EMR, which may include standard phrases and drop-down boxes, is one way to address this important yet time-consuming clinical activity. A health care practitioner should periodically review the content and style of their clinical documentation to ensure clarity, efficiency, relevance, and usefulness of the captured information. The time demands of clinical documentation have been shown to be a factor in clinical burnout as well as a barrier to a clinician gathering and incorporating research into their clinical practice, which supports evidence-based practice.[19-21] Becoming an effective and efficient writer is an art that takes practice and reflection (Box 8.4). Creating clear and relevant clinical documentation is a key element of the patient/client management and interdisciplinary communication that is vital for the provision of effective and efficient patient-centered care.

BOX 8.2 • Basic Elements of Clinical Documentation

Date of service
Patient/client identifying information (eg, name, date of birth, medical record number)
Area of report (eg, physical therapy, occupational therapy, physical medicine and rehabilitation)
Patient/client diagnostic information (eg, medical diagnosis, International Classification of Diseases [ICD] code)
Patient/client report
Examination findings
Evaluation of examination findings. If progress noted, include progress made toward established goals.
Plan of care, including goals and prescription for services (ie, intensity, frequency, and duration recommended to achieve the stated goals), if appropriate.
Identification and dated signature of the provider

Chapter 8 / Communication in Health Care

BOX 8.3 • Goal Attainment Rate

Scenario
A patient is seen in physical therapy for gait training with an assistive device. At the initial evaluation, the patient demonstrated the ability and endurance to independently ambulate over a level surface with the use of a two-wheeled walker for 20 feet before showing clinical signs of fatigue. A goal to be able to walk for 100 feet was agreed on and entered into the plan of care.

Subsequently, on review of the clinical documentation at the end of Week 3, the physical therapist notices that the patient was able to walk for 20 feet at the end of Week 1 of the plan of care, 40 feet at the end of Week 2, and 60 feet at the end of Week 3.

Question
Approximately how many more weeks will it take for the patient to achieve the goal of 100 feet?

Answer
The data show an increase of 20 feet per week, so an estimated two more weeks are needed for the patient to reach the goal of 100 feet.

Interprofessional Communication

Interprofessional communication is a common and important aspect in health care today because patients may encounter numerous health care providers during their course of treatment.[22] These providers have expertise in their respective professions, which may include physicians, surgeons, psychologists, nurses, occupational therapists, social workers, teachers, administrators, or coaches, depending on the setting of service delivery. These settings provide a structure and expectation, or utilization, of specific professional services. Acute care hospitals, outpatient clinics, schools, hospice programs, or athletic teams are environments with specific guidelines, goals, reporting requirements, and expectations for collaboration. Effective interprofessional communication is vital in each of these settings to ensure the efficient and timely delivery of services that optimize the patient, client, athlete,

BOX 8.4 • Tips for Documentation

1. Organize information into a checklist or note page (electronically or on paper) that reflects the relevant clinical information to gather during a patient encounter. This can be a standard format that is used in subsequent patient encounters, a template.
2. Review the patient's medical record or intake information prior to the visit, and record the relevant information onto the checklist or note page.
3. Record key points or objective data during the patient encounter, avoiding writing or typing sentences, because this may give the impression that the physical therapist is documenting instead of listening to the patient.
4. Review the key findings/goals/follow-up actions with the patient at the end of the encounter for clarification and agreement.
5. Complete the documentation at the point of care, transferring the notes and objective data into a clinical record at the end of the encounter (eg, electronic medical record [EMR] template, dictation, electronic note). Be concise.
6. Review the documentation for clarity and truthfulness.
7. Periodically review documentation and reflect on the relevance, clarity, and use of the information collected. Make adjustments as needed.

family, or student outcome. Yet interprofessional communication has its inherent challenges. Foremost is the hierarchy within interprofessional groups, with the physician commonly assuming the role of leader, albeit unintentionally at times.[23] This deference to a group leader to make the decisions can be a barrier to the exchange of ideas and problem-solving discussions that are important in patient/client management. It takes an intentional understanding of the role of the professionals in the group, who should all have a strong sense of professional identity, understand and contribute within their professional scope of practice, and be able to relinquish part of their autonomy for the betterment of the group decisions.[24] The group must also encourage participation and show respect for each members' contribution[24] (Box 8.5). This respect is fostered by the member's ability to provide succinct, relevant, and factual information that fosters the decisions of the group. Each member of the interprofessional group is responsible for using clear and direct verbal communication skills that contribute to the group discussion, detailed written documentation that supports the professional's contribution to the discussion, and nonverbal communication behaviors that reflect active listening and respect for all the members of the group. Interprofessional communication can happen in face-to-face encounters, or it can be facilitated through the use of electronic communication, which can be of great benefit to the patient and the organization, improving outcomes, patient satisfaction, and continuity of care.[25-27]

Patient Communication

Effective communication, both verbally and nonverbally, is paramount to providing effective and meaningful individualized care. The ability to actively listen, show concern and understanding of the patient's message, and convey information that is understandable to the patient, that is culturally and professionally appropriate, and that shows respect for the patient and their situation should be recognized as vital to the patient-therapist relationship. In addition to the style and manner of communicating with a patient, the time and place of the exchange must also be taken into consideration. A controlled environment and a sense of trust must quickly be established in order for the patient to feel comfortable and confident with sharing private information with the provider. Using open-ended questions and engaging in active listening are tools to build trust. Whether the information is on a one-to-one basis or to a group, what needs to be communicated must be anticipated to appropriately plan the interaction. The provider should anticipate the following key factors:

1. Who needs to participate in the conversation?
2. What is the level of confidentiality required?
3. What may the potential reaction to the information provided be, and, therefore, what additional support may be required (eg, social worker)?
4. How much time is to be allotted for the encounter?[28]

BOX 8.5 • Fostering Interprofessional Communication

Be friendly (show interest in other team members).
Respect others' time (start and end the meeting at the set times).
Understand your role in the group.
Provide helpful and truthful information (avoid personal opinions).
Stay within your professional scope of practice.
Be supportive and encouraging (provide positive feedback when appropriate)
Actively listen to other members.
Understand and respect cultural perspectives.
Provide and attend staff education on team collaboration and communication.

Chapter 8 / Communication in Health Care **181**

Failure to plan adequate time and an appropriate environment for important communication places an unnecessary barrier to open communication, which may lead to a lack of full disclosure by the patient or resistance by the patient and/or caregivers to suggestions offered.

Effective communication with patients is supported by clear and objective written documentation that is gathered by the provider to assist with patient education on their condition/impairment/functional limitation, and/or the response to the interventions provided. This information is used throughout the episode of care to provide patients and their families appropriate information to understand the goals of their care and to make knowledgeable decisions. Additionally, throughout the continuum of care, other providers in subsequent settings required clear and succinct information to make the transition of care more seamless. A lack of clear and timely communication can result in the delivery of substandard care, or, worse, jeopardize patient safety. Health care providers should keep this in mind as they often work according to varying standards and cultural norms that influence communication. In addition, the work environment can also impact communication through the pressures inherent in working with a lack of sufficient staff, a fast-paced high-productivity environment, which contributes to errors caused by multitasking, interruptions or distractions, memory lapses, fatigue, stress, and sleep deprivation—all potentially compromising the safety of patients.[29]

As a business owner, the responsibility to acknowledge and address communication and the barriers that impact effective communication is vital to a practice that supports patient-centered quality care. Communication on the anticipated care to be provided is only one half of the providers' responsibility. The patient should also be informed of the administrative aspects of health care and their rights and responsibilities and should be provided with a complete picture of the cost and expectations of the services offered with an opportunity to ask questions and seek clarification (Box 8.6).

Communication is an important aspect of the overall utilization of health care in the United States. It is an important aspect of care that must be developed, supported, and refined as the delivery and systems of health care develop, including the emergence of value-based health care. Value-based health care is a reimbursement model that pays

---

BOX 8.6 • Providers' Communication With Patients[29]

1. Communicate the expected cost of care.
2. Orient the patient to the care environment and equipment that may be used in treatment.
3. Discuss and obtain informed consent (which includes refusal of treatment) in the language and manner that the patient can understand.
4. Provide a written statement about the patient's rights and responsibilities in the language and manner that is appropriate for the patient or patients served.
5. Make accommodations for literacy levels, language differences, or cultural aspects of the patient.
6. Speak to the patient with respect, given the patient's age and intellectual level.
7. Keep the medical record documentation current and organized.
8. Provide truthful information.
9. Be clear with discharge or transition (from one setting to another or one provider to another) communications and plans.

---

value-based health care – a reimbursement model in health care that pays providers based on patient outcomes instead of the number of services provided

providers based on patient outcomes instead of the number or amount of services provided. An important aspect of patient outcomes is patient satisfaction, which is influenced by the amount of time spent with the patient, the quality of the verbal and nonverbal communication, and the patient's opinion about the value the health information provided and the manner in which it was delivered.[30]

Payer Communication: Coding

Documentation of the services provided to a patient must contain information that helps the provider manage the patient's episode and care, provide the relevant information on the overall care of the patient, communicate the care provided to other health care providers who are involved in the patient's care, and demonstrate the need for, and benefit of, the skilled services provided as justification of payment. This documentation must clearly identify the services provided when those services are paid for by the patient (the first party), or the provider (the second party), or a patient's health insurance company (the third party). Health insurance companies will require that aspects of the documentation are coded to allow for an efficient identification and categorization of the health information that facilitates appropriate payment for the billable services provided.

Coding the Procedure

Most third-party payment structures such as health care insurance companies incorporate their payment formula with Current Procedural Terminology (CPT) codes.[31] Established by the American Medical Association (AMA), CPT codes are five-digit codes used throughout the country by health care providers to designate the type of service or services provided. Physical therapists typically use codes in the Physical Medicine and Rehabilitation section, or 97000 codes. Examples of several CPT codes used in physical therapy can be found in Table 8.2. CPT codes are reviewed and updated annually by the AMA. To ensure that the coding and billing practices are accurate and up to date, it is recommended that all health care providers become familiar with all the codes associated with their specialty.

Table 8.2 Example of Current Procedural Terminology Codes Used in Physical Therapy	
Code	Definition
97010	Supervised modality; application of a modality to one or more areas
97110	Therapeutic exercise in one or more areas, each 15 min, therapeutic exercises to develop strength and endurance, range of motion, and flexibility
97116	Therapeutic procedure, 15 min. Gait training therapy includes stair climbing; therapist required to have direct (one-on-one) patient contact
97530	Therapeutic activities; direct (one-on-one) patient contact by the provider (use of dynamic activities to improve functional performance); each 15 min

Jannenga H. Physical therapists guide to CPT codes. WebPT. Published February 20, 2023. Accessed May 30, 2023. https://www.webpt.com/guides/cpt-codes/

third-party payment structures – the use of a third party (not the patient or provider) to pay for the health care services provided

Common Procedural Terminology – five-digit codes used throughout the country by health care providers to designate the type of service or services provided. Published by the AMA

Chapter 8 / Communication in Health Care

To enhance a code or be more specific in coding, certain modifiers are used to better define the code or the service provided. Modifiers, which are two-digit numbers or letters, help to more accurately define the CPT code used in billing and can be found in any CPT publication or online resource. Modifiers are attached to CPT codes when the code alone is not adequate to explain exactly the service or treatment provided. The modifier does not change the definition of the code but is used to denote that something has been altered owing to certain circumstances. Modifiers that are commonly used when providing physical therapy services are the 59, 22, 95, GP, CQ, and the KX modifier.

For example, *modifier 59* is used when a physical therapist needs to indicate a distinct or independent procedural service, meaning that two different procedures were performed on the same day on two different anatomic sites such as an intervention for the shoulder as well as for the knee. An example of the use of modifier 59 is as follows:

Working one-on-one with a patient, the physical therapist performs therapeutic exercises. CPT code 97110 is billed for each 15-minute increment.
Modifier 59 is only appropriate if the therapeutic exercises (97110) are performed on different regions of the body, such as the lower limb and shoulder.

Modifier 22 is used when additional work, above and beyond what is normally required, is needed. An example might be the provision of physical therapy to a patient who is non-communicative, violent, or too heavy to transfer by one person, necessitating an additional person to provide the intervention. Judgment must be used, and supporting documentation in the form of medical records and notes are required in order for modifier 22 to be paid.

Modifier 95 is used to indicate that services were provided via telehealth, synchronously through real-time audio and visual interaction (see Chapter 6 on providing a telehealth visit).

Modifier GP is used to indicate that the service was provided to the patient by a physical therapist. This modifier is frequently used in the acute care and outpatient settings where multidisciplinary teams are common. It clarifies which professional was providing the treatment. *Modifier CQ* is used when the physical therapy service has been provided solely by a physical therapist assistant (PTA) for more than 10% of the treatment time in either minutes or units.[32] This modifier clarifies the professional level of the service provider and results in a decrease in payment for that service provided by the PTA. The *KX modifier* is used in billing Medicare to indicate that a service has reached its reimbursement threshold (ie, therapy cap), yet the continued services provided are medically necessary to justify payment. It is vital that documentation justify this statement/modifier. There are other modifiers that may be appropriate in specific clinical settings or required by specific payers of service. Understanding and applying the proper codes for the services provided, ensuring that the appropriate codes are used, that the documentation supports the use of the code, and that all billable aspects of the service are properly coded for payment is an important aspect of achieving and maintaining the financial health of a practice.

Coding Other Services

The Centers for Medicare and Medicaid Services (CMS) is a federal agency within the department of Health and Human Services, which is responsible for setting the reimbursement rates at which the government pays health care providers. To ensure that claims

modifiers – two-digit numbers or letters that follow a CPT code to more accurately define the CPT code when the code alone is not adequate to explain exactly the service or treatment provided. The modifier does not change the definition of the code but is used to denote that something has been altered owing to certain circumstances

Table 8.3 Example of Level II Healthcare Common Procedure Coding System Codes Used in Physical Therapy

Code	Definition
S9131	Physical therapy; in the home, per diem
A4595	Electrical stimulator supplies; two leads per month
L1940	Ankle foot orthoses, custom fabricated
E0100	Standard cane with tip

American Academy of Professional Coders. Codify. What is HCPCS? Accessed May 30, 2023. https://www.aapc.com/resources/medical-coding/hcpcs.aspx

are processed efficiently, CMS uses the Healthcare Common Procedure Coding System (HCPCS), commonly referred to as "hicks picks" codes.[33] *Level I* HCPCS codes match the CPT codes, which are used primarily to identify medical services and procedures furnished by physicians and other health care professionals such as physical therapists. *Level II* of the HCPCS is a standardized coding system that is used primarily to identify products, supplies, and services not included in the CPT codes, such as ambulance services and durable medical equipment, prosthetics, orthotics, and supplies (DMEPOS) when used outside a physician's office. Level II codes are also referred to as alpha-numeric codes because they consist of a single alphabetical letter followed by four numeric digits, whereas CPT codes are identified using five numeric digits. Examples of several HCPCS codes used in physical therapy can be found in Table 8.3.

Coding the Disease

When billing by CPT code, it is important that the ICD code is also indicated, especially when billing Medicare/Medicaid and third-party insurers. The ICD-11 code is the International Classification of Diseases, Eleventh Revision, developed by the World Health Organization.[34] This code identifies the patient's disease (or diagnosis) for which the patient is being treated. Since the passage of the Medicare Catastrophic Coverage Act of 1988, it is required by law that the ICD code be submitted in order to receive reimbursement from Medicare. Since then, all third-party insurers have adopted this requirement. The World Health Organization periodically updates these codes and publishes them on the internet free of charge. The ICD codes and the data it provides are used for reporting on the incidence of diseases internationally, to support payment systems, service planning, and administration of quality and safety programs and are used in health services research.[34]

Billing

Once the services that were provided are documented and appropriately coded, a bill can be sent to the third-party payer. Typically, revenues are recorded as gross revenues, meaning that they reflect the amount listed on the fee schedule (Chapter 2). However, what a

Healthcare Common Procedure Coding System – published by the CMS, HCPCS (*hick picks*) match the CPT codes, which are used to identify medical services, procedures, and durable medical equipment furnished by physicians and other health care professionals

International Classification of Diseases – developed by the WHO, these codes identify the patient's disease (or diagnosis) for which the patient is being treated. An ICD code is required on a death certificate in the United States

Chapter 8 / Communication in Health Care

practice is actually paid is referred to as net revenue (ie, revenue after something has been removed). The difference between gross and net in this case is termed the contractual allowance (Chapter 2). Payments vary based on contractual agreements with various federal and state insurers or private and nonprofit insurers. For example:

> A physical therapist charges $500 for orthotics fitting and training—extremities and/or trunk; CPT code 97660. The insurance company states that they will pay only $250 for the service. If the physical therapist performs five of these services in a given week, the total gross charges for the week would be $2,500 (5 × $500). The physical therapist's net revenue would be what he actually receives in payment for the services or $1,250 (5 × $250). The difference of $1,250 is termed the contractual write-off or allowance. In this example, the contractual write-off is 50% of the gross charge, leaving 50% as payment rate or reimbursement rate.

CPT codes and HCPCS do not always capture the variations in effort, resources, and staff specialization that go into the delivery of services. The federal government, through the administration of Medicare, has attempted to capture the variation in costs associated with the delivery of services in different geographic areas around the country. Two payment programs, the Resource Based Relative Value Scale (RBRVS) and Diagnosis Related Groups (DRGs), are ways of bundling like or related services or resources associated with the delivery of services into one payment. These methodologies are viewed as a way to correct skewed financial incentives among various procedures and medical practices. For example, a physical therapist could not bill separately for services rendered to a patient who comes into the hospital for an orthopedic surgery and receives physical therapy while in the hospital. These services, the surgery, the physical therapy and nursing care, would all be bundled under one DRG, and only one bill and payment would be issued. If follow-up physical therapy is ordered once the patient has left the hospital, then the physical therapist could bill for those services.

In the early 1990s Relative Value Units (RVUs; a key factor in the RBRVS calculation) were developed by Medicare to assign a value to a particular service or type of treatment. Although there are several types of RVUs, the *work RVU (wRVU)* is the one most commonly used to measure productivity. Other RVUs include *malpractice RVU (mpRVU)* and *practice expense RVU (peRVU)*. In most cases, when a service or treatment becomes more complex or time consuming, the wRVU increases, providing one way to reduce geographic biases in payments by Medicare. No matter where in the country a practice is established, the wRVU for a particular service remains the same. These three RVUs are associated with the reasonable price or reimbursement that Medicare will pay for a unit of service or CPT code. They are contained in the formula:

$$\text{Reasonable amount} = ([wRVU \times wGPCI]) + [peRVU \times peGPCI]) + (mpRVU \times mpGPCI) \times \text{a conversion factor (CF)}[35]$$

Resource Based Relative Value Scale – a physician payment system developed by the CMS that takes into consideration the variation of resource costs for providing health care services across the country

Diagnosis Related Group – a payment system that bundles payment (ie, provides one payment) for the treatment of specific diagnoses

Relative Value Units – units that assign a value to a particular service or type of treatment. Used in the RBRVS as three measures: work, malpractice, and practice expense

In addition to the values associated with the RVUs, the Medicare payment is adjusted to reflect variations in practice expenses among various geographic regions by using a specific Geographic Practice Cost Index (GPCI). There is also a GPCI for each RVU. A conversion factor (CF) is determined annually by Congress and the CMS. Medicare also distinguishes between a facility and nonfacility practice expense RVU, based on where a service is provided. Facility locations, under the resource-based system for calculating payments, include inpatient and outpatient hospital settings, emergency rooms, skilled nursing facilities (SNF) or ambulatory surgical centers (ASC). Outpatient rehabilitation services are usually reimbursed at the nonfacility per RVU. Although the formula is complex, it is a good way to estimate appropriate revenues from services provided and does attempt to provide a fair and equitable distribution of payment based on several factors other than the organization's fee.

Box 8.7 shows the formula used in the Medicare calculations.[32] Using the Medicare formula, the higher the wRVU, the higher the pricing amount and payment. Although the formula is complex, it is a good way to estimate appropriate costs and proceeds for work performed. There is also an online calculator that make this process more efficient. It is usually available through a professional organization.[36] RVUs are linked to CPT codes. Without the proper CPT code, a bill will not be paid or not be paid correctly. It is important to correctly code for services, as wrongful coding is illegal and can lead to accusations of fraud. This is why many organizations and practices hire professional coders who have been trained and certified in proper coding. Ultimately, proper coding is based on the documentation provided by the physical therapist or other health care provider.

Independent Contractor

Billing third-party payers for professional services by a physical therapist as an independent contractor is done using an HCFA 1500 form. The HCFA 1500 is a form created

---

BOX 8.7 • Formula for Calculating Medicare Reimbursement

The formulas for calculating Medicare reimbursements are:

$$\text{Nonfacility pricing amount} = ([wRVU \times wGPCI] + [\text{Nonfacility peRVU} \times peGPCI] + [mpRVU \times mpGPCI]) \times \text{Conversion factor.}$$

$$\text{Facility pricing amount} = ([wRVU \times wGPCI] + [\text{Facility peRVU} \times peGPCI] + [mpRVU \times mpGPCI]) \times \text{Conversion factor}$$

Key
RVU—relative value unit
GPCI—geographic practice cost index
pe—practice expense
mp—malpractice expense
w—work expense

Medicare Learning Network. How to use the MPFS look-up tool. Centers for Medicare and Medicaid Services. Accessed May 30, 2023. https://www.cms.gov/files/document/physician-fee-schedule-guide.pdf

---

Geographic Practice Cost Index – a CF used in the RBRVS formula to reflect the variations in practice expense among various geographic regions in the United States

Chapter 8 / Communication in Health Care

by the Health Care Financing Administration (HCFA. Currently known as the Centers for Medicare and Medicaid Services or CMS) and approved by the AMA's Council on Medical Service. Basic information required on the HCFA 1500 includes the patient's name, address, insurance ID number, insurance company, and address. Treatment information in the form of CPT/HCPCS codes, dates of service, and diagnosis codes (ICD) are required as well. Finally, the health care provider's signature, credentials, address, and the Unique Physician Identification Number (UPIN; a number assigned by Medicare to all physicians and nonphysician practitioners) or group insurance number are also required. A Universal Billing (UB) form may also be used when physical therapists are enrolled with the third-party payer as a group, such as in a hospital setting. This is the official form used by health care providers when submitting bills to Medicare, Medicaid, and commercial third-party insurances. The UB form includes information on patient demographics, ICD, CPT, HCPCS codes, and units of service. Which form is used for billing will depend on how the physical therapist is enrolled in the insurance program.

In most instances, when working as an independent contractor, a physical therapist provides a payment invoice that is broken down by time. Unlike the insurance companies or governmental agencies, which rely on CPT coding as a way of noting services, most independent contracting is billed based on time. In order to correctly calculate an hourly rate, the physical therapist should have an estimate of the total annual cost of providing the services (see the Cost Worksheet in Chapter 1). On average a full-time employee works 2,080 hours per year, which breaks down to 40 hours per week for a 52-week year. Dividing the 2,080 hours by the total annual costs will produce the minimum hourly rate. A markup, as a percentage, is added to the actual cost of the service, to come up with an hourly rate, which includes a profit. This can ensure that the financial targets for the year are met (Box 8.8). A markup is arbitrary but should be reasonable, based on the local market and skill-level needed for the service provision, and should be something that can be easily calculated and explained (Chapter 1).

Participating With the Third Party

Understanding who is going to pay and how much they will pay for a service is vital in managing a practice's finances. Depending on the situation, payers can be the government, third-party insurance carriers, patients, or families of patients, schools, or other organizations with whom a practitioner has a contract. In each situation, it should be remembered that the patient, either owing to circumstances or by choice, has decided to participate in this type of payment structure for a certain level of health care services.

BOX 8.8 • Calculating an Hourly Rate, Including a Markup

A physical therapist has decided to become an independent contractor with the local school. The school is in need of physical therapy services for three, 8-hour days a week, for 48 weeks of the year. (This includes the extended school year program.) The physical therapist has estimated a total cost of $60,000 per year to cover the cost of time and supplies. Given the cost of living in the region and other market factors, the physical therapist has estimated a markup to be 15%. The hourly rate can be calculated as follows:

Total costs	$60,000
+ Markup (15%)	+ 9,000
Annual target	$69,000
Annual hours	1,152 (24 hours per week for 48 weeks)
Hourly rate quoted	$59.89

Each state has its own set of laws and regulations regarding health care insurance. Each insurance company also has its own rules and policies regarding covered services. It is best to check the local and state government's webpage to get specific information for a particular state regarding insurance companies. The larger national insurance companies have their own websites, which provide useful information. A private practice owner may find that when dealing with patients who have regional or local insurance coverage, additional research may be required to ensure payment is received. In most instances, the amount and type of insurance coverage is based on what the insurer (patient or patient's family) or their employer is willing to pay. Thus, it is important to become familiar with the local insurance companies and governmental rules and regulations within a particular state. The rules and regulations can be complex, and it is important to become familiar with them or to retain the assistance of someone who is familiar with them (see "Getting the Right Help" section in Chapter 6). In most cases, larger organizations and groups have dedicated personnel whose only function is to keep abreast of governmental and insurance company rules and regulations and to ensure that the practice is getting the appropriate level of reimbursement for their services.

Insurance companies and governmental agencies can also act as a referral source to a practice. By enrolling with an insurance carrier, a physical therapist becomes part of a larger network of health care providers who have access to a larger pool of potential patients. The enrollment process with an insurance company usually takes several weeks to months and requires that certain professional licenses be obtained and adequate paperwork be submitted. Once the initial round of paperwork is completed, there are only annual renewals to be done, and these are typically straightforward. The process of becoming credentialed or enrolled begins with obtaining a state license to practice. After receiving a state license, the health care practitioner can then apply for a Medicare UPIN. To enroll with Medicare, the physical therapist must contact the CMS regional office in the state where they plan to practice.[37] Typically, the application process takes 30 to 60 days. An advantage of participating in the Medicare program is that Medicare fees are 5% higher than if the health care practitioner were a nonparticipant. Once the health care practitioner has a Medicare UPIN, they can enroll in other insurance programs, both public and private. Although the process can be arduous because of the excess amount of paperwork, it is well worth it financially. On average, it can take 3 to 9 months to become credentialed with all the various insurance agencies in an area.

Summary

The health care provider, such as a physical therapist, is faced with a myriad of hurdles to navigate in order to develop a successful practice in the health care industry today. The practice owner can no longer be concerned only with patient management, but must also be able to manage finances, or at least participate in the discussion of finances, communicate effectively with a variety of people using the language of business, including billing, and participate in the administrative aspect of health care to help form well-planned, strategic business decisions for the good of the patient and the practice.

REFERENCES

1. Vermeir P, Vandijck D, Degroote S, et al. Communication in healthcare: a narrative review of the literature and practical recommendations. *Int J Clin Pract.* 2015;69(11):1257-1267. doi:10.1111/ijcp.12686
2. Liebler JF, McConnell CR. *Management Principles for Health Professionals.* 4th ed. Jones and Bartlett; 2004.
3. US Department of Health and Human Services. Office of Disease Prevention and Health Promotion. Health literacy in Healthy People 2030. Accessed June 20, 2023. https://health.gov/healthypeople/priority-areas/health-literacy-healthy-people-2030

Chapter 8 / Communication in Health Care

4. Timmins L, Kern L, O'Malley A, et al. Communication gaps persist between primary care and specialist physicians. *Ann Fam Med.* 2022;20:343-347. doi:10.1370/afm.2781
5. Shonka M, Kosch D. *Beyond Selling Value: A Proven Way to Avoid the Vendor Trap.* Dearborn Trade Publishing; 2002.
6. Spector R, McCarthy PD. *The Nordstrom Way: The Inside Story of America's #1 Customer Service Company.* John Wiley and Sons; 1995.
7. Super C, Gold RD. *Selling (Without Selling) 4 ½ Steps to Success.* American Management Association; 2004.
8. American Physical Therapy Association. *Guide to Physical Therapist Practice v 4.0.* APTA; 2023. Accessed January 28, 2023. http://guidetoptpractice.apta.org/
9. Constand MK, MacDermid JC, Dal Bello-Haas V, Law M. Scoping review of patient-centered care approaches in healthcare. *BMC Health Serv Res.* 2014;14:271. doi:10.1186/1472-6963-14-271. PMID: 24947822.
10. Levensky ER, Forcehimes A, O'Donohue WT, Beitz K. Motivational interviewing: an evidence-based approach to counseling helps patients follow treatment recommendations. *Am J Nurs.* 2007;107(10):50-58.
11. Hashim MJ. Patient-centered communication: basic skills. *Am Fam Physician.* 2017;95(1):29-34. Accessed May 2, 2023. https://www.aafp.org/dam/brand/aafp/pubs/afp/issues/2017/0101/p29.pdf
12. DHS Office for Civil Rights and Civil Liberties. A guide to interacting with people who have disabilities. US Department of Homeland Security. Accessed May 2, 2023. https://www.dhs.gov/sites/default/files/publications/guide-interacting-with-people-who-have-disabilties_09-26-13.pdf
13. Juckett G, Unger K. Appropriate use of medical interpreters. *Am Fam Physician.* 2014;90(6):476-480. PMID: 25369625.
14. Collins LG, Schrimmer A, Diamond J, Burke J. Evaluating verbal and non-verbal communication skills, in an ethnogeriatric OSCE. *Patient Educ Couns.* 2011;83(2):158-162. doi:10.1016/j.pec.2010.05.012. PMID: 20561763.
15. DiMatteo MR, Taranta A, Friedman HS, Prince LM. Predicting patient satisfaction from physicians' nonverbal communication skills. *Med Care.* 1980;18(4):376-387. doi:10.1097/00005650-198004000-00003. PMID: 7401698.
16. Lee T, Lin E, Lin H. Communication skills utilized by physicians in the pediatric outpatient setting. *BMC Health Serv Res.* 2022;22:993. Accessed January 28, 2023. doi:10.1186/s12913-022-08385-5
17. American Physical Therapy Association. Physical therapy documentation of patient client management. APTA. Accessed May 4, 2023. https://www.apta.org/your-practice/documentation
18. American Physical Therapy Association. Setting-specific considerations in documentation. APTA. Published January 31, 2018. Accessed May 8, 2023. https://www.apta.org/your-practice/documentation/defensible-documentation/setting-specific-considerations#Workers
19. Bowens AN, Amamoo MA, Blake DD, Clark B. Assessment of professional quality of life in the Alabama Physical Therapy Workforce. *Phys Ther.* 2021; 101(7):pzab089. doi:10.1093/ptj/pzab089
20. da Silva TM, Costa Lda C, Garcia AN, Costa LO. What do physical therapists think about evidence-based practice? A systematic review. *Man Ther.* 2015;20(3):388-401. doi:10.1016/j.math.2014.10.009
21. Jette D, Bacon K, Batty C, et al. Evidence-based practice: beliefs, attitudes, knowledge, and behaviors of physical therapists. *Phys Ther.* 2003;83(9):786-805.
22. Whitt N, Harvey R, McLeod G, Child S. How many health professionals does a patient see during an average hospital stay? *N Z Med J.* 2007;120(1253):U2517.
23. Lancaster G, Kolakowsky-Hayner S, Kovacich J, Greer-Williams N. Interdisciplinary communication and collaboration among physicians, nurses, and unlicensed assistive personnel. *J Nurs Scholarsh.* 2015;47(3):275-284. doi:10.1111.jnu.12130
24. Kvarnstrom S. Difficulties in collaboration: a critical incident study of interprofessional healthcare teamwork. *J Interprof Care.* 2008;22(2):191-203. doi:10.1080/13561820701760600
25. Papermaster AE, Champion JD. Exploring the use of curbside consultations for interprofessional collaboration and clinical decision-making. *J Interprof Care.* 2021;35(3):368-375. doi:10.1080/13561820.2020.1768057
26. Anderson R. Effects of an electronic health record tool on team communication and patient mobility: a 2-year follow-up study. *Crit Care Nurse.* 2022;42:23-21.
27. Block L, LaVine NA, Martinez J, et al. A novel longitudinal interprofessional ambulatory training practice: the improving patient access care and cost through training (IMPACcT) clinic. *J Interprof Care.* 2021; 35(3):472-475. doi:10.1080/13561820.2020.1751595
28. Resnik C. Communicating with skill. In: Nosse L, ed. *Management and Supervisor Skills for the Physical Therapist.* Lippincott Williams & Wilkins; 2007.
29. Joint Commission on Accreditation. Communicating clearly and effectively to patients. Joint Commission International. Published 2018. Accessed May 22, 2023. https://store.jointcommissioninternational.org/assets/3/7/jci-wp-communicating-clearly-final_(1).pdf
30. Moslehpour M, Shalehah A, Fadzlul Rahman F, Lin K-H. The effect of physician communication on inpatient satisfaction. *Healthcare (Basel).* 2022;10(3):463. doi:10.3390/healthcare10030463

31. Centers for Medicare and Medicaid Services. List of CPT/HCPCS Codes. Published March 16, 2023. Updated April 18, 2024. Accessed April 22, 2024. https://www.cms.gov/medicare/regulations-guidance/physician-self-referral/list-cpt-hcpcs-codes
32. Therapy Services. Centers for Medicare and Medicaid Services. CY 2023 therapy services updates. Accessed May 15, 2023. https://www.cms.gov/medicare/billing/therapyservices
33. U.S. Department of Health and Human Services. Centers for Medicare and Medicaid Services. HCPCS background information. Accessed on June 20, 2023. https://www.cms.gov/medicare/coding/medhcpcsgeninfo?redirect=/medhcpcsgeninfo/
34. World Health Organization. International Classification of Diseases. 11th ed. ICD-11. Adopted May 2019. Effective January 2022. Accessed May 30, 2023. https://icd.who.int/en
35. Medicare Learning Network. How to use the MPFS look-up tool. Centers for Medicare and Medicaid Services. Accessed May 30, 2023. https://www.cms.gov/files/document/physician-fee-schedule-guide.pdf
36. Medicare Physician Fee Schedule. American Physical Therapy Association. Accessed May 30, 2023. https://www.apta.org/your-practice/payment/medicare-payment/coding-billing/mppr/mppr-calculator
37. Centers for Medicare and Medicaid Services. Medicare enrollment guide for providers and suppliers. Accessed May 30, 2023. https://www.cms.gov/medicare/provider-enrollment-and-certification/become-a-medicare-provider-or-supplier?redirect=/medicareprovidersupenroll/

SECTION 3
The Plan to Succeed

CHAPTER 9

Monitoring and Measuring

KEN ERB

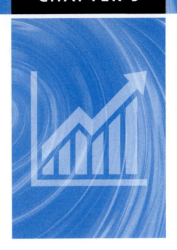

Learning Objectives

The reader will

1. Understand and identify key areas to monitor and measure by level of importance to a private practice.
2. Define key performance indicators (KPIs) in a physical therapy (PT) practice.
3. Develop skills for measuring KPIs in a PT practice.
4. Understand benchmarking and risk adjustment.
5. Know the basics of management and leading physical therapists "By the Numbers."
6. Understand how the integration of financial reports with practice accounting software KPIs, and payroll reports, can produce the highest resolution picture of a PT practice.

Vital signs, namely, blood pressure, body temperature, heart rate, respiration rate, oxygen saturation level, and pain, are what the physical therapist uses on a daily basis to monitor and measure the status of a patient. The physical therapist, as a student, learns these skills and develops them in clinical practice to guide clinical decision-making. Vital signs are so important that many people know how to measure at least a few of them through their participation in educational programs for cardiopulmonary resuscitation (CPR) certification, life guarding, or basic life support/first aid certification. Measuring the body's response to movement or exercise gives the skilled practitioner vital information on how the patient is responding to, or tolerating, a specific intervention. The expert practitioner can include more advanced tests and measures (eg, arterial blood gas [ABG] analysis, blood urea nitrogen [BUN], physiologic cost index [PCI]) to tell whether a body is functioning optimally or whether something is going on in the background that might cause a problem in the future.

PT practices function in exactly the same way. There are signs and symptoms that, when interpreted correctly, drive decision-making for the betterment of the practice. There are other measurements that tell a practice owner that although things may be going well now, the system is at risk for challenges in the future. Specific data from select measurements provide information that clarifies alternate decisions. This chapter will provide the reader with the basic fundamentals for understanding what those measurements are, how to capture and track them over time, and when to take action, if necessary. Information is also provided on specific measurement tools that a practice owner can use to understand more clearly the financial health of the practice. Finally, the chapter will focus on translating an improved understanding of fundamental measurements into actionable strategies and solutions geared toward improving performance of the PT practice.

Key Performance Indicators

Although metrics represent any measurable aspect of a business, or its performance, key performance indicators (KPIs) represent a set of measures focusing on those aspects of organizational performance that are the most critical for the current and future success of the organization.[1] They are important to a specific practice at a point in time and can therefore differ from industry to industry or individual practice to practice. What one practice considers a KPI might not be a KPI for another practice, although there are some universally important KPIs that are applicable to all PT practices. Practice metrics is any set of data that can be assembled and reviewed, that provides information on a specific area of practice (eg, patient census, marketing efforts and results, financial standing). Although certain KPIs are a subset of practice metrics, they serve as the bare minimum that a practice owner should track to understand the financial health of the practice. *These are identified in the chapter by the use of an asterisk and include the metrics of the number of new patients, visit per week, average number of visits per plan of care, arrival rate, payment per visit, profit and loss statement, cost per visit, and profit per visit.*

Metric Timing

When deciding to track a metric, the most important factor to start with is the question of *metric timing*. What time frame does the data reflect? This may seem inconsequential, but analyzing a few data can make an outlier look like the norm and subsequently drive poor decision-making. For each KPI and metric discussed in this chapter, the timelines and sample sizes provided are recommendations for a typical practice. Depending on the size of a practice, the timeline may vary in order to capture a valid sample size for making a decision. With some metrics (eg, annual or quarterly profit), the timeline is determined by financial reporting requirements. Some metrics have timelines that are best suited to different sample sizes and may vary depending on the practice. Suggested timelines for these metrics are noted as best practice. All of the metrics described in this chapter can and should be aggregated to be viewed with a larger sample size. For example, a weekly metric such as visits should also be viewed monthly, quarterly, and yearly. A metric like payment per visit may not need to be viewed weekly or monthly, but it is appropriate to aggregate the data into the quarterly and yearly statistics of the practice.

Metric Scope

When considering a metric, it is important to understand what the metric is capturing for the practice for a specific period of time and over the life cycle of the practice; the *metric scope*. For example, having a high body mass index (BMI) is not typically life threatening

key performance indicators (KPIs) – a set of measures focusing on those aspects of organizational performance that are critical for the current and future success of an organization

practice metrics – a set of data that can be collected and reviewed that provide information on a specific area of practice

Chapter 9 / Monitoring and Measuring

today but may indicate poor health and poor outcomes in the future. The scope of a BMI is measuring something that creates a risk factor for the body. Compare this to pulse oximetry, where a % SpO_2 that dips into the low 80s can indicate a severe and immediate life-threatening situation. In this chapter, the metric scope is categorized into three response time groupings: Immediate (having an effect right now, or in the coming days or weeks), Midrange (the effects of this will impact the practice in the coming weeks or months), or Long Term (the effects of this will impact the practice in the coming quarter or year).

Leading and Trailing Indicators

As the names imply, leading indicators are metrics that have some "downstream effect." A leading indicator tells you what is going to happen. How many new patients did the practice have last week? This question can predict how many visits the clinic will likely schedule in the upcoming week, making it an example of a leading indicator (Table 9.1). Conversely, trailing indicators provide information on what has happened in the past. They are helpful in providing a picture of where the practice is now compared to a past point in time and can be used, in part, to evaluate the actions taken but cannot provide information on what will happen in the future. A question such as how much money the practice made in the last quarter is a lagging indicator.

The Physical Therapy Revenue Equation

A revenue equation describes how a business makes money or revenue. In the practice of outpatient PT, the Physical Therapy Revenue Equation consists of data on the number of new patients (NP), total visit numbers (V), and the payment per visit (PPV) that result in the revenue of the practice.

New patients (NP) × Visit total (V) × Payment per visit (PPV) = Revenue ($)

Skilled nursing facilities, home care agencies, and other practice settings vary in terms of payment structure; however, given the dominance of outpatient clinics in PT practice, it is prudent to use this setting as an example. It is important to note that although payment structures change, understanding the variables associated with the production of revenue leads to the ability to individualize KPIs for practices in specific settings.

Table 9.1 Examples of Practice Indicators	
Leading Indicators	**Trailing Indicators**
New patients	Visits per month
Unique website visits	Revenue last quarter
Calls from website visits	Return on investment of marketing campaign
Attendance at a wellness clinic	Percent collection of copays

leading indicator – a metric that provides information that impacts the future

trailing indicator (lagging indicator) – a metric that provides information about past performance

Physical Therapy Revenue Equation – an equation that reflects how the number of new patients, total visit numbers, and payment for those visits impact the revenues of a business

Estimated revenue from the PT Revenue Equation is a starting point for calculating practice revenue. To bring these numbers into a higher resolution, additional information from other metrics, such as the collection rate (ie, what percentage of the fee is collected from billing), cancellation and no-show rate, and the number of new versus returning patients, provides more clarity and a better estimate of the practice's revenue.

Benchmarking

Back in the days before mass production and high-tech equipment, adjustments to correct the performance of a firearm were carried out on a workbench. Thus, the word benchmarking referred to the fine modifications necessary for a firearm to perform with accuracy. Over time, the term benchmarking evolved into the idea of businesses refining their operational standards to be in line with those of their leading competitors and/or accepted industry norms.—Nancy Seiverd[2]

Benchmarking is critical in understanding what metrics are reporting and when actions should be taken. Benchmarks acts as standards against which performance can be measured. If the industry standard (an external benchmark) is collecting 90% of all copays at the time of service and a practice is collecting 70%, and, therefore, not meeting the benchmark, then a decision should be made on why this is happening and what should be done to address the difference.

Finding external benchmarks and determining industry standards is an important exercise for practice owners. Sensitive business information is closely guarded by most small businesses. As such, the most useful benchmarking typically occurs when practices agree to participate in blinded benchmarking studies. A blinded benchmarking process protects the business owner's individual information, by way of a Nondisclosure Agreement, and aggregates and reports on the KPIs of other business owners who have agreed to participate. Professional organizations, such as the American Physical Therapy Association (APTA), are a valuable resource for finding benchmarking information for their particular industry.[3]

Just as important is the exercise of internal benchmarking. How does the practice's performance this year compare to that of last year? How many visits were delivered last year? What was the therapists' productivity? How many new patients were seen? These metrics, as well as others, are important to track and identify trends inside the practice in order to make strategic decisions for the future. Using the copay collection example, if a practice had been collecting 99% of all copays at the point of service last year but is collecting 90% this year, what changed? Did the practice lose a superstar collection person at the front desk? Did the practice decide to stop accepting credit card payments? Did a major third-party payer raise copay or deductibles for their beneficiaries? This metric is a catalyst for asking the subsequent questions to better understand the situation. In this case, the metric (90% copay collection) is important, because declining KPIs (internal benchmarking) signal a problem. Knowing and responding to this information allows a practice to fine-tune the business of health care delivery.

Monitoring and Reporting

Many businesses operate monthly, bill monthly, and track expenses monthly. Most banks and billing companies issue statements monthly, so a business can reconcile its accounts monthly. As a practical matter, internally, using a calendar-month gives a fixed interval to

benchmarking – a standard against which performance can be measured

Chapter 9 / Monitoring and Measuring

compare to from previous years (a metric called Same Store Sales). When communicating to employees, partners, and investors, speaking in monthly terms gives a common framework, a period that people can easily understand. (eg, "the practice had less revenue in the trailing 5 weeks, compared to this same 5 weeks from last year" is not as easily understood or clearly communicated as the practice had a bad April compared to last year.)

Quarterly monitoring (12 months of the year viewed in 4 quarters) provides a broader view of the practice's health. It is too long a time frame to effectively take action on most immediate scope metrics, but it is a tradition in the United States that businesses report on earnings quarterly so that their shareholders (ie, investors or fractional owners who provided the capital but don't have a hand in the day-to-day running of the business) can keep track of the business' performance.

Yearly monitoring is necessary for many reasons that exist outside the business model. Chief among these is that the Internal Revenue Service (IRS) will view a business as a yearly business. Yearly timing is too much of a lagging indicator to make immediate (or even midrange) data actionable, so most metrics follow a narrower span, allowing practice owners to act quicker and be more proactive with problems.

An alternative to the calendar year is the fiscal year. A business owner can choose any 12-month period to report financial information to the IRS. Although most businesses sync their fiscal year with the calendar year (January to December), it is not uncommon for businesses to choose to use another period (eg, April 1 to March 31) for reporting purposes. This is determined by an industry standard or when a business has a natural decrease in business activity, allowing for time to gather and write the end-of-year financial reports.

General Practice Metrics

*New Patients (NP): The Heart Rate of a Practice

> NP = Count NP or total NP (per measured period)
> Timing: Weekly
> Scope: Midrange

The human body does not exist without a heartbeat. Similarly, practices do not exist without new patients. New patients (NP) are the lifeblood of a practice. They drive the revenue equation. If the NP metric stays at zero for long, it is similar to the heart stopping for a long period of time. And that is troublesome. Having too few or too many patients also has an effect on the health of a business, similar to the conditions of bradycardia and tachycardia in a person.

Neither condition is desirable. Many people starting out in business worry that the practice will not be able to attract enough patients. But the opposite is also problematic; having too many patients to manage can make the employees too busy. In The E-Myth Revisited, Michael Gerber succinctly describes the problems of being too busy:

> The problem is not that the owners of small businesses in this country don't work; the problem is that they're doing the wrong work. As a result, most of their businesses end up in chaos—unmanageable, unpredictable, and unrewarding.[4]

> fiscal year – a 12-month period of time that a business routinely reports the financial activity of the business, typically chosen when a business has a natural decrease in business activity, allowing for time to gather and write the end-of-year financial reports

---

*A basic KPI that a practice owner should track to understand the financial health of the practice.

He goes on to describe the horrifying results:

. . .by the end of the first year 40% of (small businesses) will be out of business. Within 5 years, more than 80% of them will have failed. And the rest of the bad news is, if you own a small business that has managed to survive for 5 years or more. . .80% fail in the second 5.[4]

Gerber and others go on to define the problem that leads to this terrifying result. Too much work, too quickly, without the right growth strategy, and especially without enough (and the right kind) of help to do the work, lead practice owners not to want to be practice owners anymore (Box 9.1).

BOX 9.1 • The Steve Story: Too Many New Patients?

Steve was an excellent outpatient clinician working for a large company whose patients and friends always told him he should open his own PT practice. "Nobody does PT like you, Steve. . ." was a chorus that he had heard over and over again. He had a loyal following in his community and decided that the time was right to go out on his own and provide the care he wanted to provide, the way he wanted to provide it, and get to enjoy some of the fruits that his creative energies were generating.

So Steve searched for office space, did a rudimentary market analysis, bought some signage, and submitted his resignation. He also did 1,000 other things to get the doors open on day 1. And on day 1, the doors opened to . . . crickets. Steve was scared but still excited and confident. Low and behold, by the end of week 1, he had patients on the schedule! Some were people from the community, and others followed him from his old practice.

Steve had new patients who were generating visits on his schedule just as in the old operation. Of course, he did an amazing job. One thing Steve had when the patients were there was time and control. Time to spend with them (and bill for that time) and the freedom to spend more time doing more interventions that he never had time to apply at his old job. The patients loved it.

Steve is Steve, and the patients LOVE Steve. So they told their friends, who told their friends. Steve's "New Patient" metric soared. The schedule swelled. In the coming months, Steve decided that he needed help just to answer the phones and schedule the patients, so he hired his neighbor to help him do the billing and answer the phones. This gave him a little break, and he was able to treat his patients, and life was pretty good.

New patients continued to call, and Steve found that he was not providing the level of care he wanted for his existing patients. His schedule was very busy, with new patients and existing patients, a far cry from that first week when Steve worked only 9 hours treating patients. Steve thought of bringing on another PT but didn't really know if his practice would last. He also feared that another PT could not provide the level of care that he was providing.

By month 4, Steve was so busy that his first patient was at 7:00 am and his last patient was at 7:45 pm. He was documenting until 11:30 pm every day. He didn't want to turn people away because he didn't know if this influx of patients would last.

To make matters worse, the billing was falling way behind. His neighbor had to quit because her Dad took ill, and he began doing all the billing on his own until he could find someone else. But Steve was too busy treating patients to look for a new front office helper. Between the claim denials, the delay in payment, and the insurers paying him diluted fees, Steve was not making nearly as much on each patient as he had predicted when he set out.

Steve was making more money than when he worked for the hospital, but when he divided the number of hours he was treating patients (and the weekend time he was spending getting

Chapter 9 / Monitoring and Measuring

BOX 9.1 • The Steve Story: Too Many New Patients? (*continued*)

caught up on business) by the amount he was making, Steve calculated that he was actually making much *less* (per hour) than he did when he worked at the hospital. He was also working for a madman who demanded that he see all the patients and do all the billing and the hiring and training and 1,000 other tasks to run the business. The worst part was that this "madman boss" was Steve himself, so it made it really hard to quit. In addition, all his patients were depending on him.

There are 1,000 lessons to learn in the story of Steve. The first, of course, is that a person cannot possibly do it all alone. He cannot do everything with little or no help. He needs to hire people to help him. The problem with hiring is not that Steve thought he had no time to hire, but when it comes to "having the time to. . ." Steve could actually have predicted his predicament. He had a key metric. . .a *LEADING INDICATOR* that told him that he was going to need more clinical help. As Steve's New Patient KPI rose, he could have acted on the information and hired more help. Steve loved treating patients but hated numbers and metrics. So he didn't track them and didn't worry about them. Besides. . . what could be the problem with being too busy?!?

As you can see from this illustration, just paying attention to the most basic metric, and having some knowledge of what actions to take in response, can lead to make-or-break moments in the life of a small business owner.

New Patients (NP) is one of the most valuable metrics to an owner because it is a leading indicator. Leading indicators provide information on what may happen in the future. If the NP metric is low this month, next month the practice can plan on having lower visit totals and lower revenue (as existing patients complete their plans of care and are discharged without being replaced on the schedule by new patients). This data is actionable because the practice owner can act on the metric through advertising, visiting referral sources, emailing a list of previous patients to follow up on their current health (word-of-mouth advertising), holding an open house and inviting people to stop in and see the clinic or provide free screenings.

Visits per Week (V/wk): The Respiration Rate of a Practice

> V/wk = Count total visits or visits/weeks measured
> Timing: Weekly and monthly
> Scope: Immediate

Patient census is a list, or a count, of all of the current patients that are actively being served by the practice. The number of visits is a simple metric to track in any given time frame. In general, short, more recent, time frames are more actionable and behave more like leading indicators, whereas longer, more distant time frames behave more like lagging indicators. If a practice looks at *visits per day* and tomorrow there is a rash of illnesses or a school cancellation (an aspect of patient and employee attendance secondary to the need for child care), it can appear that the practice is in a terrible business position. Similarly, a particularly busy day with no cancellations can make it look like the practice is very busy and needs more help. When it comes to visit tracking, a weekly interval provides the most useful and accurate data. *Visits per week* gives a sufficiently large sample size to allow for the variations of one or two bad days (for instance, patients who cancel on a Monday or a Tuesday can reschedule later in the week and still be captured for tracking purposes) and provides more timely information for needed actions than monthly reports. *Visits per month* is a good interval to track to identify trends on how the practice is performing compared to previous years. This monthly metric may be too late to take corrective actions on

BOX 9.2 • More on Timing: Not All Months Are Created Equal!

One of the biggest confounding factors when looking at monthly data is that not all months are the same. Some months have 20 working days, whereas others have as many as 23 days. That's three extra days of visits, if a practice is tracking visits per month, but, more importantly, that's three extra days (15%) of generating and collecting revenue. For a company with profit margins of 15%, this is obviously significant (profit = revenues − expenses). Additionally, in a service industry such as health care, payroll timing can greatly skew the information obtained from monthly data. Does the practice pay its employees biweekly (usually every other Friday) or twice a month (on the 15th and 30th days)? The biweekly payroll frequency is by far the most common in the United States today and consists of 26 paydays in a year, instead of 24 paydays if the payday was twice a month. Twenty-six paydays per year means that in 2 months of a calendar year, there will be three Fridays that are paydays. When tracking expenses, these months will have 33% more salary expense than the other 10 months. (Remember that salary and benefits are the largest expense in a labor-intensive industry such as health care.) Considering the profit margins described earlier, it is not uncommon for PT practices to record a net decrease in profit in those months with three paydays. Of course, the practice depends on making up that loss in the other 10 months of the year.

The bottom line is that a practice owner who is looking at a Profit and Loss Statement on a monthly basis may think that the practice is performing poorly in those three-payroll months, whereas, in fact, the practice is busy, collecting plenty of cash and performing relatively well. Conversely, a practice that generates a monthly low profit margin may not have built up enough savings to cover expenses in the third pay of the month, when it comes around. Add to this the confounding variable of the number of working days in the month, and the result is that monthly metric tracking and reporting can generate confusing results. Monthly metric tracking is important for some areas of a practice, but it is also something that contains these known variables (eg, working days and atypical timed expenses), which must be acknowledged.

---

significant events that impact the daily operations of the practice or that have a long-term impact on the health of the practice (eg, a decline in the patient census, payments received, or number of new patients; Box 9.2).

Average Visits/Plan of Care: The Rate of Metabolism of a Practice

> Total visits/Total new patients = (V/NP)
> Timing: Quarterly, at a minimum
> Scope: Intermediate to long range

The KPI Average Visits/Plan of Care seeks to answer the question: On average, how many patient visits are associated with an established plan of care for a selected period of time? This metric expands the PT Revenue Equation to the following formula:

$$\text{New patients (NP)} \times \text{Patient visits/Plan of care (V/POC)} \times \text{Payment per visit (PPV)} = \text{Revenue}$$

The V/POC metric provides information on how long, on average, a patient is treated in the clinic. It is not an outcome measure. It does not show how much clinical or functional improvement the patient made. Therefore, a clinic with a low V/POC cannot state that it gets patients better faster. To validate that claim, the clinic would have to link the V/POC with an average outcomes score (using the Δ between start and finish measures) and compare it to

Chapter 9 / Monitoring and Measuring

an established benchmark of other similar clinics. This outcome change would have to be closely tracked for all of the clinic's patients, and risk adjusted (allow for the fact that some clinics see a more complicated mix of patients than others). The V/POC can vary depending on the practice for several reasons, including diagnosis mix. The diagnostic mix is the grouping of the various medical diagnoses of patients seen in a clinical setting. A practice that sees a lot of postoperative patients that require longer plans of care may have a high V/POC metric. Conversely, a practice that specializes in vestibular rehabilitation, where patients can recover quickly from the interventions provided, may have a low V/POC metric. Another factor that influences V/POC is the therapists' clinical skills and expertise in fostering compliance and understanding of the value of a plan of care to the patient.

It is important to monitor this KPI quarterly (doing so sooner may skew the data and make it unreliable) in order to investigate any variance in the expected or benchmarked target. An unexpected low V/POC value may indicate a problem with patient adherence to a plan of care, patients cancelling appointments (a negative impact on revenue), a change in the diagnosis mix, the effectiveness of a new intervention or a new provider of service. What is important is to investigate and understand the reason why the target was not met.

*Arrival Rate (AR) %: The Hematocrit Level of a Practice

> Total arrived patients/Total scheduled patients = AR%
> Timing: Weekly
> Scope: Immediate

Cancellations and no-shows represent one of the largest loss-leading categories and waste of resources in the health care system today. One estimation of the cost due to missed appointments in the health care puts the amount at 150 billion dollars annually.[5] The global pandemic only magnified this issue. Patient nonarrival (the combination of cancels and no-shows) creates a specific and unique problem for the PT practice owner. The owner has paid employees to manage and deliver services for a specific period of time with the expectations of creating a certain amount of revenue. When a patient calls to cancel an appointment, without leaving sufficient time to fill that space with another patient, the therapist must try to fill that time with other activities that are valuable to the practice. Because providing patient care is the only revenue-generating activity for most PT practices, this downtime presents a challenge for PT practices. Therapists typically use this time to perform administrative tasks like responding to insurer authorization or clarification requests, writing letters to physicians, completing documentation requirements, or collaborating with peers. Some practices encourage therapists to use this time for marketing activities such as contacting prior patients or referral sources. Although it would be optimal to improve the AR to 100%, this is simply not reasonable to expect. Patients do get ill, delayed at work, and have transportation or caregiver issues. For the practice owner who has budgeted the cost of that therapist, nonarrivals must be factored into the overall picture of service delivery, which can vary depending on the practice setting. Given that there is an acceptable threshold for every practice, AR presents an example of the importance of practice owners participating in and understanding benchmarking. If the practice's AR is 60% and the industry standard is 85%, the practice should investigate why the variance exists.

If the AR gradually drops below a benchmark, it usually points to a more systemic problem. Why are the patients not valuing the service provided enough to make it a priority

> diagnosis mix – the various medical diagnoses of patients that are seen in a clinical setting

and attend? Is there a therapist in the practice whose patients cancel more than other therapists? What is that therapist doing or saying that is making their patients reluctant to attend? These issues should be investigated and clarified. This starts by collecting data. The front office should always record the reason for the cancellation when a patient calls to cancel. When the AR drops, the practice owner can study the reasons and look for trends. The owner can also survey the patients who cancel and develop a working hypothesis for the issue and then intentionally address it. Some geographic areas do have higher cancellation rates than others, despite consistent practices, but this should never be accepted as a valid reason for a poor AR. Meeting the unique needs of the patients in a geographic or demographic area should be a top priority for any health care practice. Conversely, if there is a therapist or clinic who has a high AR, then the reason for such behavior should be investigated, identified, and replicated.

General Financial Metrics

Payment per Visit (PPV): The Blood Pressure of a Practice

Total revenue/Total visits = PPV
Suggested time frame: Monthly
Scope: Intermediate

PPV is an average of how much revenue the practice collects per visit. It's a "down and dirty" number that a practice can use to determine, on average, how much money is collected for each bulk unit of service provided to each patient over a given period of time. The term bulk unit is used here because there are subunits inside of PPV (Timed Units and Relative Value Units) that can be used to give a higher resolution picture of how the practice is being paid.

PPV is not the same as how much a practice gets paid per visit because it also includes losses from visits that did not get paid and losses from portions of visits that were paid incorrectly. If a practice wants to know how much the practice is paid per visit, the owner would run a report in the electronic medical record (EMR) system that shows Payment per Visit for Fully Paid Claims. Best practices at that point are to stratify fully paid claims by the entity who paid. PPV (fully paid) is usually important for ranking which payers pay the most and which pay the least. This information can then be combined with Cost/Visit (described later in this chapter) to drive decision-making for which payers the practice wants to do business with and which payers the practice may consider renegotiating the contract for services or discontinuing the contract altogether. This same exercise will apply to patient accounts. If a practice has a patient who has a large Patient Responsibility account and is found on the Bad Debt list of accounts not paid, the practice should identify those accounts and work with the patients to secure a fair and reasonable arrangement of payment for services rendered.

Profit and Loss Statement: The Oxygen Saturation Level of a Practice

Income − Expenses = Profit
Profit/Revenue = Profit margin
Metric timing: Monthly, quarterly, yearly
Metric scope: Intermediate to long term

If New Patients are the heart rate of a practice, then the blood is the Cash Flow, and the amount of oxygenated blood that is provided is profit. The key difference between cash flow and profit is that whereas profit indicates the amount of money left over after all expenses have been paid, cash flow indicates the net flow of cash into and out of a business.[6]

Chapter 9 / Monitoring and Measuring

These two may seem similar, but there is an important difference that needs to be understood. A business owner could have a lot of cash coming into the business through loans from the bank, but little income from patients or third-party insurers because not much business is being done. The owner is spending time marketing, doing workshops at the senior center, and visiting the local medical professionals, building up a patient/client base. The Cash Flow statement is positive. . .but the Profit and Loss statement (where loan income is not included) will be negative. This may sound like a practice that is in big trouble, and it is if this is a mature business, but when a practice is just starting out and building a patient/client base, a high Cash Flow Statement and a low Profit and Loss Statement is not uncommon. As this example illustrates, a Profit and Loss Statement is an important report, the first half of which is focused on describing revenues (how a practice generates and acquires money), whereas the second half focuses on expenses (how a practice spends the money it acquired). Subtracting the expenses from the revenues identifies the profit or loss for the business.

Profit margin is simply a representation of what percentage of all the money earned is profit. Margins are KPIs that can be compared to peers. If an owner can look at the best performing companies in a region and see that they run on 12% profit margins, whereas the owner's practice is running on a 2% profit margin, the data shows that this is worth investigating. Maybe the owner's practice expenses are too high (eg, located in a high-rent district or operates with expensive staff), or maybe the revenues are too low (volume is too little, or reimbursement is not meeting costs). The Profit and Loss Statement is an appropriate document to begin the investigation.

The best companies have large (often double-digit) profit margins that rarely swing negative. These companies can withstand swings in payment and seasonal dips in revenue. Many companies, however, operate on smaller profit margins. When revenue dips, or there are problems with the patient census (eg, during a worldwide pandemic), these companies' bottom line can swing into the negative and stay there. Where will the cash come from to pay the employees and the bills when there isn't enough incoming cash? Loans from the bank? Cash in accounts for dividend payments to investors, or will the owner not take a salary that month so that there is enough cash in the business to cover costs? A company with a slim or no profit margin, which stays there for long enough, will drain cash from all available sources. The owner who built a practice that was based on a mission (eg, to help people or to provide the best care) is now out of business (Box 9.3). Profit is not a luxury but a necessity if a business is to survive.

BOX 9.3 • A Word About Mission Statements

The practice example in the text is not supporting a mission of purely making money. A health care practice whose mission is financially motivated, or thinly veiled to be self-serving, may have a hard time both attracting customers and creating a rewarding work environment. Mission statements should clearly speak of the passion that drives the work. That said, the burden of everyone in the practice is to understand that, at the end of the day, the mission statement is underpinned by a successful business model where there is more income than expenses. No margin, no mission.

profit margin – the money that is available to a business after the expenses are subtracted from the reviews, reported as a percentage

Cost/Visit and Profit/Visit: The Caloric Intake of a Practice

Profit/Visits = Profit per visit
Expenses/Visits = Cost per visit
Metric timing: Quarterly
Metric scope: Long term

Combining the Profit and Loss Statement with visits during the same time period will produce a Profit per Visit metric. This is a useful number when considering how many visits are needed in a month to achieve the break-even point or profit margin. For example, a practice may need 400 patient visits next month to break even, 440 visits to meet the profit margin, and 480 visits to consider hiring additional staff (Box 9.4).

Probably more important than Profit per Visit is a metric that lives inside that equation, Cost per Visit. Simply dividing the expense side of the Profit and Loss Statement by the number of visits that the practice provided over that same period of time will result in the cost of providing a visit to a patient. This data is extremely useful when negotiating contracts with potential payers. If an insurer is offering a contract that maximizes the per diem payment at $92 and the practice cost per visit is $98, the real value of the contract is clearer. The Payer Mix metric will address how these Cost per Visit metrics factor into the decision-making on whether to accept certain contracts or not.

Payer Mix: The Diet of a Practice

% of revenues per insurer = Payer mix
Payer revenue/Payer volume = PPV (payer)
Metric timing: Semiannually, yearly
Metric scope: Long term

The EMR or internal accounting software should be able to break down revenue by payer. As an example, how much income comes from Medicare and how much from the local Blue Cross/Blue Shield insurance carrier is important information. As an owner examines the payer mix, the percentage of total revenue from each payer will become evident. Dividing the payer revenue by the number of visits by patients with that payer results in the Payment Per Visit by Payer. It is important that the practice's EMR accounting system is able to also provide the Fully Paid Claim, by Visit, by Insurer metric. This includes the PPV (payer) amount but also attaches any patient responsibility (eg, copay, coinsurance, deductible) that the patient paid for those visits. This high-level metric provides information on what the practice should expect to receive, in terms of revenue, for each visit, for any given insurer. This information is then used to compare the Cost per Visit for contract decision-making purposes.

BOX 9.4 • Profit Goals: The Goalposts Will Always Be Moving

It is important to have goals. It is just as important to be flexible about those goals. When an owner comes together with the team and strategically plans out what the practice is to achieve, remember that this is about making a reasonable best guess. Big Hairy Audacious Goals, or BHAGS, are fine for motivating a team and streamlining decision-making, but understand that as the practice matures, goals will likely evolve. They may become bigger or shrink, but either way, setting realistic benchmarks that are achievable is an important exercise for every business owner.

Chapter 9 / Monitoring and Measuring
203

One of the benefits and challenges of running a small business is that every business owner (to some degree) gets to decide on whom to do business with. Whether it is a patient who repeatedly cancels scheduled appointments or an insurance company that pays a low rate for services rendered, a practice can choose which businesses/payers to accept, depending on how the decision factors into the goals of the practice. Similarly to eating a healthy diet, the variety of payers whom a practice owner chooses to do business with will ultimately shape the long-term financial health of the practice. As with eating foods, if all a person does is eat junk food, the result will have a negative impact on the long-term health of the person. Similarly, if a practice accepts bad contracts with low payers, the business will have to be creative in the utilization of decreased revenues and manage the cost of providing services. This can be done for a short period of time but, just like an "All-Pizza Diet," cannot be done for the long term.

Sometimes it's a good decision to take on a low-paying contract. Practice owners who are just starting a business in a community/market, or who have a new service to provide, will choose to include lower paying insurers in the Payer Mix. This gives the practice access to new patients at a time when the NP metric is developing. Taking low-paying contracts when a practice is just starting gives the practice more opportunities to accept all patients. A practice owner who wants to market the practice by word of mouth benefits from seeing more patients because those successful experiences will be communicated among people in the community, building the practice's awareness and brand following (see Chapter 6). Those patients who have low-paying insurance may refer others who have a better paying insurance. This is where understanding Payer Mix meets **market share**. Market share is a portion of an identified population or market that purchases or has the potential to purchase a service or good from a business. If a practice is located in a community that is populated mostly by people who have a better paying insurance (a larger share of the market), then the likelihood of that patient with a low-paying insurance referring friends and family to the clinic is beneficial to the practice's business. The opposite also holds true. If patients with low-paying insurance become the predominant group in the practice, then the providers will have to increase the volume of patient visits, which will result in spending less time with each patient. This is one reason why an established practice will not have many contracts with low-paying insurance companies.

A formal market analysis is typically performed by practice owners prior to opening new locations. US census data can provide general statistics about the demographics of a particular zip code.[7,8] Most practices will attract clients/patients from a geographic radius around the clinic that includes small areas of a number of different zip codes. Easily obtained statistics like income level tend to correlate with the predominant type of insurer in an area, providing an estimate of the potential revenue and payer sources available (see Chapter 7).

Another reason to include low payers into the Payer Mix is the marketability of advertising to referral sources that the "practice accepts all insurances" or are "in the network with the local insurance plans." Removing the barrier of the common question "do you take my patients' insurance?" is an important step for practices who want referral sources to be able to refer patients automatically and routinely.

Expense Reporting: Salary—The Calories of a Practice

Health care is a labor-intensive industry where a significant percentage of a practice's expenses are in the salary and benefits paid to employees. It is important for a practice owner to understand how much money is spent on the revenue-generating staff (ie, physical therapists

> **market share** – a portion of an identified population or market that purchases or has the potential to purchase a service or good from a business

and physical therapy assistants), the front office staff, billing staff, support staff, and the practice owner. The amount of the expense is influenced by the cost of providing services (see Chapter 1 and the Cost Worksheet) and the market where the practice is located (What are the competitors paying?) If employees can make more money working for a competitor, the owner should evaluate why the employee is working in their practice? Is it because of the productivity requirements, administrative duties associated with billing and documentation, the Diagnosis Mix, or the benefits offered? Is it the personal management style of the practice owner? There are many reasons why a person chooses to work for an employer, and a practice owner should be aware of those reasons and the priority placed on them by the employees of the practice. Conversely, if a practice owner pays the employees more than the competitors, the owner should evaluate what services or benefits are being limited, financially, by this type of payment structure? Is a practice owner updating the equipment and technology needed to sustain a business? Is enough money going into marketing and community engagement? Is the business sustainable with this type of financial allocation? There are many factors that contribute to a profitable and sustainable practice. Expense management is vital to achieve a practice that will be a benefit to the people served and the employees.

Billing and Collection Metrics

Account Aging: The Body Weight of the Practice

Aged accounts = Current/30 days/60 days/90 days/120 days/>180 days
Metric timing: Every day
Metric scope: Immediate

Any PT practice that extends credit to payers is willing to wait (any amount of time) to get paid and will have Aged Accounts. An Aged Account is one that was not completely paid on the date the service was provided. If a service is provided on January 1, for which payment is not received by January 30, that account is said to be 30 days old. PT practices that operate on a cash-only basis will require the patients to pay the entire bill before they leave the office. These practices do not have Aged Accounts, but their market is targeted to a specific demographic that can afford to pay cash for services rendered. A practice that bills insurance companies and patients for services rendered will not receive 100% of the payment at the time of service delivery, like a cash-only business. Practices bill a patient's insurance company after the visit is completed. These practices send itemized bills of the service delivered to the insurer, and the insurer will eventually pay for the visit. The key word is *eventually*.

Tracking a practice's Aged Accounts is a function of a practice's billing person or department. The Account Aging report will break down the practice's accounts into 30-day increments. Although every account starts at day 1, most accounts don't make it to day 30 because, in today's electronic health care environment, the provider is communicating payment information to the payer electronically, often the same day. Whereas the payer used to send checks to the provider for the services in the mail, in today's electronic environment, payers are transferring funds to the provider's bank account by electronic payment and sending an email with an explanation of the payment back to the practice's accounting system. Those emails are called ERA (Electronic Remittance Advice) and, with the push of a button, the payments are applied to the patients' accounts. When payment is applied to a patient's account and the visit is "paid in full," the account is then removed from the Account Aging report. In today's electronic environment, this can happen in a matter of days, but it doesn't always happen this way.

For accounts between 1-day and the 30-day mark, practices expect to get paid by the payers who employ this level of electronic processing during this time period. When accounts hit the 30-day mark, it's time for the billing department to investigate (either by calling the insurer's billing relations line or online) and see why payments have not been received.

Chapter 9 / Monitoring and Measuring

BOX 9.5 • Deny, Delay, Dilute. . .a Poorly Performing Payer's Game Plan

Payers **deny** payment when they should have released the payment. They base these denials on any number of factors, from something as simple as the patient's name being misspelled in the system to something as complex as an expired preauthorization request. Denials are all too common, even for detail-oriented practices that send "clean claims" (requests for payment where all the i's have been dotted and t's have been crossed).

Payers **delay** payment. They didn't receive the claim; please resend it. They received it, but they are backlogged. Sometimes, there isn't even a reason cited for a delay; all that is stated is that the claim just hasn't been processed yet. How long does the payer have to respond to a request for payment (an insurance claim)? The length of time should be clearly stated in the language of the contract with the payer and monitored in the Account Aging report.

Payers may also **dilute**, or incorrectly pay providers. Each payer pays different amounts for each service that a physical therapist provides. These amounts are spelled out in the provider's contract with the payer. This list of Allowed Amounts, or amounts that the insurer is agreeing to pay the provider for each service is called that Insurer's provider's charge. The difference between the Fee Schedule and the amount that the insurer pays the provider is called an Insurance Adjustment. Obviously, since different payers affix different values to different services, it can be a very complex task to keep track of whether or not each claim is being paid correctly when the provider receives payment for their services. When insurers incorrectly affix payment that is not in line with their fee schedule, they are diluting the payment to the provider. An EMR/Billing System that can identify the expected payment from a specific payer with the actual payment is a valuable tool for a practice to capture this type of behavior.

EMR, electronic medical record

A good billing department establishes regular intervals at which to reexamine these claims and communicate with the insurance company to pay them. As accounts age from 30 to 60 and, eventually, 90 days and beyond, they are tracked in the Account Aging report both individually and cumulatively. When the Account Aging report is itemized, it gives the billing department a "to-do" list for the day in and day out "working of accounts" or "chasing payment." For the practice owner, looking at this report in terms of both the total amount of money owed (also called Accounts Receivable [AR]) and the time period for the outstanding Aged Accounts provides different but very important and useful information.

As a general rule, the amount in each 30-day period should drop by half. So if the current (0-30 days) AR is $20,000, the practice would expect the 31 to 60 days AR to be $10,000, the 61 to 90 days AR to be $5,000, and so forth. If these ARs do not drop accordingly, they should be investigated to determine why this is occurring. Is there one large account that is outstanding that is skewing the results? Did the billing department experience some attrition and is now working shorthanded? Is an insurer behaving in strange ways (like denying payments because they inadvertently moved the practice to be out of network)? Information from the Account Aging report will keep the practice owner up to date on this financial aspect of the practice and provide information in order to make timely decisions to solve little problems before they become big problems that impact cash flow. As accounts age, they become a risk to the business (Box 9.5).

Days That a Sale Is Outstanding (DSO): The Body Mass Index of a Practice

DSO = (Total accounts receivable [measured period]/Total billed sales [same period]) × Days in measured period

Metric timing: Monthly

Metric scope: Long term

The average length of time between when a service is performed and when the provider actually gets paid for the service can be tracked and is called Days (that a) Sale (is) Outstanding. When tracked for every patient visit, all the time, the average provides a general picture of how quickly money is collected for services rendered. Similarly to a patient's BMI, where the patient's weight is compared to height and age, the DSO metric is only good or bad when compared to other, similar practices (benchmarking). Cash practices should have an average DSO that is very low, whereas a practice that sees a high percentage of Workers Compensation, auto accident insurance, or litigation cases will be very high.

The time it takes a practice to collect the money it is owed is inversely related to the chance that the practice is going to be paid at all. Cash-only practices, which have the payer in front of them at the time of service (ie, the patient), can create a condition where the rules are very simple. Most cash-only practices use per diem (Latin; for each day) billing, where there is a flat rate for one day's bundle of PT services (simple rule). If the practice sets that rate at $100, it simply collects this amount prior to, or on the same day of, the delivery of the service. If the owner consistently gets paid by the patients (similarly to shopping at the grocery store), the DSO would be zero. DSO becomes important in cash-only practices the first time that the patient forgets that $100 bill and asks if payment can be made at the next treatment session. If the practice agrees with this request, then it is extending credit to that patient. To extend credit means to make or renew a loan or to enter into an agreement, explicit or implicit, for the payment or satisfaction of a debt or claim, regardless of whether the extension of credit is acknowledged or disputed, valid or invalid, and however arising. Practices that allow patients not to pay at the time of the service extend credit, or make loans to their patients, without ever checking a patient's creditworthiness, credit score, or history, or even asking how the patient views debt and loans. When a practice allows patients to leave the treatment session without paying for the visit, or the patient responsibility for a portion of the visit (eg, copay), they are entering into an undocumented loan agreement with that patient. They have become a bank, and not just any bank, but one that makes loans without formal agreements or consideration of the debtor's ability or willingness to pay the loan or how often the debtor defaults on loans, in general, and many other factors that actual banks use to assess and build a risk profile for potential borrowers.

Attitudes toward debt, both accepting loans and loaning money to others, are very important for a prospective practice owner to consider *prior* to starting a practice. A practice owner with a laissez-faire attitude regarding payment for services rendered will need to collect higher rates from their paying customers to make up for the losses of nonpayment or defaulted loans (what the PT industry calls bad debt). *Bad debt,* in accounting terms, is simply money that a practice is owed but has little to no chance of being collected. It can be recorded in the accounts and kept track of forever, or it can be recorded as bad debt and written off the accounting books as revenues lost.

The longer it takes a practice to collect debts, the more cases of default can be expected (Table 9.2). In the PT industry, what a bank would call default rate, or the percentage of loans that it issues that end up in default, rises in proportion to the length of time that it takes to collect the debt. Psychologically, the farther away from the purchase date, the less value the person places on the purchase, or service provided, and can result in a decreased desire or priority to pay the price of the item or service.

The longer it takes a practice to collect revenue for services rendered (ie, a high DSO), the more a practice will have to write off uncollectable debt. In essence, the practice is providing pro bono services that it did not agree to provide.

Ideally, a practice should target a low DSO and little to no bad debt. Consistent and clear communication with patients and payers regarding the expectation for payment for services rendered is vital to a financial health and longevity of a business. Similarly to a

Chapter 9 / Monitoring and Measuring

Table 9.2 Commercial Collection Agencies of America Data on the Potential Collectability of a Commercial Account[2]

Delinquency Period (mo)	Collection (%)
From Invoice Due Date	Potential
1	88.7
3	68.9
6	51.3
9	37.5
12	21.4
18	15.2
24	8.9

Seiverd N. Collectability scoring—a unique approach to benchmarking. Credit Research Foundation. Benchmarking the collectability of your accounts receivable—the Credit Research Foundation (crfonline.org). Published 2019. Accessed January 14, 2023.

patient's BMI, a high BMI is something that a patient can accept but is concerning from the point of view of the patient's long-term health. If a practice is frequently writing off bad debt, and/or maintains a high DSO, these too are concerning signs of the practice's long-term viability (Box 9.6).

BOX 9.6 • When Is It Acceptable to Have a High DSO?

The opposite of cash-only practices (where payment is made at the time of service) are those segments in the health care industry that have very slow payment processes. In Pennsylvania, for instance, Workers Compensation (WC) claims and Motor Vehicle Accident claims typically have to be sent, on paper claims, through the mail and accompanied by clinic notes. An adjuster reviews the documentation to make sure that what was provided meets certain standards (eg, Did the PT provide treatment only on the injured body part? Was the treatment geared to return the patient to work?). After deeming that the payment is warranted, the adjustor authorizes payment to the practice, and a check is issued and sent (again by mail). The check, once received, has to be logged in to the accounting software, applied to the patient's account, and physically taken to the bank for deposit by someone in the practice.

Contrast this with a health insurance company that does not require documentation review and that accepts electronic claims. (These companies will typically employ a "Pay and Pursue" model, where they make immediate payments to providers for service, and if they think there is a problem with the treatment, can ask for the money back later after performing an audit.) An insurer like this will typically send an email back to the provider, with an explanation of what they paid for the visit (how much money was sent for each line-item of service) and what the patient is expected to pay, subtracted out and communicated in that same email. This email is called an Electronic Remittance Advice, and typically, it will automatically go into the account for the patient in the EMR. (A paper copy of this explanation of what was paid is sent to the patient by mail; it is called Explanation of Benefits, or EOB.) Simultaneously, that same insurer will transfer the amount that the practice gets paid for the visit to the practice's bank account in the form of an electronic bank transfer (called an ACH payment). This electronic process can happen literally in hours or, at most, a few days. DSO for these payers could be in single digits.

Contrasting these two, it is apparent that a practice that sees a lot of WC patients, and very few commercial insurance patients, will have a relatively high DSO. Why is this OK? Because WC claims typically pay out at 150% to as much as 300% of commercial claims. Similarly,

(continued)

BOX 9.6 • When Is It Acceptable to Have a High DSO? (*continued*)

litigation claims, where the practice gets paid nothing at first but agrees to be paid out of a settlement from the patient's lawsuit, can have a high DSO. In these cases, the practice is expecting to get paid much more than with other claims. Most practices that work with patients in litigation will seek a Letter of Protection from the patient's attorney. A Letter of Protection is a document that guarantees that the practice will be paid for the services provided to the patient once the lawsuit is settled. The practice will then be paid by the attorney.

These examples highlight the need to benchmark the DSO metric with similar practices doing the same type of work. Cash-only practices and those that deal only with electronic remitting insurers can have a low DSO in single digits (3-9 days). Practices with a high percentage of WC, motor vehicle accident, and litigation work can expect their DSOs to be high. A good target to aim for in the typical In-Network practice is 18 to 28 days (taking less than a month to get paid for services rendered). Anything longer should be a cause for concern, and the practice owner should investigate the billing and collection process.

DSO, days sales outstanding, EMR, electronic medical record.

Individual Physical Therapist Metrics: Managing by the Numbers

Average Weighted Timed Units per Visits (TU/V) × RVU: A Measure of Efficiency

([Evaluations × 1.5] + Timed units)/Visits = Weighted timed units/Visit
Metric timing: Quarterly (monthly of new or low-billing therapist)
Metric scope: Intermediate to long term

Current payment models place a high value on units of service requiring direct therapist attendance more than others. Most, but not all, treatments involving direct 1-on-1 care are typically measured by how much time the therapist spends with the patient and, as such, are referred to as timed units. Two exceptions to the timed unit classification are the evaluation and reevaluation codes, which are untimed but require the direct skills of the physical therapist. The use of passive modalities, where a modality can be used in the treatment but does not require constant supervision during the application (eg, moist heat), has become marginalized while insurers have pushed reimbursement more toward direct 1-on-1 care provision.

Timed units are simply paid at higher rates than untimed units, so therapists should keep track of how many timed units are billed per day. Practice owners, similarly, need to track and communicate the Average Weighted Timed Unit to their therapists, monthly or quarterly depending on the practice's need. For instance, a manual therapist may bill a disproportionate number of Manual Therapy (97140) charges in the course of practice, whereas a sports therapist might bill more Therapeutic Exercise (97110) codes and a functional therapist may bill a lot of Therapeutic Activities (97530). Even though all three therapists, in this example, are billing the same number of timed units (using the published Medicare Fee Schedule as an example), because 97140 pays $27.45/unit, 97110 pays $29.82/unit, and 97530 pays $37.62/unit, it is clear to see how different patient populations, or practice patterns, affect the amount of revenues generated.[9] Establishing RVUs or weighting the units that therapists bill can help to reconcile different revenue/visit averages between therapists and can educate therapists on how their practice habits influence the PT Revenue Equation.

When a therapist starts with a company, the practice must take great care to educate them on the rules surrounding its third-party contracts and how coding of services provided comply with those unique guidelines. As such, reviews of these TU/V metrics tend

Chapter 9 / Monitoring and Measuring

to be performed more frequently so that the therapist can see how they compare with their peers and reconcile working hours with the time that is billed to the third-party payer. Similarly, low TU/V metrics help identify underbilling therapists who may see the same patient population as their peers, in the same time frame, but who consistently bill fewer timed units and thus generate less revenue.

Revenue/Visit per Therapist (Compare to TU/V-W): A Great Teaching Tool

Metric timing: Quarterly (in individual billing meetings)
Metric scope: Long term

An electronic billing system should be able to provide the practice owner with information on the Timed and Weighted Timed Units the therapists billed, how much revenue has been generated by therapists, and how much revenue has been collected in the name of individual therapists for a select period of time. This information is useful in evaluating the work of the therapists and the financial productivity of each therapist in the practice, thereby creating a teaching opportunity for all the therapists on the expected productivity and work efficiency for the practice.

Relative Value Units Billed per Visit (RVU/V): What Do Your Payers Think Is Most Beneficial?

Metric timing: Yearly
Metric scope: Long term

Not all timed units are billed equally. Each payer will affix a different value to different treatment codes. This should enter into the revenue per visit discussion that a practice owner has with the therapists. A therapist whose treatment patterns include codes for higher paying timed units will have a higher average revenue per visit as compared to one who uses lower paying treatment codes. Sometimes, this has to do with the therapist's patient population. Some therapists might see fewer complex cases and diagnoses that don't demand more complex (higher paying) codes. In those cases, it would be inappropriate to encourage those therapists to change their habits and illegal to change their codes, but it is useful to show them that is why their revenue per visit is lower, even when their TU/V is the same as that of their peers.

Acknowledging the fact that not all timed units are paid at the same rate, when a practice's EMR is capable of creating reports on therapists billing patterns, a new layer can be added to the PT Revenue Equation to provide a higher resolution picture of a practice's revenue generation model.

Update to the Revenue Equation:

New patients (NP) × Patient visits/Episode of care (V/POC) × Units of billed treatment (TU) × Relative net unit value (RVU) = Revenue

Visits/POC per Individual Therapist

Total patient visits/Total evaluations = V/POC-PT
Metric timing: 6 months
Metric scope: Long term

How long a patient remains engaged in his or her plan of care during a current episode is a key metric for a practice to capture and manage. Metric timing is critical and if done inappropriately, can yield skewed data (eg, To simply take a month's worth of total patient visits and divide by the number of total new patient evaluations over that same time gives a limited view of the practice's activity and does not capture the natural fluctuations of patients visits and evaluations over time.) A period of several months will provide a more valid and useful result.

Factors that can influence the V/POC-PT, beyond diagnosis mix and payer mix, include the therapist's practice habits and specific behaviors. The art of communication and education comes naturally to some therapists, whereas others require more oversight and feedback on how to perform these vital skills in the clinic. Patient-centered plans of care and engagement by the patient are vital in order to facilitate a positive outcome. If a therapist has a low V/POC, the reason should be investigated and understood by both the treating therapists and the practice owner. A low V/POC leads to low revenue and possibly poorer patient outcomes. Even therapists who are adept at educating their patients on the value of completing a POC and positively influencing patient engagement can have other habits or behaviors that can negatively impact this metric. There are many behaviors and habits that can adversely affect V/POC-PT, ranging from a therapist who has a negative attitude, insists on talking politics around the office, has an unprofessional appearance, to something as simple as having bad breath. These factors can be more challenging to address because they are aspects of a therapist's identity. It is important for the practice owner to identify those factors that impact patient care and to provide appropriate direction, support, and guidance to optimize the patient's adherence to a POC and ultimately achieve the goals of the POC (see Chapter 10).

Patient Register, Plan of Care Completion, and Patient Drop-Off %

Metric timing: Quarterly
Metric scope: Long term

How good are patients at completing the POC that is established at the initial evaluation? If the physical therapist includes the patient in the planning process on Day 1, and uses a complex and comprehensive evaluative system that yields a plan of care designed to achieve that patient's goals, why do some sources report that up to 70% of patients do not complete the agreed upon plan of care?[10] According to one of the largest physical therapy (PT) EMR providers' review of the data, approximately 20% of PT patients drop out of treatment within the first three visits, and 70% fail to complete their full course of care.[10] Possible reasons for patient drop-off run the gamut from affording the copay or cost to lack of observable progress.

On the PT side, a therapist's demeanor, habits, behaviors, and engagement can contribute to this attrition. As with all metrics, the more variables that can confound the results, the less useful the metric may be to the practice owner. In spite of this inherent variability, the metric should be tracked, analyzed, and used in part to evaluate a therapist's overall performance.

A Patient Registry is a tracking tool that collects POCs and compares them to completed visit numbers. Each new patient is entered, the predicted POC is identified, and the number of completed visits are recorded. From this data, the percentage of completed visits can be derived and aggregated by the therapist for internal comparison purposes and compared to available benchmarks. Therapists who consistently fall below the POC completion percentage of their peers can be identified and the issue investigated. The therapist may simply be setting POC that are too long, creating a condition where it's unreasonable

Patient Registry – a tracking tool that collects a practice's plans of care and compares them to the number of plans completed

Chapter 9 / Monitoring and Measuring

to expect a patient to continue to improve in that period of time, or developing POCs that are not individualized, which can result in wide variations in completion percentage based on the complexity of the case and other inherent factors associated with a lack of individualized care.

Reactivation Rate

Reactivated patients/Drop off calls = Reactivation rate
Metric timing: Every 2 to 4 weeks
Metric scope: Immediate

Drop-offs are patients that unilaterally discontinue coming in for PT. This behavior contributes to lower payment and poorer patient outcomes. Practices go to great lengths to keep their patients engaged and on course to complete their POC. Regardless of the reason, when a patient is not actively engaged with the practice but still has an open POC, it is best practice to follow up and contact the patient to understand the reason for the discontinuation. This typically happens by phone in the form of drop-off calls. Every inactive patient should receive a drop-off call, and a practice's ability to reactivate that patient can be tracked and compared to benchmarks by simply dividing reactivated patients by calls made. Reactivation Rate is a metric that reflects the effectiveness of the practice's outreach success and qualitatively provides feedback to improve the understanding of the reasons why a practice's drop-offs happen in the first place.

Marketing Metrics

Referral Source Reporting

List referrals (count)
Metric timing: Monthly
Metric scope: Long term

People seek the services of a business for a variety of reasons, and businesses strive to attract the right type of person in a variety of ways. Understanding how patients decided to choose a specific PT practice is critical to successful marketing and business sustainability.

For decades, traditional models of PT practice required physicians to prescribe PT for their patients. These prescriptions are commonly called referrals. When a physician writes a prescription for PT, in the United States, the patient can take that prescription and receive PT from a provider of their choice. As such, the referral that the physician is making is for the service of PT itself and not always for a particular physical therapist or clinic. Those referrals for PT could be fulfilled by any practice, but the patient is deciding on a particular practice for particular reasons. Those reasons are the true referral source, and a practice must identify and understand. One way this can be done is with the use of the EMR. Every EMR has a field that can be used to track a Referral Source. This is not the same as the Prescribing Physician (which may even be called Referral Source). Since the prescribing physician is necessary for some insurers (eg, Medicare), there will always be a field for it in the EMR, and its label may not be changeable. Capturing that information and training the staff on the specific field in the EMR in which to record the reason why the patient chose this particular practice is key. The marketing questions are, how did you hear about our practice (which reflects the marketing and communication efforts), and what are your reasons for choosing us (which reflect the attributes of the practice that patients are seeking)?

The second challenge to referral tracking is narrowing the dispersion of answers to a manageable level. If the practice knows that many of the new patients hear about the practice from others (ie, word of mouth), it can have a label for such a referral (eg, Friend). If the patient reports that they saw an advertisement for the practice, the label could be Ad; if the patient was referred by the physician, the label could be Physician or Physician's Office. It is recommended that a practice keep its Referral Source List (the number of options that an employee can choose in the EMR when they record the reason) to single digits. As a practice starts to evaluate the results, it can make individualized decisions about breaking these categories down further for the purpose of better understanding how patients are making the decision to access the practice (Box 9.7).

The Referral Source report can help with decisions on marketing and advertising. Over time, the data can provide information on market trends and marketing efforts that give the practice the best return on its investment.

Return on Investment (ROI)

Total cost on a marketing campaign/(# New patients from campaign × Profit per plan of care)
Metric timing: After every marketing campaign (successful or otherwise)
Metric scope: Intermediate

BOX 9.7 • Referral Source Reports

Referral Report Practice #1
New Patients for October: 46
Referral Source:
Former/Existing Patients: 8
Ad in September's Local Paper: 5
Google Search (Reviews): 7
Physician's Front Office: 3
Insurance Company List: 2
Physician Told Me to Come Here: 9
Location/Saw the Sign: 8
Other: 4

When a Referral Source report reads like this one, the practice owner gets information on how and why patients choose the practice. This type of Referral Source report shows a diversified referral source. This diversification lowers the practice's risk of a sudden decrease in new patients resulting from a referral dependency from one specific source.

Referral Report Practice #2
New Patients for October: 46
Referral Source:
Doctor Williams: 36
Google Search: 2
Doctor Williams' Front Office: 4
Friend or Family Member: 3
Other: 1

This type of Referral Source report shows a limited referral source. This lack of diversification increases the practice's risk of a sudden decrease in new patients resulting from a referral dependency from one specific source, Dr. Williams. What if something happens to Dr Williams or Dr Williams decides to use a different PT practice?

Chapter 9 / Monitoring and Measuring

When it comes to marketing opportunities, practice owners should view an opportunity as an investment in the practice. An advertisement in the local newspaper may cost $4,000 but might only result in two or three new patients. If a practice knows that it makes a profit of $400 per new patient, the return on investment (ROI) for this marketing effort is not financially prudent. Conversely, sponsorship of a local baseball team for $4,000 that results in 20 new patients would be prudent, and a better ROI.

Practice owners should be cautious of ROI predictions made by marketing salespeople who are unfamiliar with the financial metrics of PT practice. Caution should be exercised when the opening line in a conversation is: What is a new patient worth to you? Just because an owner knows the practice's metrics, it does not mean they are required to share them with someone who is trying to sell something. Because expenses vary across the industry, as do profit margins, it is difficult to compare ROI predictions even among practices in the same zip code. It would be better to ask, how much am I going to have to pay you (salesperson) to deliver a new patient to me?

A practice should evaluate its marketing efforts internally and track ROI on an ongoing basis. If a practice realizes 20 new patients from the sponsorship of one baseball team, then perhaps sponsoring the whole league would be an efficient use of resources. As a practice learns what works and what doesn't in a particular market, the practice begins to see a clearer picture of what resonates with the patients in a certain area and can search for similar marketing opportunities in that area. If a practice is having success with the baseball league, then maybe the local soccer program can be considered as the next step. If a practice is having success with advertisements in a newspaper, then other forms of communication may be worth exploring. This may sound like trial and error, because it is. If there were a one-size-fits-all PT marketing program, everyone would be using it. The unique nature of each practice's marketing strategy is reflected in the uniqueness of each market. A practice owner may think they know what potential patients are looking for in a PT service, but the owner needs to be sure. ROI tracking should be done for every marketing effort that a practice undertakes and evaluated in a timely manner, comparing and considering the value of the alternative options. Trends emerge and marketing dollars should be allocated accordingly. The long-term viability of the practice depends on it.

Cost of Acquisition (CoA)

> Total marketing budget spend/# New patients = Cost of acquisition (CoA)
> Metric timing: Yearly (during budget process)
> Metric scope: Long term

How does a practice determine how much money to spend on marketing? Zero dollars is clearly too small, and 50% of total expenses is too high. The goal is to spend just the right amount of money on marketing that maximizes the ROI. It should be done in the aggregate as well as with specific marketing projects/efforts. Remember the marketing salesperson's question: How much is a new patient worth to you? The answer to that question is found in the metric CoA. This metric can be benchmarked, as a percentage of total expenditures, with other practices in the industry and evaluated yearly to see if it is too high (possibly owing to excessive marketing costs) or too low (possibly owing to not enough money spent on marketing).

Rate of Customer Return (RCR; Unique Episode)

> Total patients with multiple POC/Total patients = Rate of return
> Metric timing: Every 5 years
> Metric scope: Very long term

One financial goal of a practice is to have the CoA of a patient lower than the profit made on that patient. Although it is desirable to have a lot of new patients, a business cannot spend $500 for the CoA of one patient who generates only $400 in profit. (The CoA should be greater than Profit per Plan of Care [POC-P].) However, the best PT practices don't just see a patient once across the span of that patient's lifetime. The patient returns at a future date for another episode of care and a new POC. It is not uncommon for a single patient to come to a PT practice 5 or 6 times over the course of the patient's lifetime, which changes the equations on the CoA and ROI. For that reason, calculating the likelihood that a patient is going to return to the practice again in the future (without having to acquire them via a new marketing effort) and estimating how many future episodes of care can be expected are valuable numbers. RCR is the percentage of patients who buy again from the practice.[6] In health care, this is different from the Reactivation Rate, which is a measure of how likely a practice is to revive a patient who has "dropped off," or unilaterally discontinued services, to resume his or her plan of care.

Lifetime Value of a Patient (LVP)

> Average of the total visits across all POC × (Profit/Visit) = Lifetime value
> Metric timing: Every 5 years
> Metric scope: Very long term

In the current environment of EMR reporting suites, it is easier to calculate the LVP than the Rate of Customer Return. Some EMRs are sophisticated enough to create a report that averages the revenue per patient across the practice, and others can break this down by POC and visits. Depending on the functionality that a practice's software can deliver, there are a number of methods that can be used to arrive at LVP such as Total Patient-specific Revenue (over a long period of time) × Profit Margin, or Total Visits × (Profit Margin/Visit). When a practice understands its profit margins, it can extrapolate the value that each new patient has over the entire course of their relationship merely by multiplying the revenue collected over that patient's lifetime by the practice's profit margin.

Understanding the net profitability of every patient across the longest interval (the "lifetime" of their relationship) helps clarify the value of every *Unique New Patient* (UNP differing from NP, which denotes an initial evaluation and new POC but could also include a patient who was previously seen by the practice for a different problem). UNP is a valuable metric to track for marketing purposes and can be cross-referenced with the Referral Source report to determine trends in how patients are finding their way to the practice.

Customer Satisfaction Metrics

Net Promoter Score (NPS®)

> Collected at intake, visit #2, and after DC for every patient
> Aggregated and segmented across providers, clinics, and across the company
> Metric timing: Reviewed monthly
> Metric scope: Long term

On a scale of 0 to 10, how likely is a patient to recommend this particular practice to a friend or colleague? This is a question that is frequently asked of patients or consumers of goods and for good reason. A wealth of research has been done on NPS in the United States.[11,12] In short, patients who answer with a 9 or 10 are considered to be promoters and are far more likely to refer others to the practice and say positive things about the practice to others. Patients who answer with a seven or eight are considered to be passive.

Chapter 9 / Monitoring and Measuring

These patients are unlikely to refer others to the practice, but they are also unlikely to say bad things about the practice to others. Patients who answer with a six to zero are considered to be detractors and are most likely not going to refer others to the practice but may also say negative things about the practice. When a detractor is identified, the practice owner has an opportunity to engage with the patient and address the concerns or problems immediately in order to limit the negative consequences of the detractor.

The NPS is an aggregation of the NPS questions of the practice. NPS is a calculation of the percentage of promoters minus the percentage of detractors. This may seem like an arbitrary number, but it has been studied and benchmarked across the business landscape in the United States. These scores range from +100 to −100 and describe businesses from those that generate tremendous satisfaction among their consumers (+100) to those whose customers are dissatisfied and have a negative opinion of the practice (−100).

Measuring customer satisfaction is a valuable tool in many industries. This can be done using the NPS scale or a host of other standardized questions designed to measure a patient's satisfaction with their experience. This information, used in the aggregate, is valuable for strategic planning and positioning the practice to meet the ongoing needs of the consumers in a particular geographic area.

Google Reviews

Qualitative review
Metric timing: Daily (twice a day if possible)
Metric scope: Immediate and long term

As social media evolves and communication using technology becomes easier, information becomes ubiquitous and readily available to patients who can become a more educated consumer. As discussed in the Referral Source section, obtaining a prescription or referral from a referral source does not necessarily mean that the patient will use a specific practice. Patients with access to social media understand that not all PT providers are created equal and they have a choice in regard to where they receive their care. Just as with other businesses, patients will consult Facebook, Angie's List, Yelp, Google, and a host of other review sites to view the experiences of others when deciding where to start PT. By far the most common of these is Google Reviews (see Chapter 6).

Much is written about how to manage Google reviews, but the biggest and most important job is to ask patients to post a Google review. The more reviews a practice has on Google, the more validity it gives to a practice, which may increase potential patient confidence and can act as a protective function against that occasional negative review. A practice that can garner a significant number of five-star reviews tends to delegitimize the claims of a few detractors.

Just as important as the number of reviews for the practice is the speed at which replies are posted to the reviewers. Potential patients look at positive reviews and negative reviews and judge the practice on how it replies to their patients. It is important to a potential patient that they see that the practice is listening to their patients and that it values their feedback, while ensuring their privacy.

Developing Multisite Physical Therapy Practices

One of the advantages that owners of multiple location practices enjoy is taking advantage of the economy of scale, defined as increasing production and revenues but efficiently using fixed costs (see Chapter 1). When a practice tracks its expenses, it does so in terms of the business activities that the expenses support. Some expenses can be shared among many providers or locations with only minimal increase in their cost (Box 9.8). These

BOX 9.8 • Purchasing Power

There are some economies of scale enjoyed by larger companies that are more difficult to break out but that still contribute to an improved bottom line. One of these is Purchasing Power. Generally speaking, vendors are very interested in selling larger quantities of their products to you, as the buyer, and, as such, are willing to reduce the prices they charge you for the more you buy. Using the site-specific example of a box of elastic bands, a solo practice owner may need only one box, so they pay the premium price for that box, just as a consumer would. A multisite owner can buy boxes for all of its sites and, as such, will hit breakpoints in pricing where the vendor is willing to make the per-unit price cheaper because that vendor is saving on his cost of acquiring additional customers, shipping (in some cases), and other related production expenses. A *breakpoint* is the number of units that a customer has to agree to buy before the vendor agrees to a lower price.

shared expenses are where many PT practices are able to generate more profit. From leveraging existing brand awareness and public relations, to shared insurance expenses, when companies are able to create more revenue with less expenses, their profit margins benefit.

The key to running a multisite practice is managing information and understanding which expenses are shared and which are directly attributable to a specific site or operation. Breaking out revenue data into what comes from which location is equally as important. This is typically something accounting or EMR software can achieve.

Revenue-generating KPIs should be attributed to the site where they were generated. As treatments are delivered and billed to the insurer by the treating therapist, the place of service is noted in the system. When payment is made on those claims, the system should attribute it as such. Most systems have easy to generate reports, called Place of Service Summary or Payments by Place of Service, that will generate the information needed to understand which clinic is generating what revenue.

Profit and Loss by Location (or Profit and Loss by Class)

Revenue by location − Expense by location = Profit or loss by location
Metric timing: Monthly
Metric scope: Intermediate

Slightly more complicated than tracking revenue is tracking the expense side of the equation for a multisite business. The key to expense allocation is understanding who benefits from every expense (Box 9.9). Is this something that the whole company benefits from, or is this something that benefits only one site? An example of a site-specific benefit would be supplies ordered by the site to be used at that site only. If Location A orders a box of elastic exercise bands and intends to use it only at Location A, that is a site-specific expense and should be broken out as such. Shared expenses are those that contribute benefit to the entire company. An example of a shared expense is yearly accounting fees. When a practice pays an accountant to prepare and file the tax return for the practice, the accountant creates a report for the entire practice and not for a specific site.

The key to tracking shared and fixed expenses lies in the input. When an expense is reported in the business accounting software, if it is a site-specific expense, that needs to be labeled as such. QuickBooks, a common small business accounting software, allows for tracking of these types of expenses using the label *classes*. Each site is set up as its own class of expense and, at the end of the month, the owner can run a Profit and Loss by Class report that will break those expenses out by the location. Revenue can be tracked this way

Chapter 9 / Monitoring and Measuring

217

BOX 9.9 • Salary Distribution

As a service business, it's important for practice owners to understand that a part of the salary of an employee will be shared between locations and that it is not always so simple to allocate this particular expense. Since salary is typically tracked outside of the EMR, and outside of the business accounting software, it is not easily included in the Profit and Loss by Location Report or the POS Summary. Payroll companies will allow a practice to allocate staff by location, so it is not hard to run reports that break out who is working where and how much they (cost) when an employee works only in one office. These Payroll by Location reports can easily allow the practice owner to split salary up by site. When employees are shared between practices, an additional report can be generated that adds back the salary cost of employees who are dedicated to specific sites.

When a company decides to task an employee to more than one site, it needs to track the hours that the employee spends in each place and add back the cost of the employee to one location, subtracting it from another. If the shared employee is a provider, the company has the choice of using a productivity metric (such as visits the PT provided at each site) to create a prorated percentage they can use to allocate that provider's cost, or hours spent at each site. Tracking by productivity is typically necessary because many physical therapists are salaried employees and will not be punching a clock at each facility when they work. Administrators, billing staff, and support staff that lend benefit to more than one office, even though they may be physically present in only one office, typically lend more time to busier offices, and, as such, lend more benefit to those operations. Distributing their cost can also be divided up using the prorated visit total for each office.

Example: A billing administrator costs $30,000/year and works for all three offices in a 300 visit/month practice. Office 1 bills 150 visits a month (50%), Office 2 bills 100 visits (33%), and Office 3 bills 50 visits per month (17%). When allocating the $30,000, Office 1 will allocate $15,000 (50%) to their cost, Office 2 will allocate $10,000 (33%), and Office 3 will allocate $5,000 (17%) to their individual expense profiles on the Site-specific Profit and Loss. Since the salary component of the profit and loss report is tracked through the practice's payroll provider as a whole number, simply splitting the payroll cost across the three clinics is not accurate. For this employee, if salary is evenly divided as a shared expense between the three clinics, the $5,000 extra that the busiest clinic demands needs to be added back into their expense report in the site-specific P&L and subtracted from the expense list of the smallest clinic.

as well. Creating the Payment by Location report from the EMR allows the practice owner to input the revenue into QuickBooks by class.

Now that the practice owner has income and expenses tracked by location in the accounting software, a Profit and Loss by Location report can be generated that will give the bottom line on how each site is performing, financially.

Place of Service Summary

Count of new patients, visits, revenue, and timed units for each location
Metric timing: Weekly
Metric scope: Immediate

A Place of Service Summary tracks all the KPIs by location. New Patients, Visits, Revenue, and Timed Units reports can all be broken out by the facility that billed for them. The Place of Service Summary can be used to identify trends, activity levels, and needs of each site, allowing for a better allocation and utilization of the practice's resources. This type of weekly

Monitoring the Market

The practice of PT in the health care market requires the practice owner not only to understand their business but also to be able to monitor and understand what is happening in the local and national markets of health care.[13] This skill allows the practice owner to strategically plan and position the practice to react or comply with changes in the health care market, proactively instead of reactively, optimizing the potential for success. Just as the owner monitors the KPI of the practice, annually reviewing data on the local market through environmental scanning activities[14] (see Chapter 1) or through reports from national agencies, such as the American Hospital Association's Annual Environmental Scan Report[15] or the Federation of State Boards of Physical Therapy Practice Analysis reports,[16] provides the owner with a general understanding of what is happening in the health care market.

Summary: Putting It All Together—How Often to Review Your Metrics. . .and What to Do About Them

All the data and metrics in the world are worthless in the hands of someone who never looks at them and/or who never makes decisions based on the data. This chapter has presented a variety of measurables and KPIs that practice owners *could* use to help them run their business. Monitoring all of these metrics all the time while balancing the wealth of other challenges of running a successful practice, and life outside of work, is not a reasonable place to start. Begin by developing a scorecard of KPIs that are most important to the practice owner to monitor weekly. Keep it simple at first. One example would be to collect metric information on New Patients, Visits, and Arrival Rate. Develop a spreadsheet that can contain the data for the month, quarter, and year.

The most important step when it comes to measuring and monitoring the practice is being intentional with the only nonrenewable resource: *The Owner's Time*. Make the decision today to set aside some time on the calendar to evaluate the measurables of the practice. Setting aside a little time every week to review the previous week's data and responding immediately to negative trends is a must. Earmark a larger block, once a month, to monitor whether the practice is on track to meet the established goals. Devote a half-day at the end of each quarter, and at least a full day after the close of the previous year, to form more broad assumptions and strategize for the future. Taking this time and reviewing metrics with the leadership team is time well spent and can give the practice owner insight that cannot be gained by only treating patients and running the day-to-day operations of a practice. The rest of the time during those days can be spent planning ways to improve bad metrics, addressing shortcomings, or risks, of the practice, and building on good numbers to leverage existing success and facilitate healthy growth.

REFERENCES

1. Parmenter D. *Key Performance Indicators (KPI): Developing, Implementing, and Using Winning KPIs*. Wiley; 2010.
2. Seiverd N. Collectability scoring. A unique approach to benchmarking. *Credit Research Foundation*. Published 2019. Accessed April 27, 2023. https://www.crfonline.org/wp-content/uploads/2019/07/CCAofA-Collectability-Scoring-A-Unique-Approach-to-Benchmarking-2Q2019-News.pdf
3. American Physical Therapy Association. Peer2Peer Networks. APTA Private Practice section. Accessed March 18, 2023. https://ppsapta.org/events/peer-2-peer/2023/

Chapter 9 / Monitoring and Measuring

4. Gerber M. *The E-Myth Revisited: Why Most Small Businesses Don't Work and What to Do About It*. Harper Collins; 2009.

5. Gier J. Missed appointments cost the U.S. healthcare system $150B each year. The Free Library. Published 2017. Accessed January 14, 2023. https://www.thefreelibrary.com/MissedappointmentscosttheU.S.healthcare system$150Beach year.-a0512289035

6. Stobierski T. Cash flow vs profit: what's the difference? Harvard Business Review Online. Published 2022. Accessed January 14, 2023. https://online.hbs.edu/blog/post/cash-flow-vs-profit#:~:text=The%20key%20difference%20between%20cash,and%20out%20of%20a%20business

7. United States Census Bureau. Accessed March 18, 2023. https://www.census.gov/en.html

8. Missouri Census Data Center. University of Missouri Center for Health Policy. Accessed March 18, 2023. http://mcdc.missouri.edu

9. American Physical Therapy Association. Outpatient therapy Medicare physician fee schedule calculator. Published 2023. Accessed March 20, 2023. https://www.apta.org/your-practice/payment/medicare-payment/coding-billing/mppr/mppr-calculator/fee-schedule-calculating-resource/mppr-calculator-instructions

10. Silva M. Predictors of retention in physical therapy: client-, disease, and treatment-related factors. Marquette University, Clement J. Zablocki Veterans Administration Medical Center. ePublication. Published 2010. Accessed March 20, 2023. https://epublications.marquette.edu/cgi/viewcontent.cgi?article=1013&context=researchexchange

11. Brooks LL, Owen R. *Answering the Ultimate Question: How Net Promoter Can Transform Your Business*. Wiley; 2009.

12. Reichheld F. *The Ultimate Question: Driving Good Profits and True Growth*. Findaway World Llc; 2007.

13. Schafer DS, Lopopolo RB, Luedtke-Hoffmann KA. Administration and management skills needed by physical therapist graduates in 2010: a national survey. *Phys Ther*. 2007;87(3):261-281. doi:10.2522/ptj.20060003

14. Schafer DS. Environmental-scanning behavior among private practice physical therapy firms. *Phys Ther*. 1991;71(6):482-490. doi:10.1093/ptj/71.6.482

15. American Hospital Association. Environmental scan. Accessed April 3, 2023. https://www.aha.org/environmentalscan

16. Federation of State Boards of Physical Therapy. Analysis of practice for the physical therapy profession: report memo 2020. FSBPT. Accessed April 3, 2023. https://www.fsbpt.org/Portals/0/documents/free-resources/PracticeAnalysis2020Memo.pdf

CHAPTER 10

Risk Management

MARK DRNACH

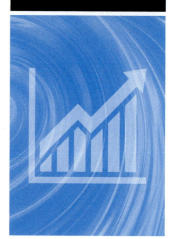

Learning Objectives

The reader will

1. Distinguish between a business risk versus an uncertainty.
2. Identify the various types of risk associated with the business of physical therapy.
3. Choose and explain the various options of dealing with an identified risk.
4. Recognize the basic options in risk management to protect a practice from experiencing a significant negative event.
5. Show how risk management is a part of quality improvement efforts of a practice.

Risk can be defined as the probability of a negative outcome or loss from an action taken. This negative outcome is often described in terms of finance (financial risk) or health (health risk) from a particular investment or behavior decision. Risk relates to a quantifiable probability of an occurrence. For example, it is known from research that there is a 30% chance of a negative health outcome associated with a certain behavior. This can be determined from research studies on a certain population where the behavior under investigation is present to some degree. A statistical probability can be calculated and provide some level of known risk associated with a decision or action. Conversely, uncertainty cannot be quantified, and the probability of its occurrence is estimated or subjectively assigned based on a belief.[1] What will patients want in the next 5 years? What will be the financial state of the local economy in the next decade? Statistical analysis of these questions, at best, uses historical data, which still leaves a certain amount of uncertainty about the future. The beliefs of economists, or other relevant experts in a particular field of study, may help with the decision-making process by offering some level of confidence in the decision, based on their opinions. Understanding risk includes understanding uncertainty.

Risk literacy is the ability to understand and evaluate risks and uncertainties and then use that knowledge to make appropriate decisions.[1] It is an important component of financial literacy (see Chapter 12) and in the management of a business or practice.[2] In health care, the management of risk is necessary to protect the employees and the financial aspect of the practice and to ensure the safe delivery of services that produce optimal outcomes of the patients served, exposing them to minimal risk. By investing in risk management, a practice is allocating a percentage of its current revenues for a future reward: sustainability. There is a belief that the greater the risk taken, the greater the reward. This principle is called the risk/reward trade-off.[3] However, risk and reward are not always proportional. In reality, it is the trade-off between the assumed risk and the *potential* reward. A physical therapist (PT) or practice owner has to identify and understand the risks associated with the practice of physical therapy, either as a proprietor or as an employee and the potential reward for undertaking those risks. The PT should be aware of the uncertainties in the health care market and understand their acceptable level of risk exposure associated with the decisions, actions, and organizational behaviors undertaken, in order to effectively manage the risks.

Identifying Risk

The first step in the process of risk management is the identification of risks associated with the practice or business (Figure 10.1). By identifying risks, a practice owner becomes aware of the potential sources of problems that may affect the practice's operations and/or reputation. These areas of risk are not limited to patient care but encompass all aspects of the business, from the administration to the contracted services retained to support operations. They can come from internal or external sources. The areas of risk can be grouped into three broad categories: Regulations, Revenues, and Reputation.

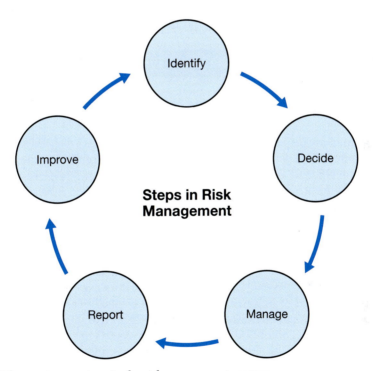

Figure 10.1 The continuous steps in the risk management process.

> **risk** – the probability of a negative outcome or loss from an action taken
>
> **uncertainty** – the probability of an event occurring that cannot be quantified and its' occurrence is estimated or subjectively assigned based on a belief
>
> **risk literacy** – the ability to understand and evaluate risks and uncertainties, and then use that knowledge to make appropriate decisions
>
> **risk/reward trade-off** – a belief that the greater the risk taken the greater the reward

Regulations

Several federal and state laws impact the structure and delivery of health care in the United States. The practice of physical therapy is defined and influenced by a number of specific federal and state laws, or statutes, that are drafted and adopted by legislative bodies and further defined and detailed in regulations created by administrative agencies to help implement the statutes (Box 10.1). These regulations establish a set of norms or standards to benchmark quality and then assess the extent to which a business meets these standards. Failure to comply with regulations may lead to sanctions such as intensified surveillance, or even revocation of license to operate (typically through a registration or licensing system).[4] Some examples can be found in the federal Medicare program that provides detailed regulations controlling the delivery and payment of services provided to Medicare beneficiaries; the requirement of informed consent and professional malpractice liability that arise from state-specific statutes and common law (ie, laws developed through court opinions); and various employment laws that influence employment arrangements or business formation requirements[5] (see Chapter 5). There are many rules and regulations that impact the delivery of health care depending on the state where the service is delivered, the type of service, and the guidelines of the payer of the service. These regulations typically address aspects of health care such as standards of practice, safety, infection control, documentation requirements, staffing levels, and the trainings of the employees[4] (Box 10.2).

BOX 10.1 • Basic Structure of the Legal System

The US Constitution is at the heart of the American legal system. All laws and legal processes must be consistent with the Constitution. Although any court can determine whether a law is constitutional, the final say on these issues rests with the US Supreme Court. The US Congress creates federal statutes such as the Social Security Act, which established the Medicare and Medicaid programs, and the Americans with Disabilities Act, which protects the rights of Americans with disabilities. These statutes can be found in the United States Code, which is a collection of all federal statutes. Often these statutes require complex rules and regulations to clarify how they apply to various situations. For instance, the Center for Medicare and Medicaid Services (CMS) is a federal agency that drafts and enforces specific rules and regulations regarding the Medicare and Medicaid programs. The process of creating (or promulgating) and enforcing these rules and regulations makes up an area called administrative law.

Each state also has its own court system, including a state supreme court, which interprets state law. For instance, most medical malpractice (professional negligence) laws are state-specific laws, developed over time by state court decisions. This is the process of common law. Just as on the federal level, individual state legislatures are responsible for creating statutory law. Each state has some form of statute, sometimes referred to as an Act, which oversees the practice of physical therapy in the state, requires a license to practice, and defines what the practice of physical therapy is in that particular state. These statutes create and empower a state agency, commonly a state board of physical therapy, to create and enforce more specific rules and regulations such as the licensing process for applicants.

Reprinted with permission from Warren B. Legal issues. In: Drnach M, ed. *The Clinical Practice of Pediatric Physical Therapy: From the NICU to Independent Living.* Wolters Kluwer Health/Lippincott Williams and Wilkins; 2008:330-338.

---

statutes – specific federal and state laws that are drafted and adopted by legislative bodies

regulations – a detailed description and requirements of a statute

common law – laws developed through court opinion

Chapter 10 / Risk Management

BOX 10.2 • Common Laws and Regulations

Health Care

Anti-Kickback and Stark Laws
Fraud and Abuse Laws
Health Insurance Portability and Accountability Act (HIPAA)
Patient Protection and Affordability Act (ACA)
Physical Therapy Practice Act
Social Security Act (for Medicare and Medicaid)
Worker Compensation Laws

Employment

Americans with Disabilities Act (ADA)
Civil Rights Act
Fair Labor Standards Act (FLSA)
Family Medical Leave Act (FMLA)
Occupational Safety and Health Act (OSHA)

A practice owner should take the time to identify the regulatory requirements for participation in a business, understand the purpose and structure of the regulations, create policies and procedures for the business that support those regulations, and have a system of employee education, system monitoring, and reporting compliance. This critical and intentional action will keep the requirements of the laws or regulations in the forefront of operations, thereby providing a structure for the practice owner to make better decisions, provide expected services, and minimize risk. There are resources available to assist in this process of identification, including federal government programs (eg, Centers for Medicare and Medicaid Services, US Department of Labor, US Small Business Administration), the American Physical Therapy Association (APTA), and the State Boards of Physical Therapy (Box 10.3). The internet also provides access to information on states' statutes, regulations, and, occasionally, summaries. Because of the risk associated with violating a law or a regulation, the practice owner should access credible resources to understand the legal issues and influences involved in the business and delivery of health care services. This can be a daunting task when starting a business. Consultation with an experienced attorney is an

BOX 10.3 • APTA Versus the Board of Physical Therapy

The board or agency controlling the practice of physical therapy in a state should not be confused with the state chapter of the American Physical Therapy Association (APTA). The APTA is a national professional organization that promotes and protects the profession of physical therapy. Individual state chapters of the APTA serve that purpose on the state level. The APTA has a Code of Ethics and Guide for Professional Conduct that all APTA members are to follow. A violation of these professional guidelines is reported to, and handled by, that state's APTA chapter. The APTA may, in response, take action against the individual's APTA membership status. In contrast, a state physical therapy board exists to protect the public and handles any violation of the state practice act and its regulations. The physical therapy board may, when appropriate, take action against the individual's license to practice physical therapy in that state.

Reprinted with permission from Warren B. Legal issues. In: Drnach M, ed. *The Clinical Practice of Pediatric Physical Therapy: From the NICU to Independent Living.* Wolters Kluwer Health/Lippincott Williams and Wilkins; 2008:330-338.

efficient means of meeting this need. Although the cost of having a question answered by an attorney may seem prohibitive, it is often far less costly than the ramifications of acting without understanding the laws and regulations that impact the practice.

Revenues

The identification and management of revenues and expenses is vital to the efficient operations of a practice. Identifying the revenues and expenses and knowing that the revenues can cover the expenses in a pay period is an important management behavior for a successful practice (see Chapter 2). Conceptualizing how the practice will be structured and the roles and responsibilities of the different jobs within the organizational structure (ie, organizational chart) will provide information to better understand how the revenues generated will support the services provided, as well as the administrative structure needed to support the safe and efficient delivery of those services. Clear written policies and procedures on gathering and reporting on the financial status of the practice through key financial reports, including the Balance Sheet, Income Statement (ie, Profit Loss Statement), Cash Flow Statement, Retained Earnings Statement, Fee Schedule, Payer Mix Report (ie, number of active patients per payer), and efficiency ratios (eg, days receivable), are fundamental in the management of revenues and expenses (see Chapter 2). The process of billing the payer of service and collecting the fees for the services delivered is also necessary to ensure timely and efficient communication and expectations between the provider and the payer. These processes may vary depending on the guidelines of a specific payer. A practice owner may hire a certified public accountant (CPA) to help with setting up the financial structure and then to periodically examine the practice's financial statements to ensure compliance with acceptable accounting practices and various US taxation and reporting requirements. These responsibilities are often internally assigned to a specific employee of the practice designated as the treasurer, controller, chief financial officer (CFO), or chief operating officer (COO). This structure has a specific position that is responsible for addressing the risk of inefficiencies in the financial aspect of the practice, helping to minimize waste, ensuing the proper allocation of revenues and expenses, and protecting the practice from fraud or embezzlement of funds.

The documentation of the services provided and the justification for payment must also be clearly described and understood by the providers. The use of an electronic medical record (EMR), specific codes for the services provided (eg, CPT, HCPCS), and other necessary documentation to comply with the payers' guidelines helps to minimize the risk of disruptions in cash flow or the recoupment of revenues from services provided (see Chapter 8). The use of an EMR and other digital devices exposes the practice to the risk of cyber threats and data breaches that could jeopardize confidential information or the efficient management of services (eg, computer crash or virus infection that shuts down the system for an extended period of time). Becoming aware of these areas of risk will allow the practice owner to better oversee and manage the systems that are vital to the creation and recruitment of revenues for the practice. In addition, the risk inherent in the market resulting from changes in the political or economic environment exposes the practice to certain risks or levels of uncertainty. Identifying these risks, through government reports, networking with local businesses and professionals, or environmental scans, can keep the practice owner generally knowledgeable of the potential risks and uncertainties in the near future in order to plan for such changes if they happen to occur.

Reputation

The reputation of the practice in the market is probably the most valuable asset of the practice. This reputation is created and supported by the image of the practice as perceived by the customers or patients, the referral sources, and other people who do business with

Chapter 10 / Risk Management

BOX 10.4 • Examples of Areas of Risk

Regulations

Violation of the State Practice Act
Failure to report suspected abuse or neglect
Breach of patient confidentiality
Committing professional malpractice

Revenues

Lack of adherence to third-party payer guidelines for payment
Committing fraud in billing practice
Misuse of codes for procedures
Underestimating costs

Reputation

Failure to obtain informed consent
Incompetent employees
Obvious structural damage to the clinic or equipment
Errors in written communication to stakeholders

the practice. Creating an image, or brand, that reflects the value of the services to those stakeholders is vital to the sustainability of the practice (see Chapters 6 and 7). This reputation is reflected in many aspects of the practice, including the physical plant, the visual organization and image of the clinical setting, the staff, the equipment that is utilized in the delivery of care, and in the communication with stakeholders. Having periodic training programs to provide education that reinforces the practice's expectations, supports the personal responsibility of the practice's reputation, as well as routine maintenance and upkeep of the physical plant and equipment are basic ways to help decrease the exposure to risks (Box 10.4). But even the most professional-looking clinic will not stay in business if the services that are provided are not of value to the patient. Maintaining the competency of the staff training through continuing education, both external and internal to the practice, providing support for credentialing and certification programs, and an explicit system to produce value-based outcomes, add greatly to the reputation of a practice.

Risk Options

Managing risk is managing variability of current operations in order to minimize the risk of future loss (eg, license to practice, finances, or reputation). After the identification of the risks associated with a practice, the practice owner then has to make a decision on what to do with that risk (see Figure 10.1). The owner could avoid the risk, accept the risk, mitigate the risk, or transfer the risk.[6]

Avoid Risk

The first option is to avoid the risk altogether. A practice can reduce its risk by avoiding certain high-risk activities (ie, not taking the risk). It may not participate with a certain third-party payer if the reimbursement and volume are not sufficient to cover costs and avoid a financial risk. It may not hire certain individuals who do not meet the standards of the company or who lack the necessary skills to provide the level of services desired, in order to avoid the risk of damaging the practice's reputation. It may choose not to offer certain interventions owing to the risk or cost associated with the safe delivery of the intervention, thus avoiding the risk of malpractice or financial loss. The practice owner may choose not to expand the practice into other markets, avoiding the financial risks associated with the cost of the physical plant, recruitment and training new staff, and the regulatory risk associated with monitoring and complying with local or state laws in the new area. The practice may choose not to take on any additional risks owning to its current limited ability to manage the risk already taken. In any of these scenarios, the owner has the option of declining to take the risk. Although risk avoidance may seem like a safe decision to make, the practice may lose the potential gain or benefit that could be achieved by accepting the risk.

Accept Risk

In health care, there is a certain level of risk inherent in the practice of physical therapy. The risks associated with PT often include the risk of harming the patient in the delivery of services, the risk of not being able to meet the financial targets of the private practice, or the risk of failing to meet the expectations of an employer. These risks should be identified and evaluated against the benefit of the action toward the desired outcome. When the benefits outweigh the risks, the PT may be more comfortable with accepting the risk. Accepting a risk is often associated with accepting a set of standards or expectations established by a governing body that provides the consumer or public with a level of trust and expected quality in the product or service provided. This quality and trust are reflected in the license to practice or in the certifications held and maintained by the provider. Whenever people, in their professional or personal lives, are presented with a choice of actions to take, the risk/reward trade-off is a common factor in the decision-making process. The reward is often the motivator, especially when the risk can be mitigated or transferred.

Mitigating Risk

Accepted risks can be mitigated by adopting policies and procedures that clearly outlined the expectations and behaviors required by the PT or employees in the day-to-day operations of the practice (Box 10.5). The creation of such policies begins with the mission statement of the practice and the organizational structure adopted to meet that mission. Mitigating risk is taking actions to prevent the risky event from occurring. This is best achieved through written, clear expectations of the employee, and routine discussions and education on the policies and procedures of the practice. Mitigating risk is not just creating policies but ensuring that the employees embrace the spirit of the policies in their day-to-day interactions with patients. It is important to monitor and report on the compliance with the adherence to policies and procedures and to take any necessary corrective actions to ensure that there is uniformity and consistency in the way the services are delivered and the practice's image, and brand, are communicated.

Transfer Risk

Another option in managing risk is to transfer the risk by purchasing insurance or outsourcing the organizational function. By purchasing insurance, the practice transfers the

> mitigating risk – taking action to prevent a risky event from occurring

Chapter 10 / Risk Management

BOX 10.5 • Basic Policies for a Business

Hiring
Probationary/Training Period
Employee Code of Conduct
Dress Code
Confidentiality
Antidiscrimination
Antiharassment
Hours of Operation
Employee Attendance
Regular and Overtime Pay
Performance Appraisal
Paid Days Off
Family and Medical Leave
Infection Control
Remote Work
Social Media
Drug and Alcohol
Firearm Regulation and Gun Control
Workplace Accommodations
Disciplinary Action
Termination

financial risk associated with an event occurring, which significantly impacts the operations of the practice, to a third-party, the insurance company. The structure is similar to the risk pooling and health insurance purchased by people for their individual needs (see Chapter 4). Common insurances in health care include malpractice insurance, which can be purchased for a business as well as an individual. Malpractice insurance protects the revenues of a practice, or a person, in the event of an adverse reaction or outcome from the care provided, which caused significant harm to the patient. Other types of insurance can protect the finances of the practice against damages to the company's property, financial loss resulting from employee negligence, unexpected medical expenses, or structural damage caused by a severe weather event (Box 10.6). The federal government also requires businesses to have workers' compensation, unemployment, and disability insurance. By having insurance, the practice transfers the financial risk to the insurance company.

The practice can also use outsourcing, or contracting services to perform specific operations for the practice. These can include the job duties associated with Human Resources, payroll, billing and collecting, and, more commonly, information technology. Outsourcing seems like a viable option in health care because the health care provider's main competency is in the diagnoses and treatments of a health condition. By outsourcing nonclinical functions, the PT has more time to provide revenue generating services. But outsourcing comes with risks. The practice is still accountable for the services provided by the subcontractor. Substandard expectations and quality, or a negative experience by a patient or employee, will have a negative impact on the practice's image and brand. Also, the control of data is transferred to the subcontractor who is responsible for data and cybersecurity, which can have a significant impact on the practice if breached.

outsourcing – contracting services to perform specific operations for the practice

BOX 10.6 • Common Insurances for a Small Business

General Liability. Protects against financial loss as the result of bodily injury, property damage, medical expenses, libel, slander, and defending lawsuits.

Professional Liability. Protects against financial loss as a result of malpractice, errors, and negligence.

Commercial Property. Protects against loss and damage of company property resulting from a wide variety of events such as fire, smoke, severe weather events, and vandalism.

The federal government requires every business with employees to have workers' compensation, unemployment, and disability insurance.

Laws requiring insurance vary by state, so visit the state's website to find out the requirements in the state where the practice is located.

US Small Business Administration. Get business insurance. Updated May 19, 2023. Accessed December 16, 2023. https://www.sba.gov/business-guide/launch-your-business/get-business-insurance#id-six-common-types-of-business-insurance

Risk Management

Risk management is a specific activity that entails identifying risks, creating strategies to protect the practice from risks, and identifying areas for improvement in operations to lessen the occurrence of certain identified risks[7] (see Figure 10.1). It is advisable for a health care professional or practice owner to seek the advice of other professionals who can provide information and guidance in the management of specific areas of risk (Box 10.7). This may provide a practice owner with a sense of certainty that the practice is somewhat protected from the negative outcome of an identified risk occurrence. The goal of risk management is to sustain the practice in a changing and uncertain health care environment, by proactively suggesting actions that minimize the practice's exposure to risks and uncertainties. In order to do so effectively, risk management has to take into consideration internal and external factors, as well as the practice's mission, goals, organizational structure, governing standards, procedures, and employee competence to ensure that the practice remains competitive and sustainable.[8] By definition, it is a participatory form of management that requires a structure that engages with a variety of stakeholders who provide useful risk judgments and perspectives that aid in proper risk management decisions.[1] These decisions deal mainly with two key areas: protection and quality improvement.

Protection

Protection against a significant negative event occurring in any business should be reflected in the organizational structure where the specific responsibilities, supervision, and reporting channels are clearly designated and the job duties relating to risk management are listed in the job descriptions. This structure gives the employees a clear idea of their specific roles and duties related to protecting the practice's brand, business, patients, and coworkers in delivering care and meeting the mission of the practice. From the financial perspective, adequate funding and time are necessary in order to educate the staff, monitor

BOX 10.7 • Key Consultants

Attorney (specializing in employment or contract law)
Certified Public Accountant
Human Resources Management Company
Information Technology Consultant

Chapter 10 / Risk Management

BOX 10.8 • Developing Policies[1]

1. Establish an organizational structure
2. Decide on recruitment and onboarding processes
3. Determine the pay and benefit package for each role
4. Establish employee retention programs
5. Prepare for audits

Betterton K. 5 steps for developing human resource policies for your start up. U.S. Chamber of Commerce. Published July 12, 2022. Accessed December 16, 2023. https://www.uschamber.com/co/run/human-resources/startup-hr-policies?cid=search

and attain reliable information associated with the identified risk, and to report and communicate information that fosters participatory management, and shared responsibility, in promoting a safe and effective work environment. Clear policies and corresponding procedures should communicate the expected behaviors to achieve the practice's goals while minimizing the risk of unlawful behaviors, loss of revenue, or jeopardizing the practice's reputation. Establishing clear policies and procedures to address risk management is only one part of the risk management process (Box 10.8). Educating, training, and monitoring compliance with the policies and procedures is the other part.

Hiring and Compliance

The first step in providing value-based, quality care is having the right employees. This begins with the hiring process (see Chapter 6). There is a risk of hiring the wrong type of person for the practice. Having a clear job description, with clear expectations of the person performing the job, and following a structured interview process, allows for a more objective and fair evaluation of the potential employee. This will help minimize the risk of accusations of discrimination or unfair hiring practices when the process is uniform and consistent with the identified qualifications and expectations of the position, compared to those of the potential employee (ie, interviewee). Once hired, the new employee will also require training and education to understand the specific policies and procedures related to the job. These are listed in an employee handbook and a policy and procedure manual for the department or clinical setting. It is important that the new employee be given adequate time to review the handbook and policy manual and document that this was done by signing a form stating that the documents have been read and understood and that the new employee will abide by those policies and procedures. This should be done at least annually or when a new policy is adopted to ensure that the employees have an understanding of the policies, procedures, and expectations of the practice.

It is appropriate to provide the new employee with a period of time in which they can assimilate into the operations of the practice. This is typically termed a probationary period: a period of time (typically in months) that is designated to the orientation and education of a new employee. This should involve a reduction in productivity expectations to allow the new employee time to learn about the operations and procedures of the job, complete any training activities associated with the delivery of health care, and acquaint themselves with the day-to-day operations of the practice. It also shows the importance of the policies and

probationary period – a period of time that is designated to the orientation and education of a new employee

procedures in supporting the uniform and efficient delivery of health care by the practice. This is done to educate the new employee and to clarify the expectations of the job.

The act of advertising, recruiting, interviewing, and orienting a new employee is a significant investment of time and money. The new employee is a valuable asset and should be viewed as such. Ongoing supervision and communication with the employee are important to ensure compliance with the expectations of the job and to decrease the risk of unlawful, unethical, or unproductive behaviors. It should not be assumed that merely by being hired, an employee would be proficient in complying with the practice's policies and procedures. Ongoing interactions, training, feedback, and recognition are important aspects of a workplace culture. The supervising employee should intentionally support and assist the new employee in becoming an active and valuable member of the team. Establishing and reinforcing expected behaviors is important in the assimilation of the new employee into the workplace culture. The supervisor should consistently follow a sequence of interactions when addressing any action by the new employee that is inconsistent with the expected performance. These steps include the following:

1. Talking to the employee in private about the identified behavior and the relevant policies and procedures pertaining to the correct or expected behavior.
2. If the behavior reoccurs, then a written corrective action plan that addresses the behavior and the expected behavior is provided along with support to correct the undesired behavior (Box 10.9).
3. If the behavior continues, then suspension or a leave of absence from the job may be warranted, with a written plan to correct the behavior and evidence of understanding (eg, certificate of completion, letter of support from the educator) before returning to work.
4. If the behavior cannot conform with the expectations of the practice, then termination is warranted.

This sequence, provided consistently, will help nurture the new employee and protect the practice's investment. It also communicates to all employees the value the practice owner places on the delivery of services by the practice. To decrease the risk of violating a regulatory standard or legal requirement; ensure that proper coding, billing, and collections are run efficiently; provide value-based care; and become a respected and integral participant in the local health care community, the practice owner must promote a workplace culture of competence, understanding, and compliance.

Employees are one of the largest investments of a practice. Allocating the appropriate resources in terms of both money and time to maintain the employer-employee relationship is important in the overall management of the practice. The risk that an employee

---

BOX 10.9 • Components of a Corrective Action Plan

1. The supervisor accurately identifies the discrepancy between performance and expectations.
2. The supervisor discusses with the employee the importance of the expectations.
3. The employee should agree that the discrepancy exists.
4. The supervisor and employee work collaboratively to develop a strategy for performance improvement.
5. The supervisor and employee agree on deadlines for improvement.
6. Clear consequences for the lack of improvement must be identified.
7. The supervisor must provide ongoing feedback, especially as improvement occurs.

Adapted from Nosse LJ, Friberg DG, Kovacek PB, eds. *Management and Supervisory Principles for Physical Therapists.* 2nd ed. Lippincott Williams and Wilkins; 2005:259.

Chapter 10 / Risk Management

will leave to set up a practice, and become a competitor, is often addressed through a non-compete clause in the employment contract. Simply stated, a noncompete clause restricts the employee from leaving the employer and starting a practice in competition with the employer. This is typically limited by geographic area or the passage of a specified amount of time before the former employee can practice in the local area. The enforceability of this type of contract clause is questionable and governed by the state where the practice is located. Enforcement varies nationally. A practice owner should consult with an attorney who specializes in employment or contract law to understand how the law applies in the state. The risk of losing a valuable employee is also addressed by creating a workplace culture that supports and motivates the employee to grow professionally and engage in the operational success of the practice. This can be achieved by providing a competitive salary and benefits, flexible work hours, and support for professional development. A practice with a bank of employees who work PRN will have more flexibility in scheduling and avoid the risk of a loss in revenues when full-time staff are absent because they are ill, on vacation, or attending an educational conference. This can also lessen the stress in the work environment when a direct care provider is absent. Additional low-cost benefits are helpful, (eg, employee of the month recognition, designated parking place, free coffee) but the attitude and respect given to all employees is a strong factor in creating a workplace culture where employees can identify with the mission and purpose of the practice and have a personal investment and desire to stay.

Safety in Operations

The safe and efficient delivery of health care services is another major area of risk. Health care decisions and interventions, by their nature, inherently contain some level of risk. Those risks should be identified and addressed in order to *do no harm* to the people who seek services from the practice.

The scheduled maintenance of the physical building and grounds should be established, funded, and followed to maintain a level of safety in utilizing the clinic site. Deferred maintenance, the act of deferring funding of basic maintenance activities on property and equipment in order to save on costs, can put the practice at an increased risk for patient or worker injury if the physical plant or equipment fails and causes harm to a person. Also, the lack of access to the physical plant caused by closure for needed repairs, or the absence of a piece of equipment used in the delivery of care, including computers, will also impact revenues and cash flow. Equipment used in the delivery of care, such as electrical stimulation units, mechanical traction tables, or supportive positioning devices, should routinely be checked and calibrated to ensure the safe and effective use of the device. Labels are commonly placed on these devices with the date of the last mechanical evaluation or unit calibration.

The behavior and competency of the employees is also an area of risk. Creating a workplace culture that fosters participatory management and collaboration allows for oversight of clinical practice and the fostering of behaviors that lead to the safe delivery of interventions, valued outcomes, and exceptional practice. The aspects of the execution of an intervention that place a patient or employee at risk should be identified and competency tested periodically. These practices generally include areas such as infection control, assisting

noncompete clause – a clause in an employment contract that restricts the employee from leaving the employer and starting a practice in competition with the employer

deferred maintenance – deferring funding of basic maintenance activities on property and equipment in order to save on costs

with patient transfers, and providing various levels of assistance with patient ambulation. In addition to the physical risk associated with these practices, the risk associated with the personal behaviors of the staff should also be identified and addressed with periodic training and education programs. These behavioral areas include topics such as harassment, discrimination, or the use of noninclusive or disrespectful language. At a minimum, annual training in these areas can help to minimize the risk of their occurrence.

It should be expected that an incident or adverse event will occur in the course of providing services. An incident is a deviation from the usual care that poses a risk of harm to the patient. An adverse event, or accident, is an incident that results in the preventable harm to a patient.[9] When either of these happens, the event should be seen not as an opportunity for punitive action but rather as a learning opportunity on how the practice responds to such events and how the consistent and efficient delivery of safe and effective services can be improved in the future. Employees should see the value of reporting inconsistencies with the delivery or outcome of services, in order to promote quality and improvement. When an unplanned event or incident occurs, there should be a reporting mechanism, documented either on paper or electronically, that captures the basic elements of the event.[10] According to the World Health Organization, there are three required elements of an incident report: description, explanation, and remedial measures[9]:

1. Description of what happened, including patient characteristics, detailed description of the incident, and location.
2. Explanation of why it happened, including perceived cause, contributing factors, and mitigating factors.
3. Remedial measures or actions that were taken as a result of the incident, including patient care, redesign process, review of the relevant policy and procedure, retraining and education of staff, or organizational changes.

The value of identifying the risk and harm associated with an event, collecting data, and evaluating the information is the starting point in the investigation into causation and prevention that promotes a workplace culture of safety, responsibility, and care. This process helps reduce the risk of future events that can have a significantly negative impact on the operations of the practice.

Protecting Information

Health and financial information are among the most sensitive areas of information that a person possesses. Creating policies and procedures that protect the security and confidentiality of the patient's personal and protected health information (PHI), stored either electronically or physically (ie, on paper), is critical for compliance with the Health Information Portability and Accountability Act (HIPAA) and to protect the practice from regulatory and reputational risks.

In addition to the advice from an information technology consultant, the Office of the National Coordinator for Health Information Technology (ONC) developed a downloadable security risk assessment (SRA) tool to help health care providers of small- to medium-size businesses conduct a security risk assessment, as required by the HIPAA Security Rule.[11] (The HIPAA Privacy and Security Rules protect the privacy and security of individually identifiable health information.) This type of risk assessment, along with the other areas of risk, should be conducted on a periodic basis in order for the practice

incident – a deviation from the usual care that poses a risk of harm to the patient

adverse event – an incident that results in a preventable harm to a patient

Chapter 10 / Risk Management **233**

owner to stay current and active in protecting the confidential information of the patients served. Employee behavior must also be monitored for breaches in confidentiality and the improper use or access of PHI. Policies on the use of the EMR and the expected behaviors that protect confidential information should be clear and strongly reinforced. Health care providers deal with very personal and private aspects of individuals. Active engagement with a patient requires trust. Breaches in confidentiality, or unauthorized disclosure of PHI, may result in legal actions, a loss of revenue, and a loss of trust, with a negative impact on the practice's reputation. Violations of confidential information can happen at any level of the organization, with any employee, but specific attention should be given to those areas of greatest risk, which include the use of, and access to, network servers, portable electronic devices, written clinical documents, and the practice's email system.[12] Overall, the safety and security of PHI is paramount. A practice owner may create a position of privacy or data protection officer to oversee the privacy practices of the business. These duties and responsibilities can also be delegated to another executive-level position in the organization, such as COO. Data breaches (personal or financial) are a serious threat to a health care practice. They present a risk of financial loss and a threat to patient safety. In view of their high prevalence and negative impact, health care organizations are purchasing cybersecurity insurance as a risk mitigating strategy.[13]

An audit is another way to protect a practice through the organized review of information and data to verify their accuracy and compliance with the requirements established by internal (policies and procedures) or external entities (eg, Internal Revenue Service). Internal audits are typically done by a member or members of the executive team. External audits are typically done by experts in a particular field, such as a CPA or a peer reviewer of clinical practice. Routine audits should be performed to ensure that the practice is complying with current regulations, that the information systems used in the practice meet security and reporting standards, that the quality of care is acceptable and congruent with current practice, and that the financial documents and processes reflect the practice's financial ability to continue into the future (see Chapter 2). Audits should provide information to help the practice identify problems or areas of vulnerability that can be addressed in a timely and organized manner to decrease the risk of an adverse event or situation occurring in the future.

Stress Testing/Situational Analysis

Stress testing or situational analysis is a hypothetical analysis and discussion where one variable (eg, patient visit numbers, reimbursement amounts, health care costs) is changed and the impact on the practice's operations is estimated and discussed. This knowledge can help the practice owner plan for specific adverse events that may happen in the future and know how much of a change in operations can be tolerated and still be able to make a profit and sustain the practice. One method is to use a spreadsheet for a common-sized comparative income statement analysis and project the estimated revenues and expenses for the next 3 years (see Chapter 2). Various scenarios can be postulated, the financial effect can be estimated, and a contingency plan can be discussed if the adverse event does occur. The following are some examples of questions to consider:

audit – an organized review of information and data to verify their accuracy and compliance with the requirements established by internal or external entities

situational analysis – a hypothetical analysis where one variable is changed and the impact on the practice's operations is estimated and discussed

1. What impact would a decrease in revenues by 10% (caused by a decrease in patient visits) have on the profit margin?
2. If Medicare reduces reimbursement by 10%, what impact will that have on gross revenues?
3. If one provider quits, how will the loss of revenue and concurrent expenses (for salary and benefits) impact the bottom line?
4. Which expense account will have to be decreased to make up for a 7% increase in rent account?

A situational analysis should be carried out when deciding on a new venture or practice expansion or if a potential threat is possible in the near future (eg, local economic downturn caused by a manufacturing plant closure, pending governmental legislation that will impact access or reimbursement). Understanding how the practice's finances can withstand a change helps the practice owner make more informed decisions regarding business operations in order to ensure that the practice remains successful in the future.

Integration

Another strategy to protect or sustain a practice is to expand the services that it offers. Horizontal integration is the expansion of a practice into a new geographic area, providing the same services that it is currently offering. This allows a practice to offer its services to more people, thereby increasing revenues, improving efficiencies through economies of scale, and possibly gaining more market share. This can be accomplished by opening a new clinic, acquiring an established clinic, or merging with an established clinic in the area. Vertical integration is the expansion of a practice through service diversification. This can be done with the current customer base or with the addition of a new one. A practice can expand by opening a gym or workout area to offer the public and former patients the opportunity to exercise; by providing pediatric outpatient services, high school athlete strength and conditioning clinics; by obtaining contracts to provide school-based or early intervention services or home care services for the older adults. This type of integration can assist with marketing efforts and foster patient loyalty by providing services in one venue (eg, an outpatient clinic for rehabilitation) and establishing a patient relationship that will lead to the patient accessing the practice's services if needed in a different venue (eg, a strength and conditioning clinic or home care services). This type of integration may lead to lower cost, improve efficiencies through economies of scale, and decrease the practice's reliance on the external payer of services. If a third-party payer lowers the reimbursement for outpatient service, the difference in revenues may be supplemented by fees in other contracts or services that the practice provides.

The concept of horizontal integration can also be applied to an independent contractor or full-time employee who works more than one job. A PT who provides home care services, early intervention services, and school-based services; teaches in higher education as an adjunct faculty member; or provides PRN services can obtain contracts to provide that *same specific service* in an extended geographic region, (eg, teaching an online course in geriatrics at several different universities or providing PRN employment at several different outpatient clinics), thereby horizontally integrating into the market. Vertical integration can be accomplished by providing a *variety of services* to a specific patient population

horizontal integration – when a practice expands into a new geographic area, providing the same services that it is currently offering

vertical integration – the expansion of a practice through service diversification (eg, providing early intervention services in the home *and* PRN PT at the local pediatric hospital *and* teaching a course in pediatrics) (see Chapter 5). Both horizontal and vertical integration by an employee or independent contractor address the risk of a loss of revenue if the employer decides to fire the employee (ie, employment-at-will doctrine, see Chapter 5) or if loss of employment occurs owing to changes in the external market.

Improvement

Risk management is an ongoing process of evaluating the employees' behaviors, the compliance with, and relevance of, the practice's policies and procedures, and the efficiency of the organizational structure, which safely moves a practice toward the achievement of the identified goals and fulfillment of its mission. It is not merely a compliance process to reduce risk but a process that refines the ability to provide efficient and safe services that optimize a patient's health or health outcome. Risk management is a key aspect of the quality improvement initiatives that a practice undertakes to continuously improve its performance (see Figure 10.1). The information gathered through a structured reporting system that includes costs (Chapter 1), financial indicators (Chapter 2), aspects of value-based care (Chapter 3) and value-based outcomes (Chapter 4), productivity data (Chapter 4), and key performance indicators and practice metrics (Chapter 9) should be tracked and shared with the appropriate stakeholders in the practice to educate the employees, reduce risk, and improve operations. Action plans should be created to clearly objectify the actions to be taken to reduce the risk, the responsible party for overseeing the implementation of the actions, and a target date for completion. This type of structure gives a clear direction to the parties responsible for achieving the objective and reducing the risk of a negative outcome for the practice (see Table 7.2 in Chapter 7). Risk management provides various learning opportunities not only to new employees but also to new practice owners that can improve individual knowledge and systems knowledge (ie, how systems work) that could ultimately improve patient care.[14] It is a valuable tool in steering a practice toward success, minimizing the exposure to risks, and growing the practice into an efficient and effective health care provider.

Summary

The PT should be aware of the uncertainties in the health care market and the risks associated with the decisions, actions, and behaviors of practice. This knowledge is necessary to effectively manage the associated risks and decrease the exposure to the inherent risks in health care. Risk is often a barrier to entering into private practice: the risk of loss. By adopting a risk management mindset, a practice can proactively and systematically promote patient and information safety as well as protect the practice's assets, market share, accreditation, reimbursement levels, brand value, and reputation.[15] Hopefully, the contents of this chapter, and other chapters in this book, will help the reader to better identify and manage the risk associated with a private practice. The reward can be great.

REFERENCES

1. Aven, T. Risk literacy: Foundational issues and its connection to risk science. *Risk Anal.* 2023. 00: 1–10. https://doi.org/10.1111/risa.14223
2. Lusardi A. Risk literacy. *Ital Econ J.* 2015. 1:5-23. doi:10.1007/s40797-015-0011-x
3. Markowitz HM. Portfolio selection. *J Finance.* 1952. 7(1):77-91.
4. Dunbar P, Browne JP, O'Connor L. Determinants of regulatory compliance in health and social care services: a systematic review protocol. *HRB Open Res.* 2021;4:13. doi:10.12688/hrbopenres.13214.3
5. Warren B. Legal issues. In: Drnach M, ed. The Clinical Practice of Pediatric Physical Therapy: From the NICU to Independent Living. Lippincott Williams and Wilkins; 2008.

6. Galai D, Robert M, Crouhy M. The Essentials of Risk Management. 3rd Ed. McGraw-Hill Company; 2023.
7. Björnsdóttir SH, Jensson P, de Boer RJ, Thorsteinsson SE. The importance of risk management: what is missing in ISO standards? *Risk Anal*. 2022;42(4):659-691. doi:10.1111/risa.13803
8. Sylwia B. The embedment of risk management in enterprise management system. *Int J Contemp Manag*. 2023;59(2):1-16. doi:10.2478/ijcm-2022-0014
9. World Health Organization. Patient safety incident reporting and learning systems: technical report and guidance. Published September 16, 2020. Accessed December 21, 2023. https://www.who.int/publications/i/item/9789240010338
10. Benin AL, Fodeh SJ, Lee K, Koss M, Miller P, Brandt C. Electronic approaches to making sense of the text in the adverse event reporting system. *J Healthc Risk Manag*. 2016;36(2):10-20. doi:10.1002/jhrm.21237. PMID: 27547874.
11. The Office of the National Coordinator for Health Information Technology. Security risk assessment tool. Version 3.4. Updated September 26, 2023. Accessed December 21, 2023. https://www.healthit.gov/topic/privacy-security-and-hipaa/security-risk-assessment-tool
12. Bahreini A. Which information locations in covered entities under HIPAA must be secured first? A multi-criteria decision-making approach. *J Healthc Risk Manag*. 2023;43:27-36. doi:10.1002/jhrm.21555
13. Kabir UY, Ezekekwu E, Bhuyan SS, Mahmood A, Dobalian A. Trends and best practices in health care cybersecurity insurance policy. *J Healthc Risk Manag*. 2020;40:10-14. doi:10.1002/jhrm.21414
14. Meydan C. Risk management. Learning from the mistakes of others. *J Eval Clin Pract*. 2014;20:505-507. doi:10.1111/jep.12165
15. NEJM Catalyst. What is risk management in healthcare? *N Engl J Med*. Published April 25, 2018. Accessed December 28, 2023. https://catalyst.nejm.org/doi/full/10.1056/CAT.18.0197

CHAPTER 11

Civic Engagement

GRACE DRNACH-BONAVENTURA

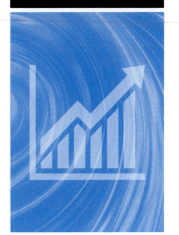

Learning Objectives

The reader will

1. Understand the basic historical and current role of the physical therapist in public health.
2. Discuss how health metrics relate to a global health agenda.
3. Identify and predict the role of social determinants of health to health outcomes.
4. Construct a basic budget and budget justification for grant funding.
5. Define service-learning and the important actions to take prior to engaging in service-learning practices.

The American Psychological Association defines **civic engagement** as "individual and collective actions designed to identify and address issues of public concern."[1] The rich history and present day role of the physical therapy profession is rooted in public health and public service. Many funding streams to support the business of health care to identify and address issues of public concern stem from understanding the national and global agenda. This includes how to use and report on health metrics to evaluate progress and population well-being through health care targets set by the United Nations. However, complex social and environmental factors can impede health at the individual level and also through business and government policies, leading to or perpetuating health disparities. Physical therapists should be prepared and educated on best practices to address these disparities as they engage in clinical practice and community efforts, such as pro bono services or service-learning activities to reduce health disparities, promote health equity, and work with community partners to provide optimal health services.

This chapter will explore the general framework in which physical therapists and physical therapy services are related to civic engagement, provide an overview of funding requirements and health metrics, and address strategies and considerations for physical therapists at the individual, business, and system levels when working with communities.

History of Physical Therapy in Public Health

Public health is the science that "promotes and protects the health of people and the communities where they live, learn, work and play."[2] Unlike physical health providers, such as nurses and physicians, who focus primarily on the treatment of individuals, public health professionals focus on prevention services to populations and aim to limit preventable health disparities and increase health equity. People in the field of public health work in a range of health care settings such as first responders, restaurant inspectors, health educators, scientists and researchers, nutritionists, social workers, epidemiologists, occupational health and safety professionals, and public policy makers.[2] Public health professionals look at health not at an individual level but from a community and systems perspective, such as increasing awareness of vaccine distribution to prevent the spread of disease, ensuring health care standards for nutrition lunch programs in schools to ensure access to healthy foods, or advocating for laws to promote healthy living, such as designated smoke-free areas or the use of helmets when operating a motorcycle.[2]

The public health profession continues to grow as a specialized field, but also overlaps with many current health care professions. The American Physical Therapy Association notes that "[t]he physical therapy profession is invested in individualized, patient-centered care, but that investment has broad societal and public health implications."[3] Historically, the practice of physical therapy has a record of civic engagement and participation in public health initiatives.

The application of physical agents and interventions has been around for ages, but physical therapy as a profession dates back to the early part of the 20th century. During the end of the 19th century and the beginning of the 20th, the Northeastern United States was dealing with a public health epidemic. The spread of the polio virus led to infections that resulted in the temporary or permanent paralysis of the infected individuals. Orthopedic surgeon Robert Lovett and physical therapists Wilhemine Wright and Janet Merrill worked together for the public good to advocate practices around rest, the importance of straightening limbs to decrease the development of muscle deformities, and to strengthen targeted muscles weakened by the disease. Lovett, Wright, and Merrill particularly advocated the importance of immobilization for children, whose movements aren't as easily controlled. The polio epidemic was one of several defining historical events that shaped the physical therapy profession and the role for the public good (see Chapter 3).[4] In 1912, individuals in the physical therapy profession formed a professional organization, first known as the American Women's Physical Therapeutic Association, now known as the American Physical Therapy Association.[5]

The US military first introduced the country to physical therapy as a result of World War I. Surgeons recognized the need for rehabilitation to increase the quality of life for the many wounded soldiers returning from war. The first physical therapists, known as "reconstruction aids," were civilian employees of the medical military who rehabilitated wounded soldiers, utilizing physiotherapy, curative workshops, and vocational therapy, to help the veteran adjust to life and return to work. The military was a key influence in standardizing procedures and evaluating the effectiveness of patient care, such as the progression of wound healing, gait analysis, and the benefit of progressive resistance exercises. After the war, these reconstruction aids returned home and dispersed into different health care sectors in their community.[6]

During World War II, with improvements in medicine, surgery, and increasing need for rehabilitation, the military noted an increase in demand for physical therapists and a formal and structured education. The military was the first to formally educate and train physical therapy assistants, who were known as "physical therapy technicians."[7]

In 1946, Congress passed the Hill-Burton Act, which gave health care facilities, such as hospitals and nursing homes funding to increase infrastructure, and, in return, the facilities

civic engagement – individual and collective actions designed to identify and address issues of public concern

public health – the science that promotes and protects the health of people and the communities where they live, learn, work, and play

Chapter 11 / Civic Engagement

would provide reasonable services to all, including those unable to pay.[8] With this law, physical therapists were able to expand further into hospitals, nursing homes, and other health care settings, increasing their services to the public.[9] In 1967, reimbursement for outpatient physical therapy services was made available through amendments to the Social Security Act.[10] Throughout the 1970s, 1980s, and 1990s, physical therapy continued to be noticed as a benefit to the public through the implementation of the Occupational Safety and Health Administration (OSHA) rules and regulations, the passage of the Education for All Handicapped Children Act (PL 94-142), the Americans with Disabilities Act and the National Center for Medical Rehabilitation Research.[7] Currently, the American Physical Therapy Association provides physical therapists information related to public health and specific population issues such as emergency preparedness, balance and falls, infectious disease control, pain management, racial and ethnic disparities, cultural competency, and nutrition.[3]

The rich history of the profession of physical therapy is rooted in the spirit of public health and civic engagement, with the mission of improving and restoring mobility for individuals to achieve optimal health. Although the early history focused on specific conditions such as war injuries and polio, as the profession progressed, so did areas of treatment and utilization. Today, physical therapists work in several areas of health care, providing evidence-based interventions and public health education, to achieve the optimal health and well-being of the individual, the family, and the public. Initiatives to promote public health through wellness and prevention programs and exercises to manage chronic pain, maintain functional independence, and participate in the workforce; optimize the ability of children with special needs to learn in the classroom; and promote workplace safety and ergonomics are just a few of the services provided by physical therapists that address public health today.

Health Metrics and Global Agenda

Similar to many health care professionals, physical therapists are an important part of the larger national and global initiatives for the public good. Understanding national and global health metrics and how they are used in outcome measures and decision making is beneficial not only in the promotion of community health but also in understanding the priorities and reporting requirements for securing federal grant monies.

Health metrics are important in monitoring and comparing population health and are used by health care professionals and policy makers to drive funding and health care initiatives. Understanding what health metrics are, how they are used for funding and global tracking, and how health metrics are tracked is important for the success of the business of health care. Health metrics can be obtained through census data registries, surveillance systems, household surveys, and health services systems such as patient files or insurance claims. For reporting to the public, many public health agencies send weekly updates to the public, such as through the World Health Organization's (WHO) Weekly Epidemiological Record or the Center for Disease Control's (CDC) Morbidity and Mortality Weekly Report.[11]

Health metrics can be used to undertake strategic planning; to evaluate services and interventions in a community; and to drive priorities in setting agendas, donor values, and

health metrics – specific health data that is used in monitoring and comparing population health and used by health care professionals and policy makers to drive funding and health care initiatives decision making.[11] In practice, measuring health metrics can be complicated. The following are a few common health metrics used in understanding the health of a community.

Population health can be defined as the "health outcomes of a group of individuals, including the distribution of such outcomes within the group. These groups are often geographic populations such as nations or communities but can also be other groups such as employees, ethnic groups, persons with a disability, prisoners, or any other defined group."[12] Public health professionals aim to prevent undesirable or negative health outcomes through several means: surveillance of disease; continued research on disease, injury, and prevention; increased community health education; advocacy for policies aimed at systemic change; and advocacy for health equity.

Morbidity and mortality describe the severity and progression of a particular event. Morbidity is the presence of an illness or disease (mild to severe), whereas mortality is the number of deaths resulting from a specific illness or disease. When reviewed together, morbidity and mortality provide the health care professionals one metric to better understand the health of a population. These metrics also allow stakeholders to more effectively prioritize health programs and allocate resources toward, and proactively manage, the potential onset of a health event.[13]

Incidence is the number of new cases of a disease occurring in a time period divided by the total number of people at risk for the disease in that time period and is typically used to study infectious diseases, acute diseases, and outbreaks.[14] Prevalence is the number of total existing cases, whether newly diagnosed or long established, divided by the total number of people in the population at the time measured; it is typically used to describe the frequency of chronic or long-lasting exposure and disease population, such as the percentage of people who have diabetes or asthma.[14]

Life expectancy refers to the number of years a person can expect to live.[15] By definition, life expectancy is based on an estimate of the average age that members of a particular population group will be when they die. An important point to bear in mind when interpreting life expectancy estimates is that very few people will die at precisely the age indicated by life expectancy, even if mortality patterns stay constant.[11] For example, very few of the infants born in South Africa in 2009 will die at 52.2 years of age. Most will die much earlier or much later because the risk of death is not uniform across the lifetime. Life expectancy is the average. In societies with high infant mortality rates, many people die in the first few years of life, but once they survive childhood, people often live much longer.[15]

Another metric associated with *life expectancy* is healthy life expectancy (HALE), which is the number of years the average individual born into the population can expect to live without a disability.[16] Measuring HALE gives insight into how people can live to older ages without experiencing extended periods of disability prior to death. From a funding and population health perspective, HALE is important because substantial resources are devoted to reducing the incidence, duration, and severity of major diseases that cause morbidity but not mortality. It is an important metric to capture both fatal and nonfatal health outcomes.

incidence – the number of new cases of a disease occurring in a time period divided by the total number of people at risk for the disease in that time period

prevalence – the number of total existing cases, whether newly diagnosed or long established, divided by the total number of people in the population at the time measured

healthy life expectancy – the number of years the average individual born into the population can expect to live without a disability

Global Targets

Health metrics are used to create a set of global goals and targets. The *Millennium Development Goals* (MDG) were adopted by the United Nations in 2000 with the aim of providing a clear strategy and evaluation of the eight goals identified to increase global well-being by 2015.[17] Several of the MDG relate to socioeconomic development and predominantly to health outcomes. The MDG were influential in providing a road map for targets and evaluation for the global agenda and served as a framework for global cooperation and international development.[18]

In 2015, new or follow-up goals related to the MDG were established using more real-time metrics and expanding global goals and targets. The United Nations released the *Sustainable Development Goals* (SDGs), which include 17 targets aimed at achieving global health.[19] SDG not only focuses on the world's poorest people, but also sets targets for countries higher on the economic growth scale to improve the lives of everyone.

The United Nations lists 17 overarching goals and a call to action to ensure overall global well-being. These 2030 goals are as follows: (1) No Poverty; (2) Zero Hunger; (3) Good Health and Well-Being; (4) Quality Education; (5) Gender Equality; (6) Clean Water and Sanitation; (7) Affordable and Clean Energy; (8) Decent Work and Economic Growth; (9) Industry, Innovation, and Infrastructure; (10) Reduced Inequalities; (11) Sustainable Cities and Communities; (12) Responsible Consumption and Production; (13) Climate Action; (14) Life Below Water; (15) Life on Land; (16) Peace, Justice, and Strong Institutions; and (17) Partnerships for the Goals.[19] Table 11.1 includes the SDGs and targets.[20]

Table 11.1 Sustainable Development Goals and Targets[20] (Excerpts)	
Goals	**Targets**
Goal 1: No Poverty	• By 2030, eradicate extreme poverty for all people everywhere, currently measured as people living on less than $1.25 a day. • By 2030, reduce at least by half the proportion of men, women, and children of all ages living in poverty in all its dimensions according to national definitions.
Goal 2: Zero Hunger	• By 2030, end hunger and ensure access by all people, in particular, the poor and people in vulnerable situations, including infants, to safe, nutritious and sufficient food all year round. • By 2030, end all forms of malnutrition, including achieving, by 2025, the internationally agreed targets on stunting and wasting in children under 5 y of age, and address the nutritional needs of adolescent girls, pregnant and lactating women and older persons.
Goal 3: Good Health and Well-being	• By 2030, reduce the global maternal mortality ratio to less than 70 per 100,000 live births. • By 2030, end preventable deaths of newborns and children under 5 y of age, with all countries aiming to reduce neonatal mortality to at least as low as 12 per 1,000 live births and under-5 mortality to at least as low as 25 per 1,000 live births. • By 2030, end the epidemics of AIDS, tuberculosis, malaria, and neglected tropical diseases and combat hepatitis, water-borne diseases, and other communicable diseases. • By 2030, reduce by one-third premature mortality from noncommunicable diseases through prevention and treatment and promote mental health and well-being.

(continued)

Table 11.1 Sustainable Development Goals and Targets[20] (Excerpts) (*continued*)

Goals	Targets
	• By 2030, ensure universal access to sexual and reproductive health care services, including for family planning, information and education, and the integration of reproductive health into national strategies and programs. • Achieve universal health coverage, including financial risk protection, access to quality essential health care services, and access to safe, effective, quality and affordable essential medicines and vaccines for all. • Substantially increase health financing and the recruitment, development, training and retention of the health workforce in developing countries, especially in least developed countries and small island developing states. • Strengthen the capacity of all countries, in particular developing countries, for early warning, risk reduction, and management of national and global health risks.
Goal 4: Quality Education	• By 2030, ensure that all girls and boys complete free, equitable and quality primary and secondary education, leading to relevant and Goal-4 effective learning outcomes. • By 2030, ensure that all girls and boys have access to quality early childhood development, care, and preprimary education so that they are ready for primary education. • By 2030, ensure equal access for all women and men to affordable and quality technical, vocational, and tertiary education, including university. • By 2030, eliminate gender disparities in education and ensure equal access to all levels of education and vocational training for the vulnerable, including persons with disabilities, indigenous peoples, and children in vulnerable situations. • By 2030, ensure that all learners acquire the knowledge and skills needed to promote sustainable development, including, among others, through education for sustainable development and sustainable lifestyles, human rights, gender equality, promotion of a culture of peace and nonviolence, global citizenship, and appreciation of cultural diversity, and of culture's contribution to sustainable development.
Goal 5: Gender Equality	• End all forms of discrimination against all women and girls everywhere. • Eliminate all forms of violence against all women and girls in the public and private spheres, including trafficking and sexual and other types of exploitation. • Eliminate all harmful practices, such as child, early and forced marriage, and female genital mutilation. • Adopt and strengthen sound policies and enforceable legislation for the promotion of gender equality and the empowerment of all women and girls at all levels.
Goal 6: Clean Water and Sanitation	• By 2030, achieve universal and equitable access to safe and affordable drinking water for all.
Goal 7: Affordable and Clean Energy	• By 2030, ensure universal access to affordable, reliable, and modern energy services.
Goal 8: Decent Work and Economic Growth	• Sustain per capita economic growth in accordance with national circumstances and, in particular, at least 7% gross domestic product growth per annum in the least developed countries. • Achieve higher levels of economic productivity through diversification, technological upgrading and innovation, including through a focus on high-value added and labor-intensive sectors.

Chapter 11 / Civic Engagement

Table 11.1 Sustainable Development Goals and Targets[20] (Excerpts) (*continued*)

Goals	Targets
	• By 2030, achieve full and productive employment and decent work for all women and men, including for young people and persons with disabilities, and equal pay for work of equal value. • By 2030, devise and implement policies to promote sustainable tourism that creates jobs and promotes local culture and products.
Goal 9: Industry, Innovation and Infrastructure	• Develop quality, reliable, sustainable and resilient infrastructure, including regional and transborder infrastructure, to support economic development and human well-being, with a focus on affordable and equitable access for all. • Significantly increase access to information and communications technology and strive to provide universal and affordable access to the internet in least developed countries by 2020.
Goal 10: Reduce Inequalities	• By 2030, progressively achieve and sustain income growth of the bottom 40% of the population at a rate higher than the national average. • By 2030, empower and promote the social, economic, and political inclusion of all, irrespective of age, sex, disability, race, ethnicity, origin, religion, or economic or other status. • Ensure equal opportunity and reduce inequalities of outcome, including by eliminating discriminatory laws, policies, and practices and promoting appropriate legislation, policies, and action in this regard. • Adopt policies, especially fiscal, wage, and social protection policies, and progressively achieve greater equality. • Ensure enhanced representation and voice for developing countries in decision making in global international economic and financial institutions in order to deliver more effective, credible, accountable, and legitimate institutions.
Goal 11: Sustainable Cities and Communities	• By 2030, ensure access for all to adequate, safe, and affordable housing and basic services and upgrade slums. • By 2030, provide access to safe, affordable, accessible, and sustainable transport systems for all, improving road safety, notably by expanding public transport, with special attention to the needs of those in vulnerable situations, women, children, persons with disabilities, and older persons. • Strengthen efforts to protect and safeguard the world's cultural and natural heritage. • By 2030, significantly reduce the number of deaths and the number of people affected, and substantially decrease the direct economic losses relative to global gross domestic product caused by disasters, including water-related disasters, with a focus on protecting the poor and people in vulnerable situations.
Goal 12: Responsible Consumption and Production	• Implement the 10-y framework of programs on sustainable consumption and production, all countries taking action, with developed countries taking the lead, taking into account the development and capabilities of developing countries. • By 2030, achieve the sustainable management and efficient use of natural resources. • By 2030, halve per capita global food waste at the retail and consumer levels, and reduce food losses along production and supply chains, including postharvest losses. • By 2030, substantially reduce waste generation through prevention, reduction, recycling and reuse.

(continued)

Table 11.1 Sustainable Development Goals and Targets[20] (Excerpts) (*continued*)

Goals	Targets
	• By 2030, ensure that people everywhere have the relevant information and awareness for sustainable development and lifestyles in harmony with nature. • Support developing countries to strengthen their scientific and technological capacity to move toward more sustainable patterns of consumption and production.
Goal 13: Climate Action	• Strengthen resilience and adaptive capacity to climate-related hazards and natural disasters in all countries. • Integrate climate change measures into national policies, strategies, and planning.
Goal 14: Life Below Water	• By 2025, prevent and significantly reduce marine pollution of all kinds, in particular from land-based activities, including marine debris and nutrient pollution.
Goal 15: Life On Land	• By 2030, combat desertification, restore degraded land and soil, including land affected by desertification, drought and floods, and strive to achieve a land degradation-neutral world. • By 2030, ensure the conservation of mountain ecosystems, including their biodiversity, in order to enhance their capacity to provide benefits that are essential for sustainable development.
Goal 16: Peace, Justice and Strong Institutions	• Significantly reduce all forms of violence and related death rates everywhere. • End abuse, exploitation, trafficking, and all forms of violence against and torture of children. • Promote the rule of law at the national and international levels, and ensure equal access to justice for all.
Goal 17: Partnerships for the Goals	**Finance** • Strengthen domestic resource mobilization, including through international support to developing countries, to improve domestic capacity for tax and other revenue collection. **Technology** • Enhance North-South, South-South, and triangular regional and international cooperation on and access to science, technology, and innovation and enhance knowledge sharing on mutually agreed terms, including through improved coordination among existing mechanisms, in particular, at the United Nations level, and through a global technology facilitation mechanism. **Capacity-building** • Enhance international support for implementing effective and targeted capacity-building in developing countries to support national plans to implement all the sustainable development goals, including through North-South, South-South, and triangular cooperation. **Trade** • Promote a universal, rules-based, open, nondiscriminatory and equitable multilateral trading system under the World Trade Organization, including through the conclusion of negotiations under its Doha Development Agenda. **Systemic issues** *Policy and institutional coherence* • Enhance global macroeconomic stability, including through policy coordination and policy coherence. • Respect each country's policy space and leadership to establish and implement policies for poverty eradication and sustainable development.

Chapter 11 / Civic Engagement

Table 11.1 Sustainable Development Goals and Targets[20] (Excerpts) (*continued*)	
Goals	*Targets*
	Multistakeholder partnerships • Enhance the global partnership for sustainable development, complemented by multistakeholder partnerships that mobilize and share knowledge, expertise, technology, and financial resources, to support the achievement of the sustainable development goals in all countries, in particular, developing countries. • Encourage and promote effective public, public-private, and civil society partnerships, building on the experience and resourcing strategies of partnerships. *Data, monitoring, and accountability* • By 2030, build on existing initiatives to develop measurements of progress on sustainable development that complement gross domestic product, and support statistical capacity-building in developing countries.

Table information was compiled through the United Nations. United Nations Department of Economic and Social Affairs. #Envision2030: 17 goals to transform the world for persons with disabilities. Accessed August 14, 2022. https://www.un.org/development/desa/disabilities/envision2030.html. Visit this site for the full listing of the Target objectives. Reprinted with the permission of the United Nations.

Activities from physical therapists mostly align with SDG 3: Ensure healthy lives and promote well-being for all ages.[19] The goal of achieving "Good Health and Well-Being" for everyone is lofty and somewhat ambiguous. To clarify goals and establish measurable health metrics, SDG creates targets and indicators for each goal. SDG 3.8 relates to monitoring universal health coverage to understand the financial burden and access to health care in a specific population. The target envisages "substantially increas[ing] health financing and the recruitment, development, training, and retention of the health workforce in developing countries, especially in least developed countries and small island developing [s]tates."[21]

Challenges and Considerations With Achieving Sustainable Development Goals

There is a complexity and interdependence on other external factors to consider, such as a country's or community's economic status, the presence of economic and social inequalities, rapid urbanization, the rising antimicrobial resistance, and the continuing societal burden of diseases, such as COVID-19 and HIV/AIDS. Furthermore, societal policies can create barriers to achieving goals. Scaling up investment in universal health care coverage is essential to achieving health and well-being for everyone, yet in many countries, including the United States, limited progress has been made in implementing universal health care. International acceptance of definitions is another limitation to achieving these goals; "well-being" as defined by one country or community may differ from how it is defined by others.

Although there has been progress in the areas of ensuring healthy lives and promoting a population's well-being, such as increasing global life expectancy, proactively addressing infections and diseases, addressing maternal mortality, and reducing deaths caused by disease such as malaria, the COVID-19 pandemic drastically slowed this progress, with 90% of countries reporting a halt in essential health services during this period. With health workers in short supply around the world, decades of progress in areas such as reproductive health, maternal health, and child health have been stalled or even reversed.

Addressing these disruptions will take several years to correct; however, health care professionals and business owners can take steps to restore the achievement of health outcomes through clear directives that act on specific health metrics.[21] Funding for such efforts may be obtained from banks or other financial institutions or may be obtained from government or private granting agencies.

Grant Funding

Health care providers looking for grant funding for innovations within their business may use health metrics, personal experience, and identified community needs to advocate for their identified health programs, services, and/or interventions. However, grants are competitive and require a clear and convincing strategy for the granter's consideration and funding. When advocating for a program, it is important to note "who" is in the granting organization and "what" is the focus of their mission and funding priorities. For example, the Bill and Melinda Gates Foundation focuses on activities and innovations around new health technologies because of the history and expertise of the Microsoft company.[22] Funders often require current health metrics to be reported, a clear description of how the funding would support a system change and achieve specific outcomes, and how the project would achieve more favorable health metrics.

To acquire funding for initiatives, a business must first identify and gather available and appropriate health metrics about their target market for the purpose of writing a proposal. In reality, there are several barriers to gathering accurate information. For example, in some rural areas in the United States, the lack of electronic data management can compromise the validity of the data available or make it prohibitively expensive to gather. Funders prefer proposals based on strongly established business practices, valid data, clear plans to address an appropriate health metric, and evidence of the business using data for business decision making. Grant funding is often prioritized based on grants with the highest action impact within a population and is most cost-effective. It is important to note a funder's restrictions when applying for a grant and to understand the requirements and restrictions for implementing the desired activities.

A funding agency, such as the Health Resources and Human Administration (HRSA) or the Substance Abuse and Mental Health Services (SAMHSA), may require the funders to target populations within a rural service area. During the application process, the agency applying agrees to certain reporting requirements, such as submitting biannual progress reports, data reports, and annual sustainability plans. Additionally, an estimated budget is an important part of the grant application (see Chapter 2). This includes the estimated costs and budget justification. It is important to be forward thinking in multiyear budgeting, such as expecting cost of living adjustments or changes in mileage reimbursement rates. An example of a proposed budget and budget justification can be found in Box 11.1.

Social Determinants of Health

The World Health Organization defines social determinants of health (SDOH) as "the non-medical factors that influence health outcomes. They are the conditions in which people are born, grow, work, live, and age, and the wider set of forces and systems shaping the conditions of daily life. These forces and systems include economic policies and

social determinants of health – the nonmedical factors that influence health outcomes

Chapter 11 / Civic Engagement

BOX 11.1 • Grant Budget Proposal and Justification: An Example

[Company Title Here]
Example Proposed Budget
2019 to 2023

Account	2019	2020	2021	2022	2023	Total
Salaries						
Fringe rate is 30.4% for all listed						
Director, [TITLE]	6,500	6,500	13K	6,500	6,500	39,000
Fringe benefits	1,976	1,976	3,952	1,976	1,976	11,856
Director, [TITLE]	0	10K	10K	5,000	5,000	30,000
Fringe benefits	0	3,040	3,040	1,520	1,520	9,120
Associate VP	12K	12K	12K	12K	12K	60,000
Fringe benefits	3,648	3,648	3,648	3,648	3,648	18,240
Administrative associate	2,000	4,000	4,000	2,000	2,000	14,000
Fringe benefits	608	1,216	1,216	608	608	4,256
Staff IV	4,300	8,600	8,600	4,300	4,300	30,100
Fringe benefits	1,307	2,615	2,615	1,307	1,307	9,151
Staff IV	4,900	9,800	4,900	4,900	4,900	29,400
Fringe benefits	1,490	2,979	1,490	1,490	1,490	8,939
Director,	9,000	9,000	9,000	9,000	9,000	45,000
Fringe benefits	2,736	2,736	2,736	2,736	2,736	13,680
Adjunct pay		22K	22K			44,000
Flat rate						0
Total	50,465	100,109	102,198	56,985	56,985	366,742

Account	2019	2020	2021	2022	2023	Total
Administrative						
Printing	920	920	920	920	920	4600
Misc. supplies	600	600	600	600	600	3000
Total	1,820	1,820	1,820	1,820	1,820	9,100
Contracted Services						
[Contract #1]	3,200	3,200	3,200	1,600	1,600	12,800
[Contract #2]	5,600	5,600	5,600	5,600	5,600	28,000
[Contract #3]	5,600	5,600	5,600	5,600	5,600	28,000
Communications	1,080	2,160	2,160	1,080	1,080	7,560
Data analyst	1,200	2,400	1,200	2,400	1,200	8,400
Web development/ support	0	5,280	2,640	1,320	1,320	10,560
Total	16,680	24,240	20,400	17,600	16,400	95,320

(continued)

BOX 11.1 • Grant Budget Proposal and Justification: An Example (*continued*)

Account	2019	2020	2021	2022	2023	Total
Travel Allowance						
Mileage	3,924	3,924	3,924	3,924	3,924	19,620
Car rental	2,322	2,322	2,322	2,322	2,322	11,610
Lodging	4,320	4,320	4,320	4,320	4,320	21,600
Meals	4,500	4,500	4,500	4,500	4,500	22,500
Total	15,066	15,066	15,066	15,066	15,066	75,330

Account	2019	2020	2021	2022	2023	Total
Meetings and Seminars						
Rental space for meetings/retreats	800	800	800	800	800	4,000
Refreshments	300	300	300	300	300	1,500
Travel reimbursement for participants	1,047	1,047	1,047	1,047	1,047	5,235
Total	2,147	2,147	2,147	2,147	2,147	10,735
Expense total	86,178	143,382	141,631	93,618	92,418	557,227
Indirect costs	8,600	14,300	14,100	9,300	9,200	55,500
Grand totals	94,778	157,682	155,731	102,918	101,618	612,727

[Company Title Here]
Example Proposed Budget
2019 to 2023

Budget Summary						
Account	2019	2020	2021	2022	2023	Total
Salaries and fringes	50,465	100,109	102,198	56,985	56,985	366,742
Administrative	1,820	1,820	1,820	1,820	1,820	9,100
Contracted services	16,680	24,240	20,400	17,600	16,400	95,320
Travel allowance	15,066	15,066	15,066	15,066	15,066	75,330
Meetings and seminars	2,147	2,147	2,147	2,147	2,147	10,735
Expense total	86,178	143,382	141,631	93,618	92,418	557,227
Indirect costs	8,600	14,300	14,100	9,300	9,200	55,500
Grand totals	94,778	157,682	155,731	102,918	101,618	612,727

Chapter 11 / Civic Engagement

BOX 11.1 • Grant Budget Proposal and Justification: An Example (*continued*)

Budget Narrative

Salaries

We are asking the endowment to fund only a portion of the person's time based on the need for that person during the various phases of the program (ie, Evaluation in year 1, Development in year 2; Implementation in year 3; Refinement and Sustainability in years 4 and 5)

Percentage of time/ phase/year	Year	1	2	3	4	5	
Director, [TITLE]	$65,000	10	10	20	10	10	
Director, [TITLE]	$50,000	0	20	20	5	5	
Associate VP	$120,000	10	10	10	10	10	
Administrative associate	$40,000	5	10	10	5	5	
Staff IV, average	$43,000	10	20	20	10	10	
Staff IV, average	$49,000	10	20	10	10	10	
Director, [TITLE]	$45,000	20	20	20	20	20	
Adjunct pay	$ 2,200/course						
Dollars/year	**Year**	**1**	**2**	**3**	**4**	**5**	**Total**
Director, [TITLE]	$65,000	6,500	6,500	13K	6,500	6,500	39,000
Director, [TITLE]	$50,000	0	10K	10K	5,000	5,000	30,000
Associate VP	$120,000	12K	12K	12K	12K	12K	60,000
Administrative associate	$40,000	2,000	4,000	4,000	2,000	2,000	14,000
Staff IV, average	$43,000	4,300	8,600	8,600	4,300	4,300	30,100
Staff IV, average	$49,000	4,900	9,800	4,900	4,900	4,900	29,400
Director, [TITLE]	$45,000	9,000	9,000	9,000	9,000	9,000	45,000
Adjunct pay	$ 2,200/course		22K	22K			44,000
Total direct pay excluding fringes							291,500

Administrative	
Printing/graphic design	Printed information for public invitations, announcements, or educational materials at an average cost of $23/hour for graphic design
Postage	For 5 d/y would be $920/y for 5 y = 4,600 Mailings to areas with limited internet access. Postage for surveys with return postage paid at an average cost of $300/y (2018 1 oz postage rate of $0.50) for 5 y = 1,500 For 5 d/y would be $920/y for 5 y = 4,600 Mailings to areas with limited internet access. Postage for surveys with return postage paid at an average cost of $300/y (2018 1 oz postage rate of $0.50) for 5 y = 1,500
Miscellaneous supplies	Includes paper, toner, pens at an average cost of $600/y for 5 y = 3,000

(continued)

BOX 11.1 • Grant Budget Proposal and Justification: An Example (*continued*)

Contracted Services	
[Contract #1]	For other [Contract #1] staff with expertise in education, health care, communication, or psychology. Current rate is $40/h. 80 h ($3,200) for year 1 (Evaluation), 80 h ($3,200) for year 2 (Development), 80 h ($3,200) year 3 (Implementation), 40 h ($1,600) years 4 and 5 (Refinement and Sustainability)
[Contract #2]	To utilize employees in [Contract #2] offices with resources in ministry formation and support. In 2017, the average salary for a [STAFF] was $45,593. Add 30.4% for fringes = $59,453. Divide by 2,080 h (FTE) = $28/h 200 h per year = $5,600
[Contract #3]	To utilize other professionals of various denominations throughout the region who are identified as leaders in the field. Calculation of cost done as listed earlier.
Communication	For other communication experts with specific skills in areas of health care knowledge. $43,000 \times 0.304 = 13,072 + 43,000 = 56,072/2,080$ (hours per year full time) = $27/h 40 h ($1080) for year 1 (Evaluation), 80 h ($2,160) for year 2 (Development), 80 h ($2,160) year 3 (Implementation), 40 h ($1,080) years 4 and 5 (Refinement and Sustainability)
Data analyst	$30/h (www.bls.gov reference) for survey design and data analysis and reporting using both qualitative and quantitative data. 40 h ($1,200) for year 1 (Evaluation), 80 h ($2,400) for year 2 (Development), 40 h ($1,200) year 3 (Implementation), 80 h ($2,400) year 4 (Refinement and Sustainability), and 40 h ($1,200) in year 5 (Refinement and Sustainability)
Web development/ support	$33/h (www.bls.gov reference) 0 h in year 1 (Evaluation), 160 h ($5,280) in year 2 (Development), 80 h ($2,640) in year 3 (Implementation), 40 h ($1,320) in years 4 and 5 (Refinement and Sustainability) to assist in the development of web-based portals for resources and communications and to assist with problem-solving when utilizing various systems, of different ages, throughout the region

Travel Allowance	
Mileage	1 time per week; 36 wk/y; 200 miles round trip; $0.545/mile = 109/trip $\times$ 36 = 3,924/y for 5 y = 19,620
Car rental	For trips over 200 miles round trip, we will rent a car at $43/d based on Enterprise Rentals in [City]. Each trip = 3 d or $129 at 2 trips/month for 9 mo = 2,322/y for 5 y = 11,610
Auto fuel	200 miles $\times$ 36 wk = 7,200 miles/y for 5 y is 36,000 400 miles (based on round trip to State Capitol, which is the center of the State) $\times$ 2/mo = 800/mo for 9 mo = 7,200/y for 5 y = 36,000 36,000 + 36,000 = 72,000 miles per year. Cars average miles per gallon = 25 miles/gallon @ $3/ gallon is 72000/25 = 2880 $\times$ $3 = $8640/y for 5 y = 43,200
Lodging	Two nights lodging, 1 time per month for 9 mo = 18 nights/year at $120/night/room/person = 2,160. For two rooms = 4,320/y for 5 y = 21,600
Meals	$50/day/person maximum. 36 one-day trips per year + 54 d for overnight trips per year = 90 d per year at $50/d = 4,500/y for 5 y = 22,500

Chapter 11 / Civic Engagement   **251**

> ## BOX 11.1 • Grant Budget Proposal and Justification: An Example (*continued*)

Meetings and Seminars	
Rental space for meetings/retreats	Average cost is $200/event. Estimate 4 per year = $800/y.
Refreshments	Allocate $75/event at 4 per year = $300

Travel reimbursement for participants:	Estimate events/year; 12 participants/event; 40 miles round trip/participant at 0.545 cents per mile = $1,047/y

Indirect Costs

Support services for accounting and finance services (including contract management and procurement services) human resources for benefit management, information technology infrastructure at the place of employment (data and voice services, network systems, and hardware upkeep). Estimated at approximately 10% of annual expenses.

Budget Justification

The program director will be responsible for managing the program staff, ensuring the fidelity of program delivery, and overseeing the ongoing evaluation of "Stay Wise, Be Safe." Duties will also include, but not be limited to, corresponding with the funding organization, corresponding with partnering centers around the New Orleans community, hiring staff, and monitoring budget compliance. The program director at will be working in a 0.5 FTE capacity. We will thus be allocating $24,000 for compensation, or 50% of $48,000, the average salary of a comparable program's director. $48,000 × 0.5 FTE = $24,000.

"Stay Wise, Be Safe" plans to employ two associate directors who will oversee different sectors of our program. The associate director of operations will manage the implementation of the program, including overseeing the delivery of our program activities and managing the CHWs at a closer level. The associate directors will be responsible for overseeing the process evaluation component of our program. They will work closely with the evaluator and the data manager during our 2-week assessment periods pre- and post intervention to analyze participant cohort trends and identify any areas of improvement. Each associate director will be dedicating 0.50 FTE to their positions within the program and will therefore be compensated with $20,000 each, which is 50% of the average comparable associate director's salary of $40,000. $40,000 × 0.5 FTE = $20,000.

Each of the six CHWs we plan to employ will be current staff members of the community home and will be responsible for overseeing participant cohorts at their assigned community center. They will assist with cultural tailoring of our program by conducting small focus groups or individual conversations during the working day. These CHWs will serve as integral components of our recruitment and retention protocols by making weekly check-ins with the participants. Because we anticipate that the CHWs will already be staff of the community center, we are offering a stipend rather than a salary. We anticipate 3 weeks of recruitment, 8 weeks of intervention, and 2 weeks of evaluation for a total of 13 weeks of work. We are offering $100 per session for each of the six CHWs. $100 × 13 weeks × 6 CHWs × 2 interventions per year = $15,600.

Because we plan to conduct ongoing process evaluations throughout the duration of our 3-year program, we will employ a Tulane Intern as an evaluator who will oversee this process. The evaluator will work closely with the data manager and the associate directors to analyze statistical trends and create evaluation plans that will assess the effectiveness of the program's

(continued)

BOX 11.1 • Grant Budget Proposal and Justification: An Example (*continued*)

activities. They will inform program development processes to ensure that "Be Wise, Stay Safe" is functioning at maximal capacity. The evaluator will be permitted to use this experience as a practicum and will be given a stipend of $2,000.

The secretary will be responsible for printing and supplying participating community centers with pamphlets, copying and printing blank facts sheets for each community center each week, keeping office supplies readily available, and answering phone calls or email with questions and comments in regard to "Be Wise, Stay Safe." A secretary's average salary is $26,000, and the secretary will be working full time, 1.00 FTE, for "Be Wise, Stay Safe." $26,000 × 1.00 FTE = $26,000.

The data manager will be responsible for working with the evaluator and assistant directors with logging and interpretation of statistics and information received from the participants in the program. The data manager will organize data and feedback, compare statistics between community centers and pre- and post sessions, and strategize improvement based on input during the off-weeks between classes. Like the evaluator, the data manager will be a Tulane intern and permitted to use this experience for their practicum. The data manager will be given a stipend of $2,000.

Fringe benefits will total 0.30 of the total salaries for both professional and nonprofessional salary totals, excluding the Tulane stipend. With total salaries equaling $91,800, fringe benefits will total $27,540. $91,800 × 0.30 = $27,540.

The graphic designer will be responsible for creating a relevant company logo and designing recruiting pamphlets for the beginning of the educational sessions. The graphic designer has an average pay of $200 per day and will be working with "Be Wise, Stay Safe" for a total of 5 days. $200 per day × 5 days = $1,000.

Open community space will be used as the environment to host the educational sessions for our participants. The average rental space is $100 per hour. At 8 weeks per educational session, with two sessions per year, community space will total $3,200 per year.

$168 × 40 weeks = $6,720. Rental of office space will be used to host working personnel and provide a concrete address for addressing and mail. The average cost of renting office space is $12,000 per year. $12,000 × 1 year = $12,000.

Two tablets will be purchased in order to collect and store data, create and store attendance logs and pamphlet updates, research, and correspond via email. These will be used by the data manager and the evaluator and returned at the end of the year. The average price of a tablet is $500. Two tablets × $500 = $1,000.

General office supplies such as paper, toner, and pens will be used daily in the office for tasks such as printing and signing documents. The average cost of office supplies per year is $600. A landline telephone will be used as a concrete number for "Be Wise, Stay Safe" and will be located at the office. This will be the contact number given to the participants and put on the pamphlet. The average cost of a telephone for one year, including monthly charges, is $800.

To hold participant retention, participants will receive prizes, such as gift cards, during the educational session. There is an average reward of $10 per participant per session. For an expected 50 participants for each of the eight sessions, conducted 2 times per year, we expect a total of $8,000. $10 × 50 participants × 8 sessions × 2 times per year = $8,000.

---

systems, development agendas, social norms, social policies and political systems."[23] These factors can be grouped into five domains: Economic Stability, Education Access and Quality, Healthcare Access and Quality, Neighborhood and Built Environment, and Social and Community Context (Table 11.2).[24] Factors within each of the domains include places where

Table 11.2 Five Domains of Social Determinants of Health[24]

Domain	Includes
Education Access and Quality	• High school graduation • Enrollment in higher education • Language and literacy • Early childhood education and development
Health care Access and Quality	• Access to health care • Access to primary care • Health literacy
Economic Stability	• Poverty • Employment • Food insecurity • Housing instability
Social and Community Context	• Social cohesion • Civic participation • Discrimination • Incarceration
Neighborhood and Built Environment	• Access to foods that support healthy eating patterns • Quality of housing • Crime and violence • Environmental conditions

Source: The Office of Disease Prevention and Health Promotion. Social determinants of health. Healthy People 2020. Accessed July 7, 2022. https://www.healthypeople.gov/2020/topics-objectives/topic/social-determinants-health/interventions-resources.

people work and live, and affect an individual's lifestyle such as access and quality of health care, access to early childhood education and development, economic stability, access to transportation, housing stability, availability of healthy foods, air and water quality.[25]

SDOH can be directly related to health outcomes, and properly addressing SDOH can lead to health equity. Several aspects of an individual's health, such as mental health and substance use can be shaped by the social, economic, and physical environments in which people live.[25] For example, in relation to income and access to care, when a household is considered to be a high-income or wealthy household, if an individual from that household has a health concern, he or she usually has access to more resources for immediate high-quality health care, accurate diagnostic testing, and effective therapies, such as physical therapy. The availability of these resources also provides the ability to address health issues early, which can prevent mild issues from becoming severe problems. On the other hand, low-income households generally have fewer resources to access when someone sustains an injury or develops a severe illness, or they may not be able to afford to seek care, whether life threatening or not. They could experience issues with transportation, co-pays, childcare, or no sick leave, from their job, preventing them from being able to access health services.[11]

An individual's level of education can also impact access to health care services. The ability to read and a higher number of years of formal education are correlated with higher health status for adults and their children. Individuals who cannot read will have difficulty with health-related activities such as learning about new exercise programs in newspapers, magazines, or other written material, comprehending written health and safety warnings on products, reading posters advertising immunization and screening campaigns, following directions on medicine bottles, or applying for benefits.[11] Care seeking may also be stalled because of a fear of judgment by others or the inability to read or complete intake forms.

Health care professionals are often educated on SDOH but can lack the ability and organizational support to transfer classroom knowledge into clinical practice to address and resolve root causes of health disparities. Even when SDOH factors are addressed properly, health care professionals can feel helpless when faced with the complexities of historically compounding societal inequities that have led to poorer health outcomes.[26] To fully support the integration of actionable outcomes related to SDOH and health equity, health care professionals need to be supported personally and through policies by the health care organization. For example, some health care agencies require SDOH screening policies in the intake paperwork, with instructions to connect the individual to a case manager or appropriate resources if applicable. Health care professionals should understand and reference SDOH data to better recognize root causes that affect population health and adjust their business models accordingly. Online tool kits, active programs, and policy resources are available from the Center for Disease Control and Prevention (CDC at https://www.cdc.gov/socialdeterminants/tools/index.htm) to assist in turning SDOH data into actionable outcomes to reduce health disparities.

Health Equity, Health Equality, and Health Disparities

Domestic and global achievements, such as innovations in health technology and the uneven distribution of health care access, lead to health disparities not only between countries but also within some of the richest countries (eg, urban vs rural health areas). Yet all people around the world are at risk for the same set of hazards, such as drug-resistant pathogens or COVID-19 infections. The general goals of global health are to create the same access to health, health care services, and health care technology around the world. However, even with the same goals in place, not every individual has the same path leading to those goals.

Health disparities are seen when avoidable differences in health status between population groups is observed.[27] Health equality is seen when every individual has access to the same standard of health care services. Health equity is present when the services available are tailored to the specific needs of the individuals, providing a fair and just opportunity for the same level of health. Health equity requires removing societal barriers such as those found through SDOH. The differences between health equality and health equity can be seen in the following example.

Each of three neighborhoods is within equal geographic distance from the fresh food market. One neighborhood has no public transportation system to access the fresh food market, and the streets are not safe after dusk. Another neighborhood is separated from the market by a river and requires a boat to go shopping. The third neighborhood has access to roads, public transportation, and active streetlights and a safe walking environment. Equality gives a one-size-fits-all approach and provides each individual in all the neighborhoods a new pair of shoes to walk to the local fresh food store. Equity individualizes the approach for fairness given each neighborhood's current situation to create access for each community, providing a bus for one neighborhood and a bridge to another. The third neighborhood did not receive services given the current ability to access the fresh

health equality – the condition where every individual has access to the same standard of health care services

health equity – the condition where health services are available and tailored to the specific needs of the individuals, providing a fair and just opportunity for the same level of health

Chapter 11 / Civic Engagement

food market. Engaging in equity does not limit or burden those neighborhoods who are advantaged but provides resources so that disadvantaged neighborhoods can have the same opportunities.[28]

Many organizations, such as the CDC and the WHO, provide guidance for health care organizations to recognize SDOH and reduce health disparities.[29] Health care professionals can take individual and collection action to identify and reduce health disparities through the following actions:

- *Name and Identify Health Disparities.* Making decisions toward health equity begins with the recognition and identification of health disparities, often found in SDOH. Although an increase in the opportunities provided will benefit everyone in the community, an intentional focus should include groups who have been historically excluded or marginalized.
- *Understand Inequitable Policies.* An organization's polices should be periodically reviewed and updated, with the intention of identifying any out-of-date or discriminatory practices. Outdated and unfair human resource or organizational policies that create barriers to health equity will continue to exclude and oppress marginalized populations until the impact of those policies are identified and changed. This barrier can also impact the number of people who may benefit from the services, employment opportunities provided, and the community outreach efforts by the health care organization.
- *Raise Awareness.* Educating the community and policy makers on the presence and impact of inequitable policies, the opportunities lost, and the financial loss resulting from the underutilization of resources helps to expand awareness of the issue and facilitate change.
- *Vote.* Sustainable change is also made at the health care systems level. Understanding the platforms and policy making agendas of those in public office, or running for public office, is the civic responsibility of each citizen in a democratic system.
- *Build Partnerships.* Strengthen business partnerships by identifying those in the community who advocate for equitable change. Forming coalitions to address the root causes of health disparities raises the likelihood of making a change.
- *Monitor Impact and Reassess Processes.* Reducing health disparities will not occur overnight and may take years, decades, and even generations to see impactful results. Celebrate and reinforce small successes, and make adjustments as needed when results aren't as expected. During the evaluation and reevaluation process, it is important to compare the marginalized groups to the advantaged groups rather than to the general population as a whole to truly achieve equity.[29]

In response to the problem of inequities in physical activity and overall health in the United States, the American College of Sports Medicine (ACSM) has developed a national road map that supports achieving health equity through a physically active lifestyle.[30] The actionable, integrated pathways that provide the foundation of ACSM's road map include the following:

- Communication. Raising awareness of the issue and magnitude of health inequities and conveying the power of physical activity in promoting health equity;
- Education. Developing educational resources to improve cultural competency for health care providers and fitness professionals as well as developing new community-based programs for lay health workers;
- Collaboration. Building partnerships and programs that integrate existing infrastructure and leverage institutional knowledge, reach, and voices of public, private, and community organizations; and
- Evaluation. Ensuring that ACSM attains measurable progress in reducing physical activity disparities to promote health equity.[30]

Providing Services to Vulnerable Populations

It is important to be particularly aware when providing health care services to vulnerable populations. Vulnerable populations can be defined as those who are at greater risk for poor health status and health care access and who experience significant disparities in life expectancy, access to and use of health care services, morbidity, and mortality.[31] Vulnerable populations can include patients who are racial or ethnic minorities, children, older adults, socioeconomically disadvantaged, veterans, immigrants, underinsured or those with certain medical conditions.[31] Some granting agencies require specific activities and outcomes related to increasing access to health services and health outcomes for vulnerable populations.

Domestic and International Outreach

Health care professionals in the United States have the opportunity to serve both domestically and internationally. This opportunity includes understanding the roles and responsibilities in domestic and international outreach. Throughout the history of colonization by Western countries, education, religion, and medicine are a few of the footprints left in countries around the world. Although the benefits of Western involvement remain, traditional cultures and practices are also present and are important to acknowledge and engage with to foster effective and respectful communication and beneficial services.

Preparing for international travel for service or pleasure or traveling domestically outside of one's traditional community (eg, to settings such as urban or Appalachian), individuals have a civic responsibility to understand the host community, culture, and people. To presume that all cultures are open and accepting of Westernized practices when entering into a community, whether international or within a country, can be detrimental to the establishment of relationships and, ultimately, a disservice to the people that were intended to be served.

White savior complex is an ideology that is acted upon when a white person, from a position of superiority, approaches a community to attempt to help or "save" a Black, Indigenous, or People of Color (BIPOC).[32] This occurs regardless of intentionality and is rooted in historical events such as colonization. Today, it is often manifested through humanitarian efforts.[32] White saviorism can lead to poorer life and health outcomes of BIPOC.[32] While working in a community, be sure to understand the prime importance of relationship building, to first listen before making decisions, and always consider what structural or systemic barriers exist to influence the well-being of the person in the host community, rather than adhering to your own individual point of view as a visitor. Thinking of the negative effects of White savior complex, reflect on the one community's response, as reflected in the excerpt To Hell With Good Intentions (Box 11.2).[33]

Service-Learning and the Role of Physical Therapy

Physical therapists can be instrumental in providing community-level interventions and services and empowering individuals to be their own health advocate. Service-learning is a structured learning experience that combines community service with preparation and

---

vulnerable populations – people at greater risk for poor health status and health care access, who experience significant disparities in life expectancy, access to and use of health care services, morbidity, and mortality

service-learning – is a structured learning experience that combines community service with preparation and reflection

BOX 11.2 • To Hell With Good Intentions

An address by Ivan Illich to the Conference on InterAmerican Student Projects (CIASP) in Cuernavaca, Mexico, on April 20, 1968.

I did not come here to argue. I am here to tell you, if possible, to convince you, and hopefully, to stop you, from pretentiously imposing yourselves on Mexicans. I do have deep faith in the enormous good will of the US volunteer. However, his good faith can usually be explained only by an abysmal lack of intuitive delicacy. By definition, you cannot help being ultimately vacationing salesmen for the middle-class "American Way of Life," since that is really the only life you know.

If you have any sense of responsibility at all, stay with your riots here at home. Work for the coming elections: You will know what you are doing, why you are doing it, and how to communicate with those to whom you speak. And you will know when you fail. If you insist on working with the poor, if this is your vocation, then at least work among the poor who can tell you to go to hell. It is incredibly unfair for you to impose yourselves on a village where you are so linguistically deaf and dumb that you don't even understand what you are doing, or what people think of you. And it is profoundly damaging to yourselves when you define something that you want to do as "good," a "sacrifice" and "help." I am here to suggest that you voluntarily renounce exercising the power which being an American gives you. I am here to entreat you to freely, consciously and humbly give up the legal right you have to impose your benevolence on Mexico. I am here to challenge you to recognize your inability, your powerlessness and your incapacity to do the "good" which you intended to do. I am here to entreat you to use your money, your status and your education to travel in Latin America. Come to look, come to climb our mountains, to enjoy our flowers. Come to study. But do not come to help.

Reprinted with permission from Illich I. To hell with good intentions (1968). In: Kendall JC, eds. *Combining Service and Learning: A Resource Book for Community and Public Service.* Vol I. National Society for Internships and Experiential Education; 1990:314-320.

---

reflection.[34] It can be an effective method of self and community learning when implemented correctly in community settings. It is important to center service-learning on the community and reflect on the value of reciprocal learning between health care professionals and community partners. Traditional definitions of "teacher" and "learner" are blurred in service-learning, because both the health care professional and the community partners play an active role in each. Proper preparation, such as understanding the community, and daily reflection on the part of the participants are important parts of the service-learning experience. Whether through service-learning or the business of health care, physical therapists should include local community partners in activities, while offering a fair compensation for their time. See Table 11.3 for a comparison of what service-learning is and what service-learning is not.[34]

Preparing for Service-Learning

Communication is defined equally by both the receiver and the person delivering the information. Thus, it is important to be mindful of how physical therapists approach and communicate from the first encounter and throughout the engagement with a community partner (see Chapter 8).

Understanding the community and establishing trust is a vital role in successful learning. Strength-based assessments are a client-led approach to fostering discussion on a

strength-based assessments – a client-led approach to identifying a community's strengths that recognizes the client's and community's ability to be a resource and partner in the endeavor

Table 11.3 What Is Service-Learning[34]

Important Elements of Service-Learning	What Service-Learning Is Not
A form of experiential education	An add-on to an existing curriculum
Addresses human and community issues and needs	An episodic volunteer program
Occurs through active participation in thoughtfully organized service	Logging a set number of community service hours in order to graduate
Includes structured reflection linking experience to learning	Compensatory service assigned as a form of punishment by the courts or by school administrators
Coordinated in true collaboration with the community	Only for high school or college students
Links to curriculum and/or co-curriculum, but must include structured time for reflection	One-sided: benefiting only students or only the community
Leads to acquisition of new skills, knowledge, leadership, and a sense of caring and social responsibility	

Information was compiled from Racine WI. The Johnson Foundation. National Service-Learning Clearinghouse.

client's and community's strengths and to illuminating the individual's and community's ability to be a resource and partner.[35] On the other end, **needs-based assessments** aim to capture the gaps, whether knowledge, physical, or systematic, that impede an individual or community from reaching optimal health outcomes.[36] Understanding both a strength-based and needs-based assessment can capture the current condition and realistic probability of an individual's ability to engage in learning and increase in a health outcome. Beginning with a strengths-based assessment mindset can not only communicate and highlight the positive resources within the community but can also be a sign of respect that acknowledges and affirms what the community has been able to build.

Prior to working with a domestic or international community, considering the following:

- *Listen.* Engage in deep listening with the community partner. Fully reflect on the stories of successes and strengths as well as challenges and perceived root causes. Engage in reflective listening before engaging in conversations around solutions or next steps.
- *Maintain Eye Contact.* Physical therapy work should always be person centered. Maintain eye contact with the community partner when listening, conversing, and during discussions. If the physical therapist is using an interpreter for support, be sure to make eye contact with the community partner when listening and giving responses rather than talking to the interpreter.
- *Learn Phrases in Local Languages.* If traveling internationally, take the time to review local phrases such as simple greetings. When working within the United States, there are additional resources to support communication across multiple languages. Nondiscrimination in Healthcare Programs and Activities under Section 1557 in the Affordable Health Care Act gives guidance around translation services and aims to reduce health disparities and protect vulnerable populations against discrimination in health care, including individuals with limited English proficiency (Section 1557).[37]
- *Identify the Local Expert (Champion):* Identifying a local expert, or champion, can increase a physical therapist's understanding of community norms and practices and

needs-based assessments – a process of capturing the gaps, whether knowledge, physical, or systematic, that impede an individual or community from reaching optimal health outcomes

increase community buy-in. People may be uncomfortable discussing health concerns and being examined by a health professional who is not a member of their group or who is insensitive to their cultural beliefs and practices. Working with a local expert can increase the learning experience for the physical therapists and understand the community's unique systems and needs.

- *Contact the International Health Care Association.* The World Confederation for Physical Therapy/Physiotherapy World (website: https://world.physio/) is just one of the professional organizations that provide a resource to member organizations in various regions of the world. Contact and collaboration with the international health care organization can promote an efficient and respectful collaboration within the global community.
- *Use Community Health Workers.* Community health workers (CHWs), including physicians and nurses, have multiple benefits for both the health care business and the community and overall goals for optimal well-being. Identify the local experts in the community who are providing health care services, people who are trained, or want to be trained in rehabilitation, to optimize the health of the community. Integrate the skills and value of CHWs in the health care plan, ensuring the professionals are also receiving a fair compensation for their services.
- *Use Training of Trainers Model.* When teaching or communicating a new skill, the Training of Trainers Model engages professionals to engage individuals or community members on key functions to be advocates on a particular skill. Physical therapists and other health professionals should effectively conduct skill-based communication and training when appropriate.[38]

Documentation

For all populations, proper documentation is a necessary component of health care services. In the traditional health care setting in the United States, this is a requirement. In other areas of the world, the requirements and safeguards may be more lax or not as important. The health care provider should always keep in mind the cultural expectations and ethical obligation that guides clinical practice regardless of the country of practice. Physical therapists should also consider the importance of documentation when providing services in untraditional settings. These untraditional settings can include verbal consultations in day-to-day conversations, services provided to family or friends, and domestic or international service-learning experiences. All types of documentation should be thorough, including services provided and time spent with the individual. Like other personal health information, service documentation should be kept confidential, written or provided in a manner that is understood by the intended audience, and secured from public disclosure.

Ethical Considerations

Collecting health metrics and conducting research is vital to monitoring progress or barriers to progress for health care professionals to best serve the intended individuals. It is also important to understand and reflect on the relationship and how power affects research policy in framing, planning, and implementation in the business of health care. Historically, many research practices have been viewed by individuals or a community as piratic, where patient or community data is extracted and used for purposes outside the context and sometimes in ways that were not in the best interest of the community being "researched."[39] All too often, researchers capitalize on people's progress, wisdom, and lived experiences, resulting in prestigious publications and esteemed grants to continue funding departments and businesses, while leaving the individuals and communities unpaid and unacknowledged. As a step toward equity in research, researchers should be intentional in the returns and recognition provided to the community during and after the research process. Some ways to include the community can be through recognition of authorship, fair wages for time, and implementing and monitoring activities, all of which result in real, unambiguous change.

Summary

The role of the physical therapists is historically and deeply rooted in the spirit of public health. Current roles and responsibilities of physical therapists are often intertwined with both the individual and population health practices. In this chapter, the responsibilities of the physical therapists in the context of both service provider and in the business of health care is discussed with a broader application to the global agenda and community needs. The MDG and SDG provide an overarching guide and vision for all health professionals to achieve the goal of health. Within those goals, understanding health metrics and reporting mechanisms is important in order to not only understand progress but also maintain funding streams. Key questions arise at this time: What metrics are appropriate both for the funder and to understand patient outcomes? Who are the funders and what outcomes do they want to see in order to maintain funding for the services? Do the funders' requirements match the need of the community and that of the individual?

A physical therapist has a unique role in balancing the goals of the business of health care and those of the community being served. Uncovering SDOH and health disparities is the first step in understanding a patient's full story that includes the strengths and barriers to improvements in care. The physical therapist can be engaged in this process by recognizing health disparities and actively participating in administrative duties such as proper documentation of the services provided, monitoring cancellation rates (which may indicate a barrier to access instead of a desire on the part of the patient), and the volume, type, and duration of services delivered to certain populations. Advocating for larger systemic changes by identifying and acting on unfavorable health metrics, participating with community organizations, and engaging in civic activities, such as voting, are appropriate methods to address the task of reducing negative SDOH and reducing health disparities.

When planning civic engagement, the physical therapist, as well as other people involved in the life of the community, can take one step forward to "[e]nsure healthy lives and promote well-being for all ages."[19]

REFERENCES

1. American Psychological Association. Civic engagement. Published 2009. Accessed July 7, 2022. https://www.apa.org/education-career/undergrad/civic-engagement
2. American Public Health Association. What is public health? Published 2021. Accessed July 7, 2022. https://www.apha.org/what-is-public-health
3. American Physical Therapy Association. Public health and population care. Accessed July 7, 2022. https://www.apta.org/patient-care/public-health-population-care
4. Rogers N. Polio and its role in shaping American physical therapy. *Phys Ther.* 2021; 101(6): pzab126. doi:10.1093/ptj/pzab126
5. American Public Health Association. APTA history. Accessed July 7, 2022. https://www.apta.org/apta-history
6. Bonfiglioli Stagni S, Tomba P, Viganò A, Zati A, Benedetti MG. The First World War drives rehabilitation toward the modern concepts of disability and participation. *Eur J Phys Rehabil Med.* 2015;51(3): 331–336. Accessed July 7, 2022. https://www.researchgate.net/profile/Anna-Vigano-2/publication/275895 409_The_First_World_War_drives_rehabilitation_toward_the_modern_concepts_of_disability_and_ participation/links/5c9b242a92851cf0ae9a0725/The-First-World-War-drives-rehabilitation-toward-the-modern-concepts-of-disability-and-participation.pdf
7. Moffat M. The history of physical therapy practice in the United States. *J Phys Ther Educ.* 2003;17(3):15–25.

Chapter 11 / Civic Engagement

8. Health Resources & Services Administration. Hill-Burton free and reduced-cost health care. Published March 2022. Accessed July 7, 2022. https://www.hrsa.gov/get-health-care/affordable/hill-burton

9. Above & Beyond Physical Therapy. Evolution of physical therapy. Published February 3, 2018. Accessed July 7, 2022. https://www.aboveandbeyondtherapy.com/evolution-of-physical-therapy/

10. Cohen W, Ball R. Social Security Amendments of 1967: summary and legislative history. *Social Security*. Published February 1968. Accessed April 26, 2024. https://www-origin.ssa.gov/policy/docs/ssb/v31n2/v31n2p3.pdf

11. Jacobsen KH. *Introduction to Global Health*. Jones & Bartlett Publishers; 2014.

12. Institute for Healthcare Improvement. Population health. Accessed July 7, 2022. http://www.ihi.org:80/Topics/Population-Health/Pages/default.aspx

13. Hernandez JB, Kim P. Epidemiology morbidity and mortality. In: *StatPearls*. StatPearls Publishing. Published October 9, 2021. Accessed July 7, 2022. http://www.ncbi.nlm.nih.gov/books/NBK547668/

14. Center for Disease Control and Prevention. Principles of epidemiology – Lesson 3 – Section 2. Published December 20, 2021. Accessed April 26, 2024. https://archive.cdc.gov/#/details?archive_url=https://archive.cdc.gov/www_cdc_gov/csels/dsepd/ss1978/lesson3/section2.html

15. Ortiz-Ospina E. "Life Expectancy" – What does this actually mean? Our World in Data website. https://ourworldindata.org/life-expectancy-how-is-it-calculated-and-how-should-it-be-interpreted. Published August 28, 2017. Accessed July 7, 2022.

16. Cheng W, Luo Y, Wang H, Liu X, Fu Y, Ronco C. Survival outcomes of hemoperfusion and hemodialysis versus hemodialysis in patients with end-stage renal disease: a systematic review and meta-analysis – abstract. *Blood Purif.* 2022;51(3):213–225. doi:10.1159/000514187

17. United Nations Development Programme. The Millennium Development Goals Report 2015. Published April 17, 2017. Accessed July 7, 2022. https://www.undp.org/publications/millennium-development-goals-report-2015

18. Waage J, Banerji K, Campbell O, et al. The Millennium Development Goals: a cross-sectoral analysis and principles for goal setting after 2015. The Lancet and London International Development Centre Commission. *Lancet.* 2010;376(9745):991–1023. doi:10.1016/S0140-6736(10)61196-8

19. United Nations Development Programme. Sustainable development goals. Accessed July 7, 2022. https://www.undp.org/sustainable-development-goals

20. United Nations Department of Economic and Social Affairs. #Envision2030: 17 goals to transform the world for persons with disabilities. Accessed August 14, 2022. https://www.un.org/development/desa/disabilities/envision2030.html

21. World Health Organization. Global Health Workforce statistics database. Accessed July 7, 2022. https://www.who.int/data/gho/data/themes/topics/health-workforce

22. Bill & Melinda Gates Foundation. The future of progress. Accessed July 7, 2022. https://www.gatesfoundation.org/goalkeepers/report/2022-report/#Intro

23. World Health Organization. Social determinants of health. Accessed July 7, 2022. https://www.who.int/health-topics/social-determinants-of-health

24. The Office of Disease Prevention and Health Promotion. Social determinants of health. Healthy People 2020. Accessed July 7, 2022. https://www.healthypeople.gov/2020/topics-objectives/topic/social-determinants-health/interventions-resources

25. Center of Disease Control and Prevention. About social determinants of health (SDOH). Published March 10, 2021. Accessed July 7, 2022. https://www.cdc.gov/socialdeterminants/about.html

26. Andermann A. Taking action on the social determinants of health in clinical practice: a framework for health professionals. *CMAJ.* 2016;188:E474-E483. doi:10.1503/cmaj.160177

27. Centers for Disease Control and Prevention. Health disparities. Accessed July 7, 2022. https://www.cdc.gov/healthyyouth/disparities/index.htm

28. Centers for Prevention MN. Health equity animated: equity vs equality. Published May 21, 2018. Accessed July 7, 2022. https://www.youtube.com/watch?v=tZd4no4gZnc

29. Chin MH, Clarke AR, Nocon RS, et al. A roadmap and best practices for organizations to reduce racial and ethnic disparities in health care. *J Gen Intern Med.* 2012;27(8):992-1000. doi:10.1007/s11606-012-2082-9

30. Hasson R, Brown DR, Dorn J, et al. Achieving equity in physical activity participation: ACSM experience and next steps. *Med Sci Sports Exerc.* 2017;49(4):848–858. doi:10.1249/MSS.0000000000001161

31. Waisel DB. Vulnerable populations in healthcare. *Curr Opin Anaesthesiol.* 2013;26(2):186–192. doi:10.1097/ACO.0b013e32835e8c17

32. Murphy C. White savior complex is a harmful approach to providing help—here's why. Health website. Published September 20, 2021. Accessed July 7, 2022 https://www.health.com/mind-body/health-diversity-inclusion/white-savior-complex

33. Illich I. To hell with good intentions. In: Kendall JC, ed, Combining Service and Learning: *A Resource Book for Community and Public Service*. Vol 1. National Society for Internships and Experiential Education: 1990:314–320.

34. Johns Hopkins Bloomberg School of Public Health. What is service learning? Accessed July 7, 2022. http://source.jhu.edu/publications-and-resources/service-learning-toolkit/what-is-service-learning.html
35. McCashen W. Communities of Hope: A Strengths-Based Resource for Building Community. St Luke's Innovative Resources; 2004.
36. Thyer B. *The Handbook of Social Work Research Methods*. SAGE Publications; 2009.
37. U.S. Department of Health & Human Services. Rights (OCR) O for C. Section 1557 of the Patient Protection and Affordable Care Act. Published July 22, 2010. Accessed July 7, 2022. https://www.hhs.gov/civil-rights/for-individuals/section-1557/index.html
38. Centers for Disease Control and Prevention. Understanding the training of trainers model. Healthy Schools. Published June 20, 2019. Accessed August 14, 2022. https://www.cdc.gov/healthyschools/tths/train_trainers_model.htm
39. Tilley L. Resisting piratic method by doing research otherwise. *Sociology*. 2017;51(1):27–42. doi:10.1177/0038038516656992

CHAPTER 12

Financial Literacy

MARK DRNACH

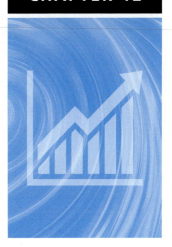

Learning Objectives

The reader will

1. Define financial literacy, and connect this concept with decisions made with personal finances.
2. Categorize wants versus needs with good or bad debt given a person's life situation.
3. Describe the basic components of a paycheck.
4. Develop, appraise, prioritize, and monitor a personal financial budget.
5. Develop a basic understanding of debt management and the role of interest rates on debt.

Financial literacy is an understanding of the skills, resources, and knowledge needed to process information and make decisions that have both business and personal financial consequences.[1] Basically, it is knowing how to manage your money taking into consideration the financial aspects, both long term and short term, of those decisions. By gaining financial literacy, a person will develop the critical thinking, refined judgment, and other skills necessary for making informed decisions both on a personal and on a business level.[2] Making sound and informed financial decisions has implications for an individual's sense of well-being and security, especially as they age.[3] A lack of understanding can impact the management of personal and/or business income and expenses, managing debt, building savings, planning for retirement income, choosing investments, or making personal financial portfolio/investment selections.[2] Financial literacy is of growing importance in an increasingly global, complex, and at times turbulent financial world. Understanding the basic principles and practices of finances is key in achieving financial success (See Chapters 1 and 2).

Financial Literacy

According to the US Financial Literacy and Education Commission, there are five principles of financial literacy.[4]

1. *Earn/Bringing in the cash*. Understand the details of a paycheck and annual income.
2. *Save and invest/Growing the cash*. "Pay yourself first" by putting a specific amount of money into a savings account. After the savings account has been addressed, a person may want to invest in other financial products (eg, financial portfolios, individual stocks). When investing, decide on the level of risk (the probability of losing money on an investment) the investment product provides.

3. *Protect/Maintaining the cash.* Keep an updated record of financial, investment, and insurance statements. Have an emergency fund (to cover approximately 3 months of monthly expenses) to pay for unexpected expenses, such as a new refrigerator, major car repairs, or unplanned trip for family or personal reasons. Understand the current insurance needs (eg, health, home, auto, life) and what the plans cover and what they don't. Be cautious with "get rich quick" schemes. Chasing opportunities that don't fit into a financial plan or structure can be costly.
4. *Spend/Managing cash outflows.* Create and follow a budget. Before making a major purchase, pause and decide if this is a *want* or a *need*. Be sure that the purchase is a good value by shopping around and comparing the price and content of other options. Purchase insurance plans (health, vision, dental, prescription drugs) that meet current needs. Take full advantage of benefits offered by an employer (eg, retirement matching dollars, no cost vision, or dental yearly exams).
5. *Borrow/Cash in that has to be paid back.* Not all debt is bad. Borrowing money enables essential purchases, such as going to college or buying a home. Borrowing money to invest in education or to purchase an asset, such as a house, that has the potential to increase the borrower's net worth, is considered to be good debt. Bad debt is money borrowed (with a high interest rate) for something that is a *want* and not a *need* and tends to depreciate over time, becoming less valuable and not adding to a borrower's net worth. When considering borrowing money and taking on debt, make sure there is a plan to manage the repayment of the debt.

These aspects of financial literacy are not inherently intuitive to most people. Formal education on financial literacy and the financial knowledge of the parents are known to be a significant factor in shaping the financial literacy of the person.[2] Educated parents have better access to economic resources, are likely to understand and manage their finances, and are likely to impart that information to their children. Financial literacy is not only the knowledge of financial concepts but also the skills, motivation, and confidence to apply such knowledge in order to make decisions to improve a persons' financial well-being. A person needs both the knowledge and the skills to be financially literate.[5] According to Lusardi, it is important to understand the following three concepts in most financial decision-making:

1. Understanding math to do interest rate calculations and understanding interest compounding.
2. Understanding inflation.
3. Understanding risk diversification.[5]

These concepts have been used to create a standard set of questions to measure the financial literacy of a person, referred to as the Big Three financial literacy questions[6] (Box 12.1).

This simple screen of a person's knowledge can help identify areas of deficiency and lead to a targeted approach to improve the person's financial literacy.

---

financial literacy – a decision-making process in which individual use a combination of skills, resources, and contextual knowledge to process information and make decisions with knowledge of the financial consequences of that decision

good debt – borrowed money that has the potential to increase a person's net worth

bad debt – borrowed money (with a high interest rate) for something that is a *want* and not a *need* and tends to depreciate over time without adding to the borrower's net worth

Chapter 12 / Financial Literacy

BOX 12.1 • The Big Three Financial Literacy Questions

1. Suppose you have $100 in a savings account and the interest rate was 2% per year. After 5 years, how much do you think you would have in the account if you left the money to grow?
   a. more than $102
   b. exactly $102
   c. less than $102
   d. do not know
   e. refuse to answer
2. Imagine the interest rate on your saving account was 1% per year and inflation was 2% per year. After 1 year, how much would you be able to buy with the money in this account?
   a. more than today
   b. exactly the same as today
   c. less than today
   d. do not know
   e. refuse to answer
3. Please tell me whether this statement is true or false. "Buying a single company's stock usually provides a safer return than a stock mutual fund."
   a. true
   b. false
   c. do not know
   d. refuse to answer

Answers.

1. A
2. C
3. B

From Lusardi A, Mitchell OS. Financial literacy around the world: an overview. *J Pension Econ Financ.* 2011;10(4): 497-508. Copyright © 2011 Cambridge University Press. Reproduced with permission.

Needs and Wants

Fundamental to the concept of financial well-being is an understanding of the difference between a need versus a want. Maslow presented a human-centered theory on motivation that categorized a human's basic needs in a hierarchical fashion, where the appearance of one need rests on the prior satisfaction of another[7] (see Chapter 1). People need the basic necessities of life such as food and water, shelter, work, a means of transportation, and a safe living environment. The money that a person earns is then spent on acquiring and maintaining these basic necessities.

Wants are things that a person desires or would like to have. People want a certain type of food or bottled water or a certain type of shelter or dwelling such as an apartment, condominium, or a house; they want to work for a specific company or in a specific type of business; they want a certain type of transportation or automobile; and they want to live in a specific geographic region or environment. Wants can add a level of enjoyment or happiness to life, a sense of contentment and achievement, but they are not necessary for survival. So before making a substantial purchase, the buyer should pause and ask: Is this a need or a want? Does this purchase add value to my net worth or detract from it? Is this expense necessary at this time? Some people make a purchase to fulfill a basic need and have no additional income to purchase a want. Their decision to purchase a need will

Table 12.1 Allocations Based on a Net Monthly Pay of $5,000			
Allocation	*Living Expenses*	*Savings*	*Expenses for Wants*
80/20	$4,000	$1,000	$0[a]
50/30/20	$2,500	$1,000	$1,500
70/20/10	$3,500	$500	$1,000

[a]Taken from living expenses.

be based on the availability, understanding, and the price of the good or service. This can impact the health services or insurance policies that are purchased, leading to variations in care or insurance coverage owing to socioeconomic factors that influence the purchase of a need versus a want (see Chapter 11). The purchase of a want is not a bad thing but should be done with an understanding of the value the item brings to the buyer and be within the buyer's budget.

There are several methods for budgeting income for needs and wants. These methods can range from an 80/20 rule, where 80% is allocated for expenses and 20% for savings, the 50/30/20 rule; where 50% is allocated toward needs/expenses, 30% toward wants, and 20% toward savings or debt repayment; or a 70/20/10 rule for the allocation of living expenses, including wants (70%), debt repayments (20%), and savings (10%).[8] The allocation method used will depend on the individual circumstances of the person (Table 12.1).

The allocation of income in a monthly budget is based on the amount of net income the person has available. A sole proprietor or independent contractor will have to deduct the self-employment tax from the monthly income received (see Chapter 5). If the person is an employee, there will be certain deductions taken from the paycheck that will impact the "take home pay" or net pay. Understanding the mandatory and voluntary deductions from a paycheck is fundamental to understanding the allocation of available funds.

The Paycheck

Many new employees focus on the annual salary that is offered to them to work as an employee for an entity and may be surprised when they receive their first paycheck, because the amount anticipated is not what is received once taxes and other deductibles are applied. If an employee is offered a salary of $50,000 per year, paid every other week, that is, 26 paydays per calendar year, the amount per pay would be anticipated to be $1,923. (50,000/26 = 1,923). That would be the gross pay, before mandatory taxes and voluntary payroll deductions are subtracted (Box 12.2). After the subtraction, the resulting amount of money would be the net pay.

The practice of taxing citizens of the United States stems back to the English Parliament, which implemented several taxes, such as a Sugar Act of 1764, that imposed taxation on American citizens who had no representation in the English Parliament. This was a major factor in the American Revolution. After achieving independence from England, the United States continues to collect taxes from workers' pay, known as an income tax, to help pay for the Revolutionary War debt. This was inconsistently applied until the ratification of the 16th Amendment to the United States Constitution in 1913, which legalized the use of personal income tax for federal government expenditures.[9] This Amendment also introduced the familiar 1040 form, which is used today. Tax dollars collected by the federal government are used to pay for the operations of the federal government and to fund federal programs (eg, national defense, the Centers for Disease Control and Prevention, Medicare, Social Security). Payroll taxes for Social Security are collected under the authority of the Federal Insurance Contribution Act (FICA), which fund the Social Security program and

Chapter 12 / Financial Literacy

267

BOX 12.2 • Paycheck Deductions

Mandatory payroll tax deductions include the following:
- Federal income tax (depends on earnings and W2 information)
- Social Security tax (6.2% up to the annual maximum)[a]
- Medicare tax (1.45%)[a]
- State income tax (varies depending on the state)
- Various local taxes and fees (such as city, county, or school district taxes, or an occupational tax).

Voluntary payroll deductions may include the following:
- Health insurance premiums
- Retirement plan contributions (401k, 403b, IRA plans)
- Health Saving Account contributions
- Dental, vision, or life insurance deductions

[a]Internal Revenue Service. Topic no. 571, Social Security and Medicare withholding rates. Updated April 7, 2023. Accessed August 31, 2023. https://www.irs.gov/taxtopics/tc751

---

the Medicare program.[10] Both the employee and the employer are required to contribute to the FICA taxes through payroll deductions.

Federal income tax is based on the amounts of income earned in a calendar year and the situation of the individual, such as single, married, and number of dependents (ie, a person who depends on the tax payer for a specific amount of financial support). The amount of federal tax deducted from a paycheck depends on the allowances claimed on the Internal Revenue Service's (IRS) W-4 form.[11] The W-4 form is an employee's withholding allowance certificate, which records the status of the employee as well as the number of dependents in the household (available at https://www.irs.gov/forms-pubs/about-form-w-4). Information reported on the W-4 form directs the employer to withhold the correct amount of federal income tax from an employee's paycheck. If too little is withheld, the employee will generally owe money to the federal government at the end of the year, possibly including a penalty. If too much money is withheld, a refund will generally be due to the employee. That refund does not collect interest during the year, so the federal government is getting the employee's money interest free for the year. The employee also does not have that money to purchase essential needs or desired wants. Some people over withhold to be certain that they owe nothing and/or use it as a savings plan for the year, albeit one that doesn't grow with interest. This strategy may be better in a low interest rate environment as opposed to a high interest rate environment. It is important to try to keep either the payment or refund as low as possible. The employee should complete a new W-4 form when changes to personal or financial situations would change the entries on the form (eg, marriage, divorce, adding or removing dependents). This will ensure that the appropriate amount of taxes is deducted from a paycheck and optimize the amount of income received.

States also have the authority to tax their citizens income, but not all states do so. Those that do not tax income receive monies from taxes on other items such as tax on sales of goods or property owned. State monies are used for state programs such as funding Medicaid, public education, and the fire, police, and health agencies in the state.

In addition to taxation, other monies can be deducted from an employee's paycheck. These include deductions for health care premiums, retirement contributions, and health

---

W-4 form – an IRS form, also called the employee's withholding allowance certificate, that directs the employer to deduct money from an employee's paycheck based on the information provided on the form

Budgeting

The first step toward properly managing finances is preparing a budget. A budget is a financial statement of the estimated income and expenditures covering a specified future period of time such as a month, 6 months, or a year. It is an important process that establishes an allocation of income toward personal financial goals and provides data on how income and expenses are used in a given period of time (see Chapter 2). It is important to remember that budgets are pro forma statements, meaning that they are a best guess of what is going to happen in the future. Therefore, changes in the budget, either for a business or a person, are not necessarily bad. Budgeting is a dynamic process that allows a person to see how they are spending money and then make timely decisions on personal behaviors/expenditures in order to meet a financial goal such as saving for retirement, going on vacation, or purchasing a house. By monitoring expenditures, typically on a monthly basis, decisions can be made to better align spending and saving behaviors toward personal financial targets (eg, 70/20/10 rule).

The budgeting process begins with the identification of personal financial objectives (Box 12.3). This process of recording the objective, either on paper or electronically, can help set the framework in which financial decisions are made. If the goal is to pay off debt in 5 years, save enough money for a down payment on a house in 7 years, or save a specific amount of money per year for travel, starting with the end goal allows the person to make realistic allocation decisions with the finite amount of income coming in each month or year. Once one or a few personal financial objectives are identified, the next step is to identify the monthly income. This income will come from a primary source, the full-time job, and often from a secondary source, which could be either a significant other's contribution to the household budget or a second source of income generated by working either part time or PRN (as needed) (see Chapter 5). Income diversification provides income from two or more sources to the monthly income received. This can be an *active source of income*, where the person generates the income from actively working to earn it, or a *passive source of income,* where the person's income is not provided by the primary employer but is earned through other means, which do not require too much effort once the system is established, such as interest on investments, rent received from property owned, or income from online businesses or products sold. The total estimated monthly income is then identified, before taxes and other deductions. By identifying the income before deductions, the allocation of mandatory and voluntary deductions can be evaluated. The mandatory taxes such as Medicare, Social Security, Federal Withholding (based on the information on the W-4 form), and state and local taxes and fees are then deducted. These mandatory deductions are required, whereas voluntary deductions do not always apply to a person's life situation. An example is a person who does not require corrective lenses to see clearly. How often would that person go to the optometrist for an examination? Is the total amount of annual insurance premiums more than the cost of a periodic examination? It depends on the persons' individual situation.

---

budget – a financial statement of the estimated income and expenditures covering a specified future period of time such as a month, 6 months, or a year

pro forma – a term used with financial statements to denote a best guess or estimate of what is going to happen in the future

income diversification – income from two or more sources

Chapter 12 / Financial Literacy 269

BOX 12.3 • Personal Financial Planning: The Budget

a. Personal financial objective
b. Estimated monthly income
   Primary source
   Secondary source
   Gross monthly income
   Deductions
   Mandatory deductions (taxes)
       Medicare = 1.45%
       Social security = 6.2%
       Federal withholding tax (single) = 22%
       State = 4%
       Local (including fees) = 2%
   Other voluntary deductions
       Health insurance
       Dental insurance
       Vision insurance
       Life insurance
       Disability insurance
   Total take home monthly pay
c. Expenditures
   Rent or mortgage
   Loans
   Education
   Auto
   Credit card debt
   Other
       Insurance
       (in addition to what the employer provides)
   Professional liability
   Life insurance
   Disability insurance
   Long-term care insurance
   Gasoline
   Food
   Utilities
   Water
   Gas for heating or AC
   Sewage
   Electric
   Phone/cell
   Internet
   Medical or dental expenses
       (incl. prescriptions or copays)
   Gifts to charity
   Entertainment (eg, dining out)
   Total monthly expenditures
d. Revenues − Expenses

(continued)

BOX 12.3 • Personal Financial Planning: The Budget (*continued*)

e. Monthly savings
   Emergency fund
   Retirement fund
   General savings
   Investment fund

The same applies to life insurance. The need for life insurance should be predicated on the financial need of those left behind if the person dies unexpectedly. Who will need that financial support? How much will they need? It depends on the person's individual situation. *Term life insurance* is bought and paid for during a specific term of a person's life (eg, 10-20 years), such as when a person has a family or others who are financially dependent on them. This policy will pay the beneficiaries when the person dies but is valid only during the *term* that is paid into, typically on a monthly basis. Once payments are stopped, the term has ended, the insurance ends, and there is no further financial benefit. *Whole life insurance* or permanent life insurance also provides a payout to the beneficiaries when the insured person dies but is kept for a person's whole life, not for a specific term or period of life. Whole life insurance policies typically have a cash element that can be withdrawn by the policy owner at a certain point but reduces the death benefit to the beneficiaries. The premiums for term life are generally lower than for those of whole life.

The voluntary insurance programs should be evaluated for their usefulness and applicability to the person paying for them. It is important to take the time to evaluate what the insurance program has to offer during the enrollment period (see Chapter 4) that is available and to make an informed decision based on the needs and desires of the person, the amount of risk a person is willing to take, and the cost between the insurance premium and the cost for paying cash for the service if, or when, it is delivered.

Purchasing property or a house is a significant investment in a person's life. Often, people take out a mortgage to pay for such assets. This could be considered good debt if it enhances one's quality of life and/or has the potential for the asset to increase the net worth of the person. Monthly mortgage payments are generally a fixed cost (ie, fixed-rate mortgage) and do not vary month by month (see Chapter 1). Some mortgages (ie, adjustable-rate mortgage) do vary at specific time intervals, depending on the terms of the mortgage, but are generally fixed for a period of time. Mortgage and other loan payments have to be deducted from the monthly income. Consistent repayment of loans helps to improve a person's credit score, which many institutional lenders use to evaluate the risk of lending money to a person. It is important to repay loans in a consistent and timely manner.

Other types of insurance plans may be appropriate for a person. Additional life insurance, disability insurance, or long-term care insurance may be appropriate to have in addition to what the employer provides. This will provide the person with insurance that will stay in place if or when the person's employment changes. A licensed health care provider should have personal professional liability insurance to cover any unforeseen liability issue that arises outside of their place of employment. Liability insurance provided by the employer covers the actions of the persons when they are acting as an employee. Other actions outside of the work environment, where the health care provider is acting within the scope of practice, may open the health care provider to a financial risk in the event of an adverse outcome (Chapter 10). Having insurance to cover for any adverse events that may result from these encounters is prudent and protects the health care provider's personal assets.

Next in the budgeting process is the allocation of variable costs or expenses (Chapter 1). These costs vary depending on their usage and should be monitored for their effect on the overall budgeting of the monthly income. Shopping around for appropriate internet or

Chapter 12 / Financial Literacy

BOX 12.4 • General Guideline for Budgeting

- Have a system of recordkeeping of income and expenses (a budget).
- Pay yourself first in the allocation of income, after taking deductions.
- Use your employer's matching contributions to retirement funds; it is free money.
- Save for an emergency fund to cover the 3 to 6 months of expenses.
- Buy life insurance for your stage of life.
- Limit the cost of a house to no more than 4 times your annual salary.
- A mortgage payment is approximately 10% of the cost of the loan. Make sure it fits into your budget.
- Evaluate spending monthly and monitor every payday. For other investments, monitor quarterly.
- Have a least an annual meeting with a financial advisor.
- Control your variable costs/expenses.

cell phone services, gasoline prices, which can vary by state or station, and the prudent use of utilities, helps to keep these expenses at their lowest cost, allowing the person to maximize discretionary income. This is the income that is available after the mandatory and voluntary deductions are made: the income for nonessential items. The allocation of discretionary income should go toward an emergency fund to allow for the payment of monthly expenditures if the flow of income is disrupted for any reason (typically 3-6 months of expenses) and other funds to be used for future needs (eg, retirement, savings, or investment). These funds are often those that a person should allocate income to first (ie, pay yourself first) before those variable expenses listed previously.

Allocating income to a savings account first is a form of self-investment to obtain a future financial position. It reflects a priority on how income is used and determines the amount of income that is available for the remaining budget (Box 12.4). By working with a budget, a person gains a better understanding of how monthly income is spent and a more realistic understanding of how much income is needed and allocated to meet a financial goal within a specific timeline.

Debt Management

Approximately one in three Americans feel constrained by their debt, that is, their debt and debt payments prevent them from adequately addressing other financial priorities.[12] This can be a significant financial concern for the new graduate from higher education, especially if a student took out a loan, either from the federal government or from a private entity (eg, bank), to pay for the education. How does one basically manage debt? The first step in the process is to *identify a financial objective* that the person would like to achieve within a specific period of time. This is necessary in order to develop a framework in which the person can objectively allocate income, at a reasonable level, to achieve a financial goal, in a reasonable amount of time. Once the financial objective is clear, the next step is to *understand the current finances* of the individual. This would be the income from all sources and all expenses incurred in a specific time period, typically 1 month. Setting up and using a proper recordkeeping system for identifying income and categorizing expenses is basic to understanding and appropriately managing resources (Chapter 2). Also reflecting on the expenses for *needs* versus *wants* is helpful in identifying and shaping spending

discretionary income – income that is available after the mandatory and voluntary deductions

habits. Impulse buying, a spontaneous, unplanned purchase, often done with online, in retail, or in grocery store shopping, can have a detrimental effect on an adopted budgeting method.[13] Marketing concepts are used to entice the consumer to purchase a specific product. With that in mind, the consumer should pause and make an informed decision on the personal relevance of the information presented about the product, the *need* versus the *want* for the product, and the added value the product brings to the person's life. Impulse buying is not necessarily a bad behavior but should be identified as the choice that is being made at the moment and managed so it does not significantly impact the budget. (eg, you go to the grocery store and see a food item that is not on your list of items to purchase, and you decide to purchase it because you like it and now desire to have it. There is no *need* for the item but you *want* to purchase it, and the amount of income spent does not significantly impact the budget.) Impulse buying behavior, when done frequently and for significant amounts, can build up and be a major expense in the monthly budget. It is reported that over 80% of American adults have reported impulse buying, with 44% of them later regretting their decision.[14] To manage debt, minimize the costs that add to a person's overall debt, manage expenses, and reflect on buying habits.

Impulse buying is probably not the biggest expense in a person's budget. More likely, it is a loan repayment taken out for the purchase of an education degree or a mortgage for a house or for the purchase of a car. There are basically two types of loans, *secured* and *unsecured*. A secured loan is backed by an asset of the borrower, such as a house, property, or car. If the borrower cannot pay back the loan (ie, default) the lender can take the asset that backed the loan. An unsecured loan is not backed by an asset of the borrower and therefore comes with an increased cost and interest rates. A credit card is a type of unsecured loan. Failure to pay back an unsecured loan can result in the assignment of additional fees, involvement of a collection agency, damage to a credit score, or legal actions taken against the borrower. Both types of loans assign an interest rate to the amount of the loan called the principal.

To understand debt management, a person should understand the practice of charging interest on the amount of money borrowed. Interest is the monetary charge by the lender for the loan. If a borrower takes out a loan for $100,000 (the principal), for 1 year at a 7% interest rate, the interest charged would be $7,000 for the $100,000 loan. The lender would make $7,000 on the loan, which is the incentive for lending money. What if the term, or length, of the loan was for 10 years, with all of the principal due at the end of the loan term (ie, at the end of the 10th year)? The amount of interest to be paid would be $7,000 times 10 or $70,000. If the borrower makes a monthly payment, that payment will reduce the principal amount, on which interest is based, thereby lowering the total amount of interest charged over the course of the 10 years; much less than $70,000. Loan agreements typically list the monthly payment expectation, breaking down the payment into the principal payment plus the interest payment, which will vary with the age of the loan. In this $100,000 example, the total monthly payment (principal + interest) would be $1,161. The total interest paid over the term of the loan would be $39,330, with a total repayment of $139,330.[15] If the borrower only pays the interest each month, after 10 years they would still owe $100,000. If the borrower pays the monthly payment plus an additional $100 per month,

impulse buying – a spontaneous, unplanned purchase

secured loan – a loan that is backed by an asset of the borrower

unsecured loan – a loan that is not backed by an asset of the borrower

principal – the amount of money that is borrowed, not including interest or fees

interest – the monetary charge by the lender for the loan

Chapter 12 / Financial Literacy

which would go toward lowering the principal balance and interest charged, the loan would be paid off 1 year earlier, and the borrower would save $4,700 in interest payments.[15] The preceding example applies a simple interest rate calculation. In reality, the lender will advertise their loans with an annual percentage rate (APR), expressed as an interest rate, which includes the interest on the loan plus the lender's fees and reflects the total annual cost for the loan. This is typically higher than the simple interest rate and the real effective rate that the borrower pays. The lender is not obligated to include all of the fees in the APR and it is therefore important that the borrower be clear on what is included in the APR and any additional fees or costs associated with the loan. The Truth in Lending Act requires lenders to tell, in writing, the loan's APR and other financial specifics about the loan (eg, the total amount financed, additional charges, the total amount that will be paid).[16]

Credit cards are another source of debt. Eighty-two percent of adults in the United States had a credit card in 2022 and were nearly evenly split between the people who paid off their balances each month and people who carried balances forward from month to month.[17] The average credit card debt per borrower in 2022 was approximately $5,900,[18] with the average APR ranging from 16% to 24%.[19] This is a significant expense in a monthly budget that can be managed through savings, deferred spending, paying off credit card balances monthly, and shopping for the best APR and credit card benefits that align with personal goals (eg, airline points, travel protection, cash rewards). An interesting aspect of credit card debt is that the interest is typically compounded daily, as opposed the monthly or annually, and it is this compounding method that costs the borrower the most in interest paid for a given interest rate. Compounding interest is the application of an interest charge at a specified period of time (eg, daily) to the principal amount, thereby increasing the principal's value.

If a person has a $5,000 credit card balance at an annual APR of 24%, the daily interest rate would be 0.00065% (24% APR/365 days/year = percent per day). That would mean that $3.25 ($5,000 × 0.00065 = $3.25) is added to the outstanding balance on that day; $5,000 + $3.25 = $5,003.25. The next day, the interest is calculated on this new balance. The pennies will add up. Although the interest is compounded daily, the lender may only credit it to an account at a certain time, such as weekly or monthly. Most credit card companies also provide a grace period on purchases made by the cardholder.[20] If the balance is paid in full by the due date, the card holder avoids paying interest on the money borrowed for the purchase. If the balance is not paid in full, the cardholder will be charged interest on the unpaid portion of the balance due. That unpaid balance also activates the charging of interest on any new purchases made in the new billing cycle. In almost every circumstance, carried credit card debt is bad debt resulting from the high interest rate charged and the compounding method. The bottom line is to pay the balance of your credit cards monthly.

One way to manage the costs of a student loan is to refinance the loan when interest rates are more favorable to the borrower. By *refinancing* the loan, the old loan is paid in full, and the new loan is acquired with a lower interest rate and different term (ie, length of time to repay).

Before refinancing, make sure that the new loan will save money in the long term. Having a new loan with a lower interest rate but a longer term may result in a higher payout in the end. Ideally, the borrower wants a new loan with the lower interest rate and a shorter term to pay off the loan. Also, if the old loan was from the federal government

annual percentage rate (APR) – the total cost for a loan, including the interest rate and institutional fees

compounding interest – the application of an interest charge at a specified period of time (eg, daily) to the principal amount, thereby increasing the principal's value

and the new loan is from a private institution/bank, the borrower no longer has a government loan and may not be eligible for any government loan forgiveness program that is available.[21] Some student loans provided by the federal government may be eligible for a federal *loan forgiveness* program (eg, Public Service Loan Forgiveness). A typical requirement for these programs is that the borrower has a history of consistently making payments on time, over a number of years (eg, 10-20 years).[22,23] Federal student loans may have the option of income-driven repayment plans.[24] This is another option for the borrower to explore, although availability is often subject to legislation or other government action that is subject to change. In these plans, the borrower's monthly payments are based on income and can be more manageable. *Consolidating* student loans is different than refinancing. When consolidating several loans into one new loan, the lender typically takes the weighted average of interest from all the loans and creates one interest rate for the new loan. Although this consolidation leaves the borrower with one payment to make in a month, it does not necessarily provide the borrower with the lowest interest rate, and/or the borrower may pay more in interest over time. Also, debt consolidation does not address the underlying debt management problem. The services of a professional financial adviser can be helpful.

Personal Financial Advisors

Individuals seek the aid of financial advisors for many reasons but mainly to satisfy a set of needs. These needs include acquiring "peace of mind," having access to the opinions of an expert, and delegating financial decisions[25,26] (Box 12.5). These needs can be addressed by advice and assistance with planning, which is a strong predictor of wealth accumulation. Those who plan tend to arrive at retirement with 2 to 3 times the amount of wealth than those who do not plan.[6] It is also known that the assistance of a financial expert can have a significant impact for those with lower levels of financial literacy.[2] Seeking advice on a financial plan should come from several different professional advisors according to a person's needs and wants. The advice of an accountant, attorney, insurance agent, investment specialists, and/or a financial planner may be necessary to provide the assistance and support to develop a comprehensive financial plan with realistic financial goals. It may take time to develop a good working relationship with these advisors, but it is helpful in an ever changing, and at times complex, financial and insurance environment. Similarly to health care providers, there are generalists and specialists in certain areas of insurance and finance (eg, certified public accountant or CPA, certified financial planner or CFP, certified insurance counselor or CIC). Each may have something different to offer depending on the person's current situation, acceptable level of risk, and financial goals. Having the right professional help—that really care about doing the right thing for the client as opposed to their financial interest alone—is important to achieve financial stability, which requires dedication to the process of accounting, budgeting, planning, and monitoring. With the changing global economic landscape, people are increasingly responsible for their personal financial planning and the utilization of their resources throughout their lifetime.[5] Having professionals to assist in this responsibility can provide some level of comfort, understanding, and control.

One aspect of financial planning that a professional advisor can provide is risk diversification. **Risk diversification** is a strategy to manage the risk of losing money by

risk diversification – a financial allocation strategy to manage the risk by investing in several different assets and/or business sectors within a financial portfolio

Chapter 12 / Financial Literacy

BOX 12.5 • Benefits of a Professional Advisor

Guidance—A professional advisor can provide a framework and suggestions when establishing a plan or adjusting a financial plan based on your current situation and goals. They are helpful in monitoring the performance of established plans for the relevance to your current situation and providing options when and if necessary.

Resources—A professional advisor can provide you with options and recommendations depending on the resources you have available. These resources may change when you receive a promotion with a pay raise; have a significant increase in your income from a secondary source; have additional expenses, such as a child or dependent; or experience a significant decrease in resources from a loss of employment or other income sources. Financial security is achieved through the efficient use of resources that you have available at any specific time.

Environment—A professional advisor typically keeps track of changes that are occurring or anticipated in tax laws, federal or state laws and regulations, insurance regulations, or some other outside factor that may impact a financial plan. Personally keeping up to date on these issues can be daunting if not impractical for many people. Achieving financial goals can be done through the efficient and timely use of resources.

Consistency—Working with a professional advisor and making consistent financial decisions in line with personal factors and goals is a significant part of achieving future financial success. Developing a long-term relationship with someone who understands your current situation, goals, and comfort level of risk can provide a level of comfort and confidence in the decisions made in financial planning.

Knowledge—Financial decisions are based on behaviors learned from families and/or historical practices. Working with a professional advisor can expand a person's knowledge of the different aspects of finance, insurance, and investment that will help develop a person's knowledge base and provide comfort with the decisions made.

Stability—To achieve financial success takes a lot of work to build the foundation. Creating a plan, monitoring the aspects of the plan, making decisions that grow resources and/or provide security to a person's assets, and knowing when to take action on aspects of the plan, owing to resource and/or situational changes, provide stability for sustained growth and movement toward your financial goal.

Source: Nelson J. Making structured personal financial decisions. In: Nosse LJ, Friberg DG, eds. *Management and Supervisory Principles for Physical Therapists.* 3rd ed. Wolters Kluwer Health/Lippincott Williams and Wilkins; 2010:463-476.

investing in several different assets (eg, stock, bond, cryptocurrency) and/or business sectors (eg, semiconductors, automobiles, digital streaming services) within a financial portfolio. This allocation of funds limits the effect of any one asset's or business sector's behavior on the overall portfolio's financial performance. By diversifying the investments, when the value of one area drops, the rise in value of the other areas can balance or minimize the effect. A financial adviser is helpful in this area of financial management by providing the investor with information and options to better understand and identify the level of risk the investor is willing to take, given the investor's personal life situation and financial goals.

In addition to the personal relationship, people have the ability to obtain advice and perform financial transactions on mobile devices through the internet, which has made access to financial services readily available (eg, banking, stock trades). People who use their mobile devices for making financial transactions have the benefit of the ease of access, available information, and options to make a decision whenever and wherever it is desired. The use of automated financial advice, a computerized online program that provides financial advice with minimal human interaction, is also available and typically at a lower cost than a human adviser. These systems, called robo advisors, follow an algorithm to understand the investors preferences, level of acceptable risk, and financial goals.[27] They can also reduce some of the behavioral bias that can be found in human financial advisors.[28] On the negative side, robo advisors will not know the client as well as the human adviser who can provide more individualized advice on setting and managing financial goals, counseling during market turndowns, or providing options during changes in the client's personal situation.[28] Although online access to financial services are available the purchaser should understand that having a working monthly budget, a comfortable level of savings for emergencies and retirement, and clear obtainable financial goals, should be established. Investments (ie, individual stock purchases) are typically done for a long-term return or a financial payout in the future. Having a sound financial plan in place for the short term (ie, monthly) guards against the accumulation of unmanageable debt and allows for the growth of savings to invest when appropriate. Gaining and applying knowledge of finances is necessary in achieving goals, especially when the process aids in the identification of patterns of overconsumption or situations that may create difficulty with money management.[29] Monitoring and adjusting a budget helps to shape the saving and spending habits of the person.

Monitoring

Identifying income/revenues and expenses and then creating a budget to target financial goals are the foundations of financial management. An active engagement in the budgeting process and a commitment to adhering to the budget are important to move a financial position toward a targeted goal. Remember that budgeting is a dynamic process that will change as life situations change. Having a basic understanding of economics (Chapter 2), accounting (Chapter 1), the classification of income, the behavior of expenses (Chapter 1), and budgeting support the strategic management of finances. It is prudent to review a budget at least monthly. Identify the variances to the budget and understand the reason for the variance. Developing a habit of monitoring a budget and working with the budget to meet short-term financial goals will ultimately lead to financial security in the long term (Box 12.6).

One goal of budgeting and financial management could be to monitor the percentage change in the gross annual income compared to the annual rate of inflation, as reported by the Consumer Price Index (CPI). The CPI is a measure of the average change over time in the prices paid by urban consumers for an identified collection of goods and services.[30] It is a common indicator of inflation reported by the US Bureau of Labor Statistics (www.bls .gov), which provides a national CPI as well as a CPI for various geographic regions in the country.[31] Ideally, the percentage growth in a person's annual income should keep up with the annual growth rate of inflation, often provided through an annual cost of living adjustment (COLA) to the employee's pay, or, for the private practitioner, through an increase in gross income from primary or secondary sources that keep the total gross income at or above the rate of inflation. By comparing the growth in annual gross income (from all sources) to the rate of inflation (ie, geographic CPI), a person can have a better understanding of the purchasing power of the income earned over the years. This feedback can be an evaluation of past decisions made and have a positive impact on

robo advisor – a computerized online program that provides financial advice with minimal human interaction

Consumer Price Index (CPI) – a measure of the average change over time in the prices paid by urban consumers for an identified collection of goods and services

Chapter 12 / Financial Literacy

BOX 12.6 • Seven Steps in Monitoring a Budget

1. Record a list of income/revenue and expenses.
2. Establish financial goals.
3. Create a budget with monthly income and expenses.
4. Review the budget at least monthly, identifying the variances in budget.
   a. Identification of a hidden or unexpected expense
   b. Identification of an underbudgeted expense
   c. Identification of a spending behavior
5. Decide how to manage the variance: reallocate expenses, change spending behavior.
6. Allocate any unexpected income (eg, if the employer pays employees every other week, then there will be 2 months in the calendar year when the employee will receive three paychecks) with the same distribution established for the budget (eg, 70/20/10 rule).
7. Meet at least annually with advisors (eg, financial, insurance, employer human resource officer) to review and discuss investment options or insurance needs for the current time. Make adjustments as needed.

future decisions in financial management. Having a positive and proactive financial attitude and a financial awareness of the management of income and expenses is the most important determinant of successful personal financial planning.[32]

Summary

Financial literacy is not inherently intuitive to most people. It comes mainly from the influence of the environment in which they grew up and the observations of their parents' financial behavior. Gaining an understanding of the basic aspects of accounting, economics, and budgeting provides objective data that is used to better understand how income is generated and how it is spent. Understanding other aspects of money, such as taxes, debt, credit, interest, and inflation, provides information on external factors that deplete or add to the income earned. Through an active process of financial planning, including budgeting and monitoring, people can have a better understanding of how to control their expenses and how to plan for financial success.

REFERENCES

1. Mason C, Wilson R. Conceptualizing financial literacy. *J Consum Aff*. 2000;39.
2. Deb R. Financial literacy: a brief systematic literature review. *NMIMS J Econ Public Policy*. 2020;V(2).
3. Kadoya Y, Khan M, Hamada T, Dominguez A. Financial literacy and anxiety about life in old age: evidence from the USA. *Rev Econ Household*. 2018;16(3):859-878. doi:10.1007/s11150-017-9401-1
4. US Financial Literacy and Education Commission. My money five. Accessed August 29, 2023. https://www.mymoney.gov/mymoneyfive
5. Lusardi A, Michell OS. Financial literacy around the world: an overview. *J Pension Econ Finance*. 2011;10(4):497-508. doi:10.1017/S147474721000448
6. Lusardi A, Mitchell OS. Financial literacy and planning: implications for retirement wellbeing. In: Mitchell OS, Lusardi A, eds. *Financial Literacy: Implications for Retirement Security and the Financial Marketplace*. Oxford University Press; 2011:1739.
7. Maslow AH. A theory of human motivation. *Psychol Rev*. 1943;50(4):370-396. doi:10.1037/h0054346
8. VanSomeren L. The 50/30/20 rule of thumb for budgeting. The Balance. Updated June 15, 2022. Accessed August 30, 2023. https://www.thebalancemoney.com/the-50-30-20-rule-of-thumb-453922
9. National Archives. The 16th amendment to the US Constitution: Federal Income Tax (1913). Accessed on August 30, 2023. https://www.archives.gov/milestone-documents/16th-amendment
10. Social Security Administration. What is FICA? Publication No. 05-10297. Updated May 2023. Accessed August 30, 2023. https://www.ssa.gov/people/materials/pdfs/EN-05-10297.pdf

11. Department of the Treasury. Internal Revenue Service. Employee's Withholding Certificate. Published 2023. Accessed August 30, 2023. https://www.irs.gov/pub/irs-pdf/fw4.pdf
12. Hasler A, Lusardi A, Mitchell OS. How the pandemic altered Americans' debt burden and retirement readiness. *Financial Planning Rev.* 2023;6(1):e1156. Accessed September 19, 2023. doi:10.1002/cfp2.1156
13. Habib MD, Qayyum A. Cognitive emotion theory and emotion-action tendency in online impulsive buying behavior. *J Manag Sci.* 2018;5(1):86-99. doi:10.20547/jms.2014.1805105
14. McDermott J. The problem with impulse spending. Updated January 7, 2021. Accessed September 2, 2023. https://www.finder.com/impulse-buying-stats
15. Calculator.net. Student Loan Calculator. Simple student loan calculator. Accessed September 3, 2023. https://www.calculator.net/student-loan-calculator.html?cloanamount3=100%2C000&cmonthlypay3=1%2C161&cinterestrate3=7&cpayoffoption=extra&cadditionalmonth=100&cadditionalyear=0&cadditionalonetime=0&ctype=3&x=Calculate#repayment
16. U.S. Federal Trade Commission. Truth in Lending Act. Accessed September 4, 2023. https://www.ftc.gov/legal-library/browse/statutes/truth-lending-act
17. Board of Governors of the Federal Reserve Commission. Economic well-being of U.S. households in 2022. Research and Analysis. Published May 2023:44. Accessed September 4, 2023. https://www.federalreserve.gov/publications/files/2022-report-economic-well-being-us-households-202305.pdf
18. Hornymski C. Average credit card balances up 13.2% to $5,910 in 2022. Experian. Published March 27, 2023. Accessed September 4, 2023. https://www.experian.com/blogs/ask-experian/state-of-credit-cards/
19. Elite Personal Finance. Average credit card interest rates and APR of September 2023. Updated March 11, 2023. Accessed September 4, 2023. https://www.elitepersonalfinance.com/average-credit-card-interest-rates/
20. Consumer Financial Protection Bureau. What is a grace period for a credit card? Updated August 26, 2020. Accessed September 5, 2023. https://www.consumerfinance.gov/ask-cfpb/what-is-a-grace-period-for-a-credit-card-en-47/
21. U.S. Department of Education. Federal Student Aid. Student loan repayment. Accessed September 5, 2023. https://studentaid.gov/manage-loans/repayment
22. U.S. Department of Education. Federal Student Aid. Public service loan forgiveness (PSLF). Accessed September 5, 2023. https://studentaid.gov/manage-loans/forgiveness-cancellation/public-service
23. Fraticelli T. Physical Therapy Loan Forgiveness. Options for the Physical Therapist. *PT Progress.* February 19, 2020. Updated April 20,2024. Accessed April 22, 2024. https://www.ptprogress.com/physical-therapy-loan-forgiveness/
24. U.S. Department of Education. Federal Student Aid. Choose the federal student loan repayment plan that is best for you. Accessed September 5, 2023. https://studentaid.gov/manage-loans/repayment/plans
25. Rossi AG, Utkus SP. The needs and wants in financial advice: human versus robo-advising. Published January 3, 2020. Accessed September 11, 2023. https://ssrn.com/abstract=3759041 or doi:10.2139/ssrn.3759041
26. Nelson J. Making structured personal financial decisions. In: Nosse L, Friberg D, eds. *Managerial and Supervisory Principles for Physical Therapists.* 3rd ed. Lippincott Williams and Wilkins; 2009:473-474.
27. Ganatra M. What is a robo-advisor and how does it work? Forbes Advisor. Published November 29, 2021. Accessed September 12, 2023. https://www.forbes.com/advisor/in/investing/what-is-a-robo-advisor-and-how-does-it-work/
28. Abraham F, Schmukler S, Tessada J. Robo-advisors: investing through machines. World Bank Research and Policy Briefs No. 134881. Published February 26, 2019. Accessed September 19, 2023. https://ssrn.com/abstract=3360125
29. Ahn SY, Nam Y. Does mobile payment use lead to overspending? The moderating role of financial knowledge. *Comput Human Behav.* 2022;134. doi:10.1016/j.chb.2022.107319
30. US Bureau of Labor Statistics. Consumer price index. Accessed September 14, 2023. https://www.bls.gov/cpi/
31. US Bureau of Labor Statistics. Consumer price index. Regional resources. Accessed September 14, 2023. https://www.bls.gov/cpi/regional-resources.htm
32. Khanal S, Thapa BS, Nepal SR. Determinants of personal financial planning: a survey among business graduates in Nepal. *Batuk.* 2022;8(1):31-47. doi:10.3126/batuk.v8i1.43503

Index

Note: Page numbers in italics denote figures; those followed by a t denote tables; those followed by a b denote display boxes.

A

ACA (*see* Patient Protection and Affordable Care Act)
Academy of Neurologic Physical Therapy, 83
Accept risk, 226
Accident, definition of, 232
Account Aging report, 204–205, 205b
Account, definition of, 26
Accountable care organizations (ACO), 72
Accounting
    accrual basis, 30
    assets, 28–29
    cash basis, 30
    chart of accounts, 26–28, 26–27t
    credits, 28
    debits, 28
    definition of, 24
    double entry, 28
    equity, 29
    expenses, 31
    liabilities, 29
    principles, 24–25
    revenues, 30–31
Accounts payable, 29
Accounts receivable, 28
Accreditation, 95
Accrual basis, of accounting, 30
Accrued expenses, 29
Acid test ratio, 41
ACO (*see* Accountable care organizations)
ACSM (*see* American College of Sports Medicine)
Action minded, entrepreneurship skill, 130–131
Action plan, 154, 155t
Active source of income, 268
Acute care setting, 93–95
    examination, 95b
    infections seen in, 97b
    physical therapy interventions used in, 96b
    traveling therapist, 93, 94b
ADA (*see* Americans with Disabilities Act of 1990)
Adverse event, 232
Agency for Healthcare Research and Quality, 19
Agent of the employer, 91
AMA (*see* American Medical Association)
American College of Sports Medicine (ACSM), 255
American Hospital Association's Annual Environmental Scan, 12
American Institute of Certified Public Accountants, 25
American Medical Association (AMA), 182
American Physical Therapy Association (APTA), 53, 92, 223, 238, 239

American Physiotherapy Association (APA), 52
American Revolution, 266
American Women's Physical Therapeutic Association, 52
Americans with Disabilities Act, 58, 91, 239
Annual percentage rate (APR), 273
APA (*see* American Physiotherapy Association)
APR (*see* Annual percentage rate)
APTA (*see* American Physical Therapy Association)
AR (*see* Arrival Rate)
Arrival Rate (AR), 199–200
Audit, 233
Average total cost, 16
Average Visits/Plan of Care, 198–199
Average Weighted Timed Units per Visits (TU/V) 3 RVU, 208–209
Avoid risk, 225–226

B

Bad debt, 264
Balance sheet, 23, 32t, 33
Benchmarking, 194
Beneficiary, definition of, 66
Bill and Melinda Gates Foundation, 246
Billing, 184–188
    and collection, 46–47, 204–208
        Account Aging report, 204–205, 205b
        Days That a Sale Is Outstanding, 205–208, 207–208b, 207t
    independent contractor, 186–187, 187b
    participating with the third party, 187–188
Biomedical model, 52
Biopsychosocial model, 55
BIPOC (*see* Black, Indigenous, or People of Color)
Black, Indigenous, or People of Color (BIPOC), 256
Blackboard™, 109
The Blue Cross Blue Shield Association, 52
Bordon, Neil, 160
Brand, definition of, 159
Brand ambassadors, 135
Branding
    definition of, 134
    key elements, 159b
Break-even analysis, 18–19, 19t
    graphic representation of, *19*
Break-even cost method, 17–18
Budgeting, 268–277, 269–270t
    debt management, 271–274
    definition of, 36
    monitoring, 276–277, 277b
    personal financial advisors, 274–276, 275b
    process, 37–39, 38t
    proposal and justification, 251–252b
Bundled, definition of, 69

279

280   Index

Business plan
    components of, 140–141, 142b
    definition of, 140
Business structure, 90

C

Canvas™, 109
Capitalism, 4–5
CAPTE (*see* Commission on Accreditation in Physical
    Therapy Education)
CARF (*see* Commission on Accreditation of
    Rehabilitation Facilities)
Carnegie Foundation, 52
Cash basis, of accounting, 30
Cash flow statement, 23, 33–35, 35t
CEA (*see* Cost-effectiveness analysis)
Centers for Medicare and Medicaid Services (CMS), 96,
    183, 184
Centers for Medicare and Medicaid Services Innovation
    Center, 72
Certified public accountant (CPA), 25, 224
Chart of accounts, 26–28, 26–27t
Children's Health Insurance Program (CHIP), 72
CHIP (*see* Children's Health Insurance Program)
Civic engagement
    grant funding, 246, 247–252t
    health metrics/global agenda, 239–246
        global targets, 241–245, 241–245t
        sustainable development goals, challenges and
            considerations with, 245–246
    public health, physical therapy in, 237–239
    social determinants of health, 246–255, 253t
        health equity, health equality/health disparities,
            254–255
    vulnerable populations, providing services to,
        256–260
        documentation, 259
        domestic and international outreach, 256, 257b
        ethical considerations, 259–260
        service-learning/role of physical therapy,
            256–259, 258t
Civil Rights Act of 1964, 91
Civil War, 51–52
Clinical decision-making, 73–74
    health insurance, 73–74
        frameworks, 74–76
        frequency and duration of services, 78–80, 78
        steps in, 76–78
Clinical practice guideline (CPG), 83, 83b
Clinical reasoning, 79
Clostridium difficile, 97b
CMS (*see* Centers for Medicare and Medicaid Services)
CoA (*see* Cost of acquisition)
Code of Ethics, 92
Coding other services, 183–184, 184t
Coding the disease, 184
Coding the procedure, 182–183, 182t
Coinsurance, 67
Comfortable being uncomfortable, entrepreneurship
    skill, 132
Command economy, 5
Commercial Property, 228b

Commission on Accreditation in Physical Therapy
    Education (CAPTE), 109
Commission on Accreditation of Rehabilitation Facilities
    (CARF), 93, 98
Common law, 222, 223b
Common-size ratios, 41
Common-size statement, 39, 40t
Communication, in health care
    basic elements of, 174–182
        interprofessional, 179–180, 180b
        nonverbal, 176b, 177
        patient, 180–182, 181b
        verbal, 174–175, 176t
        written, 177–179, 178b, 179b
    billing, 184–188
        independent contractor, 186–187, 187b
        participating with third party, 187–188
    definition of, 257
    as entrepreneurship skill, 134
    payer, 182–184
        coding other services, 183–184, 184t
        coding the disease, 184
        coding the procedure, 182–183, 182t
Comparative statements, 39, 40t
Competitive market, 11–12
    focusing on specific aspects, 12–13
Compounding interest, 273
Consumer Price Index (CPI), 12, 276
Contracting services, 227
Contractual allowances, 25
Copayments, 67
Corporation, 90
Cost, 13–17
    break-even analysis, 18–19
    cost-effectiveness analysis, 19–20
    pricing, 17–18
Cost-effectiveness analysis (CEA), 19–20
Cost of acquisition (CoA), 213
Cost of living, 171
Cost/visit and profit/visit, 202, 202b
COVID-19 pandemic, 245
CPA (*see* Certified public accountant)
CPG (*see* Clinical practice guideline)
CPI (*see* Consumer Price Index)
CPT codes (*see* Current Procedural Terminology codes)
Credit cards, 273
Credits, 28
Current Procedural Terminology (CPT) codes, 182, 186
Current ratio, 41
Curriculum vitae, sample, 166–167b
Customer satisfaction metrics, 214–215
    Google Reviews, 215
    Net Promoter Score (NPS®), 214–215

D

Days That a Sale Is Outstanding (DSO), 205–208,
    207–208b, 207t
Debits, 28
Debt management, budgeting, 271–274
Deductible, definition of, 66
Deferred maintenance, 231
Demand, 8–9

Index

Demand-supply balance, 11
Demographics, 155
    information sources, 156b
Department of Health, 20
Developing multisite physical therapy practices,
        215–218, 216b
    Place of Service Summary, 217–218
    Profit and Loss by Location/Profit and Loss by Class,
        216–217, 217b
Diagnosis mix, 199
Diagnosis Related Groups (DRGs), 185
Digital marketing, 163
    email, 164
    mobile, 164
    Pay-Per-Click, 164
    Search Engine Optimization, 164
    social media, 163–164
Direct access, to physical therapy, 57
Direct costs, 14
Disability, definition of, 70b
Disability insurance, 228
Discretionary income, 271
Documentation, 259
    definition of, 80
    health insurance
        daily, utilization of, 80, 82
        outcome/result, 82–83, 83b
        terminology, 81b
Domestic/international outreach, 256, 257b
Double entry accounting system, 28
DRGs (see Diagnosis Related Groups)
Drop-offs, 211
DSO (see Days That a Sale Is Outstanding)

E
Early Intervention, IDEA, 103–105, 177–178
Economics
    basic principles
        elasticity of demand, 9–11
        scarcity, 6–7
        supply and demand, 8–9
        value and utility, 7–8
        wants and needs, 5–6
    competitive market, 11–12
        focusing on specific aspects, 12–13
    cost, 13–17
        break-even analysis, 18–19
        cost-effectiveness analysis, 19–20
        pricing, 17–18
    definition, 1
    of health care, 2–3
        capitalism, 4–5
        role of government, 3–4
Economy of scale, 11–12
Education for All Handicapped Children Act of 1975,
        103, 105, 239
Education of the Handicapped Act Amendments, 57
Effective communication, 181
Efficiency ratios, 41
Elasticity of demand, 9–11
Electronic medical records (EMRs), 174
Email marketing, 164

Employee, 90–93, 230, 232, 233
    interview questions, 92b
    unique feature of, 91
Employment-at-will doctrine, 91
Employment options
    business structure, 90
    employee, 90–93, 230, 232, 233
        interview questions, 92b
        unique feature of, 91
    independent contractor, 88
        contract, 88–90, 89b
        vs. sole proprietor, 90
    setting options
        acute care hospital, 93–95, 95b, 96b
        higher education/faculty, 108–109
        home health agency/home care, 99–100,
            100b, 101b
        hospice, 101–103, 101b, 102b
        Individuals with Disabilities Education Act, 103–107
        inpatient rehabilitation, 95–98, 97b
        outpatient rehabilitation/clinic, 98–99, 98b, 99b
        skilled nursing facilities, 107–108
EMRs (see Electronic medical records)
English Parliament, 266
Entitled service, 56
Entrepreneur, definition of, 130
Entrepreneurial resilience, 131–132
Entrepreneurship
    business plan, components of, 140–141
    creating and keeping great team, 146–147
    practice in digital age
        electronic communication, 137–138
        social media marketing, 137b, 138–139
        virtual visits, 139–140
        web page, 136–137, 136b
    profit center, 145
    skills and attributes, 130
        action minded, 130–131
        branding/marketing, 134–135
        comfortable being uncomfortable, 132
        communication, 134
        finance, 132–133
        leadership, 131
        resilience/tenacity, 131–132
        willingness to work hard, 132
    Small Business Administration, 135–136, 135b
    staff selection, 141, 143–145, 143
    subcontracting, 147–148
    tips
        direct access, 150
        first impressions matter, 150–151
        getting right help, 148, 148b
        grit matters, 148
        honesty and ethics, 149
        monitor spending, 149–150
        practitioner of choice, 150
        private pay/insurance-based reimbursement, 149
    vendor relationships, 145–146
Environmental scanning, 12
Equity, 29
Esteem needs, 5
Ethical considerations, 259–260

F

Facebook™, 138
Fair Labor Standards Act (FLSA), 91
Family-centered approach, 103
Family Educational Rights and Privacy Act (FERPA), 109
FAPE (*see* Free and appropriate public education)
FASB (*see* Financial Accounting Standards Board)
Federal income tax, 267
Federal Insurance Contribution Act (FICA), 266
Fee for service, 18, 68
Fee schedule, 17, 46
FERPA (*see* Family Educational Rights and Privacy Act)
FICA (*see* Federal Insurance Contribution Act)
Finance, entrepreneurship skill, 132–133
Financial Accounting Standards Board (FASB), 24
Financial analysis, 39
    financial ratios, 39–42
    performance indicators, 42–43
    productivity, 43–44, 45t
Financial literacy, 263–277
    budgeting, 268–277, 269–270t
        debt management, 271–274
        monitoring, 276–277, 277b
        personal financial advisors, 274–276, 275b
    needs and wants, 265–266, 266t
    paycheck, 266–268, 267b
Financial ratios, 39–42
Financial reporting, objectives of, 31–32
Fiscal year (FY), 32, 195
Fixed assets, 29
Fixed costs, 14–15
Flat fee, 17
Flexner, Abraham, 52
Flexner Report, 52
FLSA (*see* Fair Labor Standards Act)
For cause, employment, 91
Free and appropriate public education (FAPE), 57, 105
Fund accounting, 25
Fundamental financial statements, 23, 36t
    balance sheet, 23, 32t, 33
    cash flow statement, 23, 33–35, 35t
    definition of, 31
    income statement, 23, 33, 34t
    retained earnings statement, 23, 35–36, 36t
FY (*see* Fiscal year)

G

GAAP (*see* Generally Accepted Accounting Principles)
GDP (*see* Gross Domestic Product)
General financial metrics, 200–204
    cost/visit and profit/visit, 202, 202b
    expense reporting, 203–204
    payer mix, 202–203
    payment per visit (PPV), 200
    profit and loss statement, 200–201, 201b
General Liability, 228b

General practice metrics, 195–200
    Arrival Rate (AR), 199–200
    Average Visits/Plan of Care, 198–199
    New Patients (NP), 195–197, 196–197b
    Visits per Week (V/wk), 197–198, 198b
Generally Accepted Accounting Principles (GAAP), 24
Geographic Practice Cost Index (GPCI), 186
Gerber, Michael, 195, 196
GME (*see* Graduate medical student education)
GoDaddy™, 136
Good debt, 264
Good Health and Well-Being, 245
Google Reviews, 215
Google Voice™, 138
Government insurance, 68
GPCI (*see* Geographic Practice Cost Index)
Graduate medical student education (GME), 56
Grant funding, 246, 247–252t
Gross Domestic Product (GDP), 12–13
Guide for Professional Conduct, 92

H

HALE (*see* Healthy life expectancy)
HCFA (*see* Health Care Financing Administration)
HCO (*see* Health care organizations)
HCPCS (*see* Healthcare Common Procedure Coding System)
Health and financial information, 232
Health care, 203
    call to change, 58–60, *59*
        paternalism to partnership, 60
        value-based care, 60–62, 61b
    federal and state laws, 56–58
    hospital, early development of, 51–53
    physical therapist, early development of, 51–53
        treatment, 53–56
    physician, early development of, 51–53
Health care, communication in
    basic elements of, 174–182
        interprofessional, 179–180, 180b
        nonverbal, 176b, 177
        patient, 180–182, 181b
        verbal, 174–175, 176t
        written, 177–179, 178b, 179b
    billing, 184–188
        independent contractor, 186–187, 187b
        participating with third party, 187–188
    payer, 182–184
        coding other services, 183–184, 184t
        coding the disease, 184
        coding the procedure, 182–183, 182t
Health care, economics, 2–3
    capitalism, 4–5
    role of government, 3–4
    supply and demand relationship, 11
Health Care Financing Administration (HCFA), 186–187
Health care organizations (HCO), 25
Health care professionals, 254
Health care providers, 175
Health disparities, 254–255
Health equality, 254–255
Health equity, 254–255

Index

Health insurance
  clinical decision-making, 73–74
    frameworks, 74–76
    frequency and duration of services, 78–80, 78
    steps in, 76–78
  communicating with payer, 83–84
  components of, 66–68
  documentation
    daily, utilization of, 80, 82
    definition of, 80
    outcome/result, 82–83, 83b
    terminology, 81b
  productivity, 73
  questions to consider when purchasing, 68b
  types of, 68–73, 70–72b, 70t
Health Insurance Portability and Accountability Act (HIPAA), 138
Health insurance, presence of, 2
Health literacy, 174
Health Maintenance Organization Act of 1973, 68
Health metrics/global agenda, 239–246
  global targets, 241–245, 241–245t
  sustainable development goals, challenges and considerations with, 245–246
Health Resources and Human Administration (HRSA), 246
Healthcare Common Procedure Coding System (HCPCS), 184
Healthy life expectancy (HALE), 240
Hell With Good Intentions, 256, 257t
Hill-Burton Act, 238
Hill-Burton Hospital Construction Act, 56
HIPAA (*see* Health Insurance Portability and Accountability Act)
HIV/AIDS, 245
HOAC II (*see* Hypothesis-Oriented Algorithm for Clinicians II)
Home Care services, 178
Home health agency/home care, 99–100
  assessment information set, 101b
  documentation requirements, 100b
Horizontal integration, 234
Hospice care, 101–103
  diagnoses in, 101b
  physical therapy interventions, 102b
Hospital, early development of, 51–53
HR (*see* Human Resource)
HRSA (*see* Health Resources and Human Administration)
Human Resource (HR), 92, 227
Human Services Public Health Service, 20
Hypothesis-Oriented Algorithm for Clinicians II (HOAC II), 76, 76b, 77

I

ICF (*see* International Classification of Functioning, Disability, and Health)
ICR (*see* Indirect cost rate)
IDEA (*see* Individuals with Disabilities Education Act)
IEP (*see* Individualized Education Program)
IFSP (*see* Individualized Family Service Plan)
Implicit costs, 13–14
Implicit/implied contract, 88

Impulse buying, 272
Incidence, 240
Incident, 232
Income diversification, 268
Income statement, 23, 33, 34t
Independent contractor, 88, 186–187, 187b
  contract, 88–90, 89b
  vs. sole proprietor, 90
Indirect cost rate (ICR), 14
Indirect costs, 14, 251
Individual physical therapist metrics, 208–211
  Average Weighted Timed Units per Visits (TU/V) 3 RVU, 208–209
  Patient Register/Plan of Care Completion/Patient Drop-Off %, 210–211
  Reactivation Rate, 211
  Relative Value Units Billed per Visit (RVU/V), 209
  Revenue/Visit per Therapist (Compare to TU/V-W), 209
  Visits/POC per Individual Therapist, 209–210
Individual with a disability, definition of, 91–92
Individualized Education Program (IEP), 57
Individualized Family Service Plan (IFSP), 57, 104
  elements of, 104b
  transition plan, 104–105
Individuals with Disabilities Education Act (IDEA), 57, 103–107, 178
  developmental skills checklist, 116–119
  early intervention, 103–105, 104b
  physical therapy evaluation, 112–115
  regular education, 107
  school-based evaluation, documentation, and outcome forms, 120–129
  special education, 105–106
    related services, 105
Inpatient rehabilitation, 95–98, 97b
Instagram™, 138
Insurance-based models, business tips, 149
Intangible assets, 28
Integration, 234–235
Interest, 272
Internal Revenue Service (IRS), 88
International Classification of Diseases, 184
International Classification of Functioning, Disability, and Health (ICF), 55, 74–75, 75
Interprofessional communication, 179–180, 180b
Inventories, 28
IRS (*see* Internal Revenue Service)

J

JCAHO (*see* The Joint Commission on Accreditation of Healthcare Organizations)
Job description, 144, 144b
The Joint Commission on Accreditation of Healthcare Organizations (JCAHO), 94–95

K

Kenyon's pediatric focused algorithm, 77, 77b
Key performance indicators, 192–193
  leading and trailing indicators, 193, 193t
  metric scope, 192–193
  metric timing, 192

L

Law of demand, 9
Law of diminishing marginal utility (*see* Marginal utility)
Law of supply, 9
Leadership, 131
Leading/trailing indicators, 193, 193t
Learning management system (LMS), 109
Liabilities, 29
Life expectancy, 240
Lifetime Value of a Patient (LVP), 214
Limited liability corporation (LLC), 90
LinkedIn™, 138
Liquid assets, 29
Liquidity ratios, 41
LLC (*see* Limited liability corporation)
LMS (*see* Learning management system)
Love needs, 5
LVP (*see* Lifetime Value of a Patient)

M

Macroeconomic policies, 2
Managed care organization (MCO), 69
Marginal analysis, 7
Marginal cost, 16
Marginal utility, 7–8
Market, definition of, 156
Market economy, 5
Market equilibrium, 11
Market or going rate, 17
Market penetration, 158
Market positioning, 158
Market segmentation, 156, 157t
Market share, 158, 203
Marketing
    action plan, 154, 155t
    basics of, 155–159, 156b
        demographics, 155, 156b
        market, definition of, 156
        market penetration, 158
        market positioning, 158
        market segmentation, 156, 157t
        market share, 158
        niche market, 158
        target market, 157, 157t
    budget, 141
    definition of, 134, 153
    digital, 163
        social media, 163–164
    mix, 160
        packaging, 161
        personnel, 163
        physical evidence of effectiveness, 161–162
        place, 160–161
        price, 160
        processes, 162
        product, 160
        promotion, 161
    options for, 134–135
    personal marketing mix, 168, 168b
        passion, 169
        payment, 170–171

place, 170
        practice, 169–170
    plan, 141
    SWOT analysis, 154, 154t
    yourself, 165–167
        personal SWOT analysis, 168
Marketing metrics, 211–214
    cost of acquisition, 213
    lifetime value of a patient, 214
    rate of customer return, 213–214
    referral source reporting, 211–212, 212b
    return on investment, 212–213
Marketplace plans, benefits of, 72b
Markup method, 18
McMillan, Mary, 52
MCO (*see* Managed care organization)
MDG (*see* The Millennium Development Goals)
Measuring customer satisfaction, 215
Medicaid, 68, 70, 71, 177
    mandatory services, 71b
    for the IDEA-related services, 106
Medically necessary, 83
Medicare, 25, 43, 68, 69–70, 177, 267
    parts of, 70t
Medicare Catastrophic Coverage Act, 106
Merrill, Janet, 238
Methicillin-resistant *Staphylococcus aureus* (MRSA), 97b
Metric scope, 192–193
Metric timing, 192
Microeconomic principles, 2
The *Millennium Development Goals* (MDG), 241
Mitigating risk, 226, 227b
Mobile marketing, 164
Modifier 22, 183
Modifier 59, 183
Modifier 95, 183
Modifier CQ, 183
Modifier GP, 183
Modifiers, 183
Monitoring, and measuring
    benchmarking, 194
    billing and collection metrics, 204–208
        Account Aging, 204–205, 205b
        Days That a Sale Is Outstanding (DSO),
            205–208, 207–208b, 207t
    customer satisfaction metrics, 214–215
        Google Reviews, 215
        Net Promoter Score (NPS®), 214–215
    developing multisite physical therapy practices,
        215–218, 216b
        Place of Service Summary, 217–218
        Profit and Loss by Location/Profit and Loss by
            Class, 216–217, 217b
    general financial metrics, 200–204
        cost/visit and profit/visit, 202, 202b
        expense reporting, 203–204
        payer mix, 202–203
        payment per visit (PPV), 200
        profit and loss statement, 200–201, 201b
    general practice metrics, 195–200
        Arrival Rate (AR), 199–200

Index

Average Visits/Plan of Care, 198–199
New Patients (NP), 195–197, 196–197b
Visits per Week (V/wk), 197–198, 198b
individual physical therapist metrics, 208–211
Average Weighted Timed Units per Visits (TU/V)
3 RVU, 208–209
Patient Register/Plan of Care Completion/Patient
Drop-Off %, 210–211
Reactivation Rate, 211
Relative Value Units Billed per Visit (RVU/V), 209
Revenue/Visit per Therapist (Compare to TU/
V-W), 209
Visits/POC per Individual Therapist, 209–210
key performance indicators, 192–193
leading and trailing indicators, 193, 193t
metric scope, 192–193
metric timing, 192
marketing metrics, 211–214
cost of acquisition (CoA), 213
Lifetime Value of a Patient (LVP), 214
Rate of Customer Return (RCR), 213–214
Referral Source reporting, 211–212, 212b
return on investment (ROI), 212–213
monitoring the market, 218
physical therapy revenue equation, 193–194
and reporting, 194–195
Monitoring, budgeting, 276–277, 277b
Monopoly, 11
Morbidity and mortality, 240
MRSA (*see* Methicillin-resistant *Staphylococcus aureus*)

N

Nagi Model of Disablement, 74, *74*
National Center for Medical Rehabilitation Research, 239
Needs-based assessments, 258
Needs, definition of, 5
Net Promoter Score (NPS®), 214–215
New Patients (NP), 195–197, 196–197b
Niche market, 158
Noncompete clause, 231
Nonverbal communication, 176b, 177
Notes payable, 29
NP (*see* New Patients)

O

OASIS (*see* Outcome and Assessment Information Set)
Occupational Safety and Health Administration (OSHA),
93, 239
Office of the National Coordinator for Health
Information Technology (ONC), 232
ONC (*see* Office of the National Coordinator for Health
Information Technology)
Operating margin ratio, 41–42
Opportunity cost, concept of, 6
Organizational chart, 143, *143*
OSHA (*see* Occupational Safety and Health
Administration)
Out-of-pocket maximum, 67
Outcome and Assessment Information Set (OASIS),
100, 178
Outsourcing, 227

Owner's equity statement (*see* Retained earnings
statement)
Ownership (*see* Equity)

P

Parson's assumptions, 54–55, 55b
Passion, 169
Passive source of income, 268
Paternalism to partnership, 60
Patient-centered care, 175
Patient communication, 180–182, 181b
Patient Driven Payment Model (PDPM), 72, 108
Patient Protection and Affordable Care Act (ACA),
59, 66, 71
Patient Register/Plan of Care Completion/Patient
Drop-Off %, 210–211
Patient Registry, 210
Pay-Per-Click (PPC), 164
Paycheck, 266–268, 267b
Payer communication, 83–84, 182–184
coding other services, 183–184, 184t
coding the disease, 184
coding the procedure, 182–183, 182t
Payer mix, 202–203
Payment per visit (PPV), 200
Payment per Visit for Fully Paid Claims, 200
PDPM (*see* Patient Driven Payment Model)
PED (*see* Price elasticity of demand)
People-first language, 175
Performance indicators, 42–43
Personal financial advisors, 274–276, 275b
Personal marketing mix, 168, 168b
passion, 169
payment, 170–171
place, 170
practice, 169–170
Personal SWOT analysis, 168
Physiatrist, 53
Physical therapist
early development of, 51–53
treatment, 53–56
Physical therapist assistant (PTA), 183
Physical therapy evaluation, 112–115
Physical Therapy Practice Act, 56
Physical therapy, practice of, 12
Physical therapy revenue equation, 193–194
Physical therapy, role of, 256–259
Physician, early development of, 51–53
Physiologic needs, 5
Place of Service Summary, 217–218
PNF (*see* Proprioceptive Neuromuscular Facilitation)
Point-of-service plan (POS), 69
Population demographics/trends, 13
Population health, definition of, 240
POS (*see* Point-of-service plan)
PPC (*see* Pay-Per-Click)
PPO (*see* Preferred provider organization)
PPV (*see* Payment per visit)
Preauthorization, 47
Preferred provider organization (PPO), 69
Premium, definition of, 66

Prevalence, 240
Price elasticity of demand (PED), 9–10
Price on profit, impact of, 10
Pricing, 17–18
Principal, 272
Privacy, 138
Private insurance, 68, 71
Private pay model, business tips, 149
PRN employment, 87
Pro forma, 268
Probationary period, 229
Productivity, 43–44, 45t, 73
Professional Liability, 228b
Profit and loss by class, 216–217, 217b
Profit and loss by location, 216–217, 217b
Profit-and-Loss Statement, 133, 145, 200–201, 201b
Profit center, 145
Profit margin, 201
Profitability ratios, 41
Proprioceptive Neuromuscular Facilitation (PNF), 54
Protecting information, 232–233
PTA (*see* Physical therapist assistant)
PtEverywhere™, 138
Public goods, 3
Public health, physical therapy in, 237–239
Public Law 94-142, 57
Public record, 170

Q
Quarterly monitoring, 195

R
Rate of Customer Return (RCR), 213–214
RBRVS (*see* Resource Based Relative Value Scale)
RCR (*see* Rate of Customer Return)
Reactivation Rate, 211
Reconstruction aides, 51–52
Referral Source reporting, 211–212, 212b
Reflective practice, 78
Regulations, 222–224, 222b, 223b
Rehabilitation Act of 1973, 58, 107
Related services, special education, 105
Relative Value Units (RVUs), 185
Relative Value Units Billed per Visit (RVU/V), 209
Reporting, monitoring and, 194–195
Reputation, 224–225, 225b
Resilience/tenacity, entrepreneurship skill, 131–132
Resource Based Relative Value Scale (RBRVS), 185
Retained earnings statement, 23, 35–36, 36t
Return on assets, 42
Return on investment (ROI), 212–213
Revenue, 30–31, 224
   management, 45–46
     billing and collections, 46–47
     fees, 46
Revenue/Visit per Therapist (Compare to TU/V-W), 209
Righting reflex, 175
Risk diversification, 274
Risk identification, 221–225, *221*
   regulations, 222–224, 222b, 223b

reputation, 224–225, 225b
revenues, 224
Risk literacy, 220
Risk management
   identifying risk, 221–225, *221*
     regulations, 222–224, 222b, 223b
     reputation, 224–225, 225b
     revenues, 224
   improvement, 235
   protection, 228–235, 229b, 230b
     hiring and compliance, 229–231, 230b
     integration, 234–235
     protecting information, 232–233
     safety in operations, 231–232
     stress testing/situational analysis, 233–234
   risk management, 228–235
     improvement, 235
     protection, 228–235, 229b, 230b
   risk options, 225–227
     accept risk, 226
     avoid risk, 225–226
     mitigating risk, 226, 227b
     transfer risk, 226–227, 228b
Risk options, 225–227
   accept risk, 226
   avoid risk, 225–226
   mitigating risk, 226, 227b
   transfer risk, 226–227, 228b
Risk pooling, 66
Risk/reward trade-off, 220
Robo advisors, 276
ROI (*see* Return on investment)
RVUs (*see* Relative Value Units)

S
Safety needs, 5
SAMHSA (*see* Substance Abuse and Mental Health
   Services)
SBA (*see* Small Business Administration)
SBDC (*see* Small Business Development Center)
Scarcity, 6–7
School-based services, 177–178
SCORE (*see* Service Corps of Retired Executives)
SDGs (*see* Sustainable Development Goals)
SDOH (*see* Social determinants of health)
Search Engine Optimization (SEO), 164
Secured loan, 272
Self-actualization needs, 5
Self-employment tax, 88
Selling, definition of, 153
Semivariable costs, 16
SEO (*see* Search Engine Optimization)
Service Corps of Retired Executives (SCORE), 141
Service-learning, 256–259, 258t
Setting options, employment
   acute care hospital, 93–95, 95b, 96b
   higher education/faculty, 108–109
   home health agency/home care, 99–100, 100b, 101b
   hospice, 101–103, 101b, 102b
   Individuals with Disabilities Education Act, 103–107

Index

Early Intervention, 103–105, 104b
  regular education, 107
  special education, 105–106
 inpatient rehabilitation, 95–98, 97b
 outpatient rehabilitation/clinic, 98–99, 98b, 99b
 skilled nursing facilities, 107–108
SIM (*see* Subscriber Identify Module)
Skilled nursing facilities, 107–108
Skills, entrepreneurship
 action minded, 130–131
 branding/marketing, 134–135
 comfortable being uncomfortable, 132
 communication, 134
 finance, 132–133
 leadership, 131
 resilience/tenacity, 131–132
 willingness to work hard, 132
Sliding scale fee schedule, 47
Small Business Administration (SBA), 135–136
 road map, 135b
Small Business Development Center (SBDC), 141
SMM (*see* Social media marketing)
Social determinants of health (SDOH), 246–255, 253t
 health equity, health equality/health disparities,
  254–255
Social media marketing (SMM), 163–164
Social Security, 266
Social Security Act, 56, 69
Social Security Administration, 70
Sole proprietorship, 90
Special education, 105–106
SquareSpace™, 136
SSI (*see* Supplemental security income)
State Boards of Physical Therapy, 223
Statement of Operations (*see* Income statement)
State's Practice Act, 47
Statutes, 222
Strength-based assessments, 257
Stress testing/situational analysis, 233–234
Student, without disability, 107
Subcontracting, 147–148
Subscriber Identify Module (SIM), 164
Substance Abuse and Mental Health Services
 (SAMHSA), 246
Substitution, 10
Supplemental security income (SSI), 56, 70
Supply, 8
Supply and demand curve, 8
Sustainable Development Goals (SDGs), 241,
 241–245t, 245
 challenges and considerations with, 245–246
SWOT analysis, 154, 154t

T

Target market, 157, 157t
Tax Equity and Fiscal Responsibility Act of 1982, 101
Term life insurance, 270
Third party, participating with, 187–188
Third-party payment structures, 182
Tips, business

direct access, 150
 first impressions matter, 150–151
 getting right help, 148, 148b
 grit matters, 148
 honesty and ethics, 149
 monitor spending, 149–150
 practitioner of choice, 150
 private pay/insurance-based reimbursement, 149
Total cost, 16
Transfer risk, 226–227, 228b
Transition plan, 104–105
Traveling therapist, 93, 94b

U

UCR (*see* Usual, customary, and reasonable rate)
Unbundled, definition of, 68
Uncertainty, 220
Unemployment, 228
Unemployment rate, 13
Uniform Certified Public Accountant Examination, 25
Unique New Patient (UNP), 214
Unit of service (UOS), 12, 16
UNP (*see* Unique New Patient)
Unsecured loan, 272
UOS (*see* Unit of service)
US Bureau of Labor Statistics, 276
US Financial Literacy and Education Commission, 263
US military, 238
Usual, customary, and reasonable rate (UCR), 17, 46
Utility, 7–8

V

Value, 7
Value-based care, 162
 steps for, 162b
Value-based health care, 181
Value-based outcomes, 72
Vancomycin-resistant *Enterococcus* (VRE), 97b
Variable costs, 15–16
Variance analysis (*see* Financial analysis)
Vendor relationships, 145–146
Verbal communication, 174–175, 176t
Vertical integration, 234
Visits per Week (V/wk), 197–198, 198b
Visits/POC per Individual Therapist, 209–210
Vocational rehabilitation, 58
Voluntary insurance programs, 270
VRE (*see* Vancomycin-resistant Enterococcus)
Vulnerable populations, providing services to, 256–260
 documentation, 259
 domestic and international outreach, 256, 257b
 ethical considerations, 259–260
 service-learning/role of physical therapy,
  256–259, 258t

W

W-4 form, 267
Want, definition of, 6
White savior complex, 256
WHO (*see* World Health Organization)

Index

Whole life insurance, 270
Willingness to work hard, entrepreneurship skill, 132
Wix™, 136
Workers' compensation, 228
Workers' compensation laws, 57
World Health Organization (WHO), 74, 232, 239
World War I, 52, 238
World War II, 53, 238

Wright, Wilhemine, 238
Written communication, 177–179, 178b, 179b

X

X (formerly Twitter)™, 138–139

Y

Yearly monitoring, 195